AF803039

Alcohol and Cancer

Samir Zakhari · Vasilis Vasiliou · Q. Max Guo
Editors

Alcohol and Cancer

Springer

Editors
Samir Zakhari, Ph.D.
Director
Division of Metabolism and Health Effects
National Institute on Alcohol Abuse
and Alcoholism
National Institutes of Health
5635 Fishers Lane, Room 2031
Bethesda, MD 20892-9304
USA
szakhari@mail.nih.gov

Vasilis Vasiliou, Ph.D.
Professor and Director of Toxicology
Graduate Program
Department of Pharmaceutical Sciences
University of Colorado Denver
C238-P15 RC2, Room P15-3111
12700 East 19th Avenue
Aurora, CO 80045
USA
Vasilis.Vasiliou@ucdenver.edu

Q. Max Guo, Ph.D.
Division of Metabolism and Health Effects
National Institute on Alcohol Abuse and
Alcoholism
National Institutes of Health
5635 Fishers Lane, Room 2031
Bethesda, MD 20892-9304
USA
qmguo@mail.nih.gov

ISBN 978-1-4614-0039-4 e-ISBN 978-1-4614-0040-0
DOI 10.1007/978-1-4614-0040-0
Springer New York Dordrecht Heidelberg London

Library of Congress Control Number: 2011934679

© Springer Science+Business Media, LLC 2011
All rights reserved. This work may not be translated or copied in whole or in part without the written permission of the publisher (Springer Science+Business Media, LLC, 233 Spring Street, New York, NY 10013, USA), except for brief excerpts in connection with reviews or scholarly analysis. Use in connection with any form of information storage and retrieval, electronic adaptation, computer software, or by similar or dissimilar methodology now known or hereafter developed is forbidden.
The use in this publication of trade names, trademarks, service marks, and similar terms, even if they are not identified as such, is not to be taken as an expression of opinion as to whether or not they are subject to proprietary rights.

Printed on acid-free paper

Springer is part of Springer Science+Business Media (www.springer.com)

Preface

Chronic alcohol consumption is a major health problem worldwide, and may lead to addiction and damage of almost every organ of the body. The World Health Organization (WHO) Global Burden of Disease has concluded that approximately 1.8 million people die each year due to alcohol (3.2% of all deaths). One of the most significant diseases caused by chronic alcohol consumption is cancer. According to the International Agency for Research on Cancer (IARC) in Lyon, France, alcohol is considered a carcinogen for the oral cavity, pharynx, larynx, esophagus, liver, colorectum, and the female breast. Worldwide, a total of approximately 389,000 cases of these cancers representing 3.6% of all cancers (5.2% in men and 1.7% in women) are derived from chronic alcohol ingestion.

The fact that alcohol causes cancer is not new. The first observation that alcohol is responsible for esophageal cancer was published by the French pathologist Lamu in Paris in 1910. It took a long time until 1978 when the National Institute of Health (NIH) organized a workshop on this topic due to the fact that more and more epidemiologic data appeared demonstrating the causal relationship between alcohol and certain types of cancer. However, at this time mechanisms of alcohol-mediated carcinogenesis were almost completely unknown.

A second workshop in 2004 took into account the increasing literature on possible mechanisms by which ethanol and/or its first metabolite acetaldehyde stimulates carcinogenesis. The results of this workshop were published in ALCOHOL. A further step forward in bringing this important issue to the scientific public was the workshop held in Lyon at the IARC in February 2007 which ended in a clear statement that alcoholic beverages are carcinogenic and that acetaldehyde is a causal factor in esophageal carcinogenesis published in the April issue 2007 of LANCET ONCOLOGY.

Considering this historic development, it was time for a more detailed look at the effect of alcohol on carcinogenesis in a broader perspective, including epidemiology, biochemistry as well as molecular and cell biology. On June 8–9, 2010, the Division of Metabolism and Health Effects of the National Institute of Alcoholism and Alcohol Abuse (NIAAA) has invited a panel of experts to discuss this important issue. As a result, Dr. Sam Zakhari and his colleagues presented a comprehensive book on alcohol and cancer with major emphasis on molecular mechanisms, including the effect of alcohol metabolism on cancer, the effect of ethanol on epigenetics, intracellular signal pathways, retinoic acid metabolism, protein homeostasis, inflammation, immune surveillance, and stem cells. This book could have come at no better time. The contents of this book is carefully designed and analytically presented, summarizing an up-to-date knowledge on this topic with the most recent literature until summer 2010. The book "Alcohol and Cancer" edited by Sam Zakhari, Q. Max Guo, and Vasilis Vasiliou is a comprehensive and unique summary on a topic of general and specific interest to a broad readership, including oncologists, basic cancer researchers, gastroenterologists, hepatologists, and other specialists dealing with cancer. It will undoubtedly become an international landmark.

Dr. Sam Zakhari works at the NIH since 1986. He is Director of the Division of Metabolism and Health Effects of the NIAAA, Bethesda, MD, USA. He is an internationally well-known expert in the field of alcohol metabolism and alcohol associated toxicity, having worked in this field for decades. It is he and his coworkers who guarantee for the high standard and quality of this book. I wish to thank the authors for presenting an outstanding summary on a most important issue and I am convinced that this book receives the international recognition which it deserves.

Heidelberg
October, 2010

Helmut K. Seitz, MD, PhD, AGAF

Contents

About the Contributors

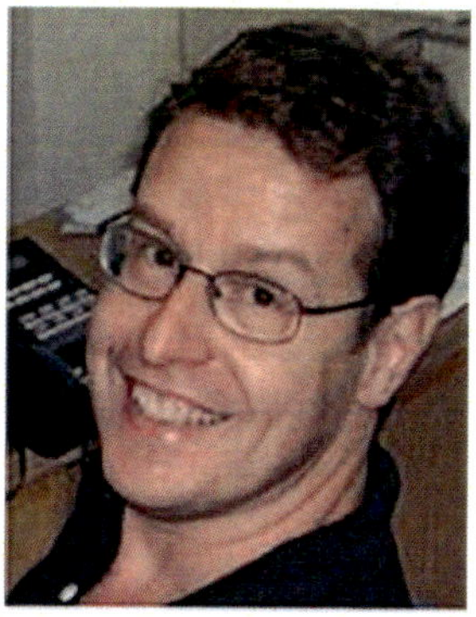

Phillip J. Brooks, Ph.D
Neurobiology, University of North Carolina at Chapel Hill, 1990
Postdoc: Rockefeller University
Started at NIH: 1994

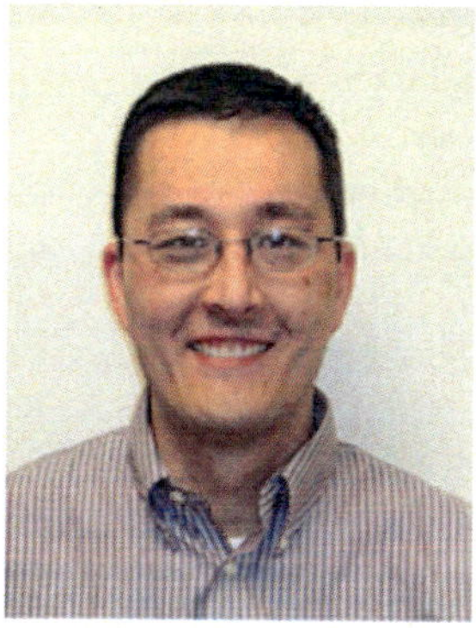

William C. Dunty, Jr., PhD
Cell and Developmental Biology, University of North Carolina at Chapel Hill, 2002
Postdoc: National Cancer Institute
Started at NIH: 2003

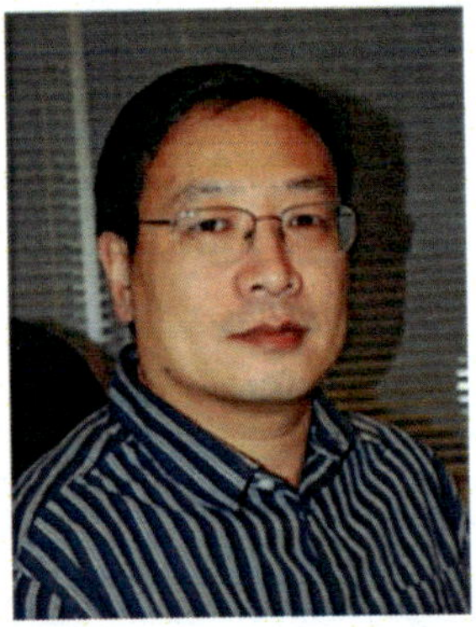

Zhigang (Peter) Gao, MD
Henan Medical University, 1988
Postdoc: Johns Hopkins School of Medicine
Started at NIH: 2005

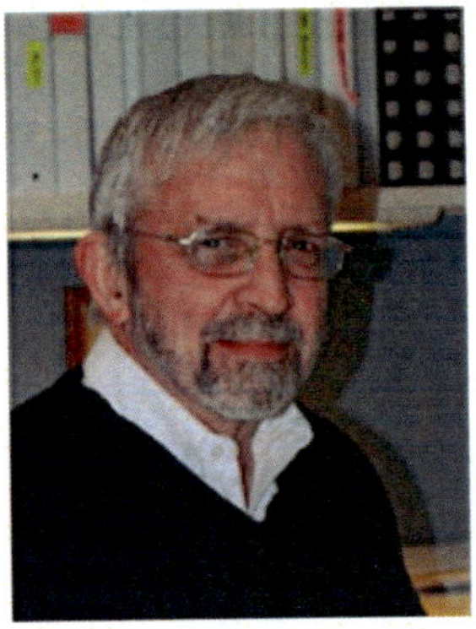

R. Thomas Gentry, PhD
Behavioral Neuroendocrinology,
Univ. of Massachusetts at Amherst, 1976
Postdoc: Rockefeller University
Started at NIH: 1996

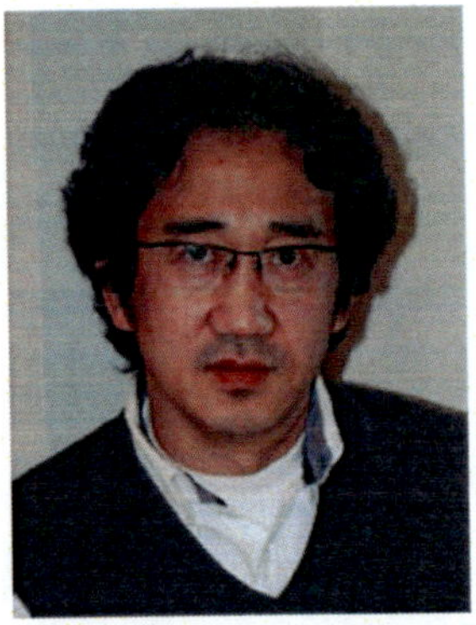

Q. Max Guo, PhD
Biochemistry, RNA Splicing,
Ohio State University, 1992
Postdoc: University of California
at San Francisco
Started at NIH: 2002

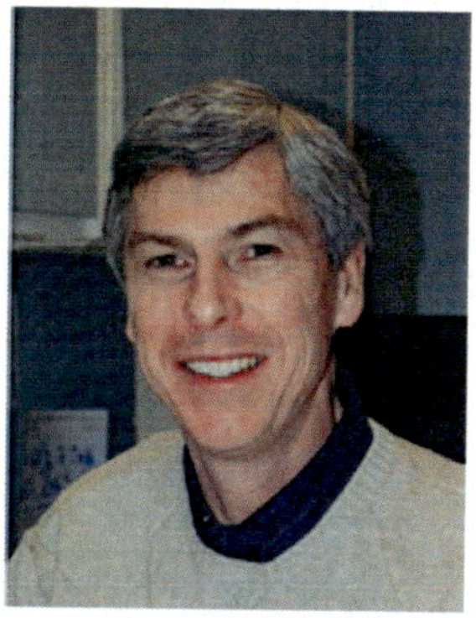

Dale Hereld, MD, PhD
Biochemistry, Cell, and Molecular Biology;
Johns Hopkins University, 1989
Postdoc: Johns Hopkins University
Started at NIH: 2008

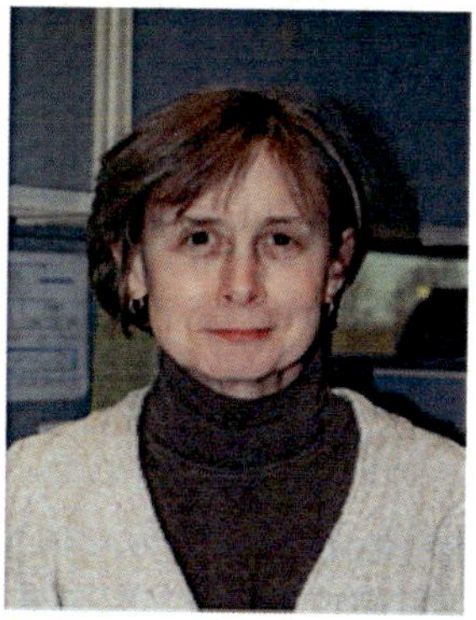

M. Katherine Jung, PhD
Physiological Chemistry,
Ohio State University, 1982
Postdoc: Friedrich Miescher Institute, Basel
Started at NIH: 2007

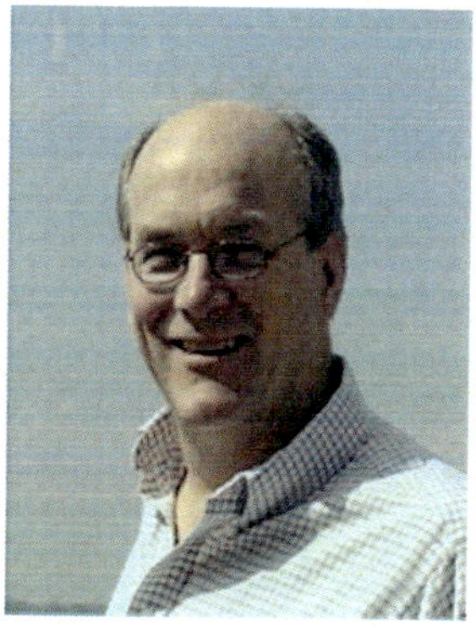

Gary Murray, PhD
Chemistry, University of Waterloo,
Canada, 1977
Postdoc: National Institutes of Health
Started at NIH: 1977

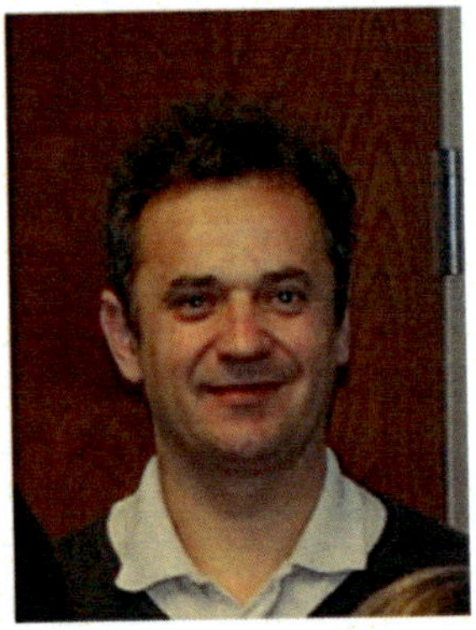

András Orosz, PhD
Biochemistry and Molecular Biology,
University of Szeged, Hungary, 1991
Postdoc: National Cancer Institute
Started at NIH: 2008

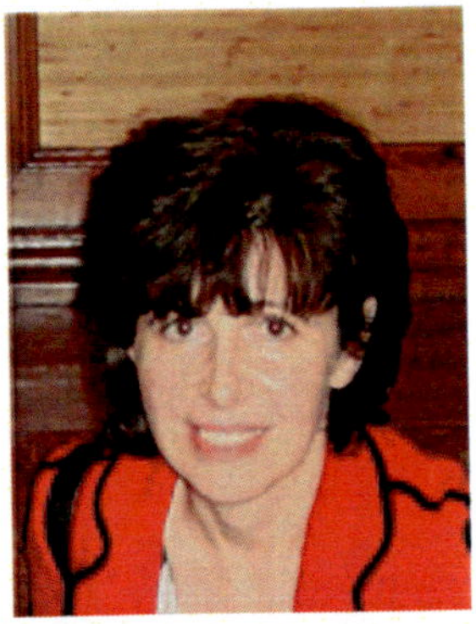

Svetlana Radaeva, PhD
Cell and Developmental Biology, Koltzov
Institute, Russian Academy of Sciences, 1992
Postdoc: German Cancer Research Center,
Heidelberg
Started at NIH: 2000

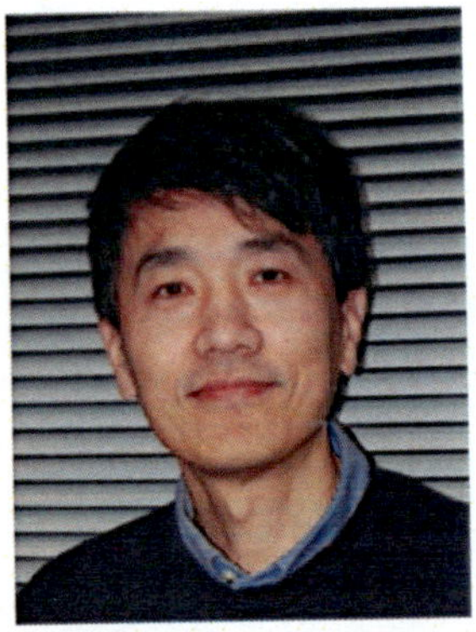

H. Joe Wang, PhD
Molecular Genetics,
Ohio State University, 1994
Postdoc: University of California
at San Francisco
Started at NIH: 2007

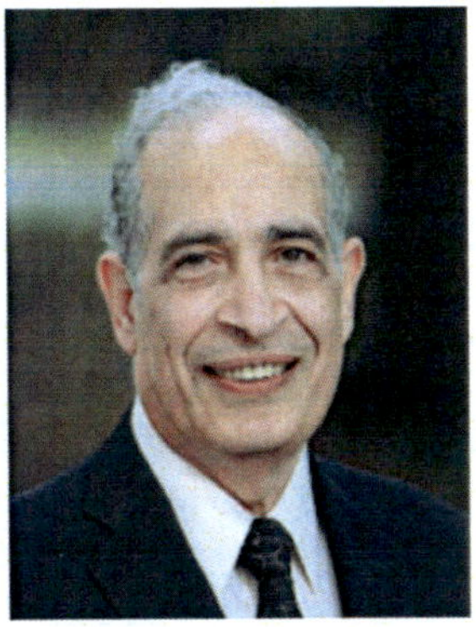

Samir Zakhari, PhD
Pharmacology, Czechoslovak Academy of Sciences, 1975
Postdoc: University of Pennsylvania School of Medicine
Started at NIH: 1986

Contributors

Phillip J. Brooks, PhD Division of Metabolism and Health Effects, National Institute on Alcohol Abuse and Alcoholism, National Institutes of Health, Bethesda, MD, USA

William C. Dunty, Jr, PhD Division of Metabolism and Health Effects, National Institute on Alcohol Abuse and Alcoholism, National Institutes of Health, Bethesda, MD, USA

Zhigang (Peter) Gao, MD Division of Metabolism and Health Effects, National Institute on Alcohol Abuse and Alcoholism, National Institutes of Health, Bethesda, MD, USA

R. Thomas Gentry, PhD Division of Metabolism and Health Effects, National Institute on Alcohol Abuse and Alcoholism, National Institutes of Health, Bethesda, MD, USA

Q. Max Guo, PhD Division of Metabolism and Health Effects, National Institute on Alcohol Abuse and Alcoholism, National Institutes of Health, Bethesda, MD, USA

Dale Hereld, MD, PhD Division of Metabolism and Health Effects, National Institute on Alcohol Abuse and Alcoholism, National Institutes of Health, Bethesda, MD, USA

M. Katherine Jung, PhD Division of Metabolism and Health Effects, National Institute on Alcohol Abuse and Alcoholism, National Institutes of Health, Bethesda, MD, USA

Gary J. Murray, PhD Division of Metabolism and Health Effects, National Institute on Alcohol Abuse and Alcoholism, National Institutes of Health, Bethesda, MD, USA

András Orosz, PhD Division of Metabolism and Health Effects, National Institute on Alcohol Abuse and Alcoholism, National Institutes of Health, Bethesda, MD, USA

Svetlana Radaeva, PhD Division of Metabolism and Health Effects, National Institute on Alcohol Abuse and Alcoholism, National Institutes of Health, Bethesda, MD, USA

H. Joe Wang, PhD Division of Metabolism and Health Effects, National Institute on Alcohol Abuse and Alcoholism, National Institutes of Health, Bethesda, MD, USA

Samir Zakhari, PhD Division of Metabolism and Health Effects, National Institute on Alcohol Abuse and Alcoholism, National Institutes of Health, Bethesda, MD, USA

Chapter 1
Alcohol as a Human Carcinogen

Philip J. Brooks

The determination and classification of chemicals as human carcinogens are formally carried out by national and international agencies. The International Agency for Research on Cancer (IARC) (http://www.iarc.fr), which is part of the World Health Organization, is tasked with the evaluation and classification of human carcinogens. This chapter discusses the IARC process, and the classification of ethanol and acetaldehyde as human carcinogens.

Outline of an IARC Working Group Evaluation

Once a particular agent is selected for review by the IARC Secretariat, the IARC staff recruits experts in different aspects of the agent under study. Individuals having conflicts of interest that would prevent them from making an unbiased evaluation are excluded from the process. Different areas of the evaluation include exposure data, studies of cancer in humans (cancer epidemiology), studies of cancer in experimental animals, and mechanistic data. Members are then assigned to critically review the literature in their areas of expertise and prepare a written summary of the findings prior to the meeting. The Working Group meeting itself takes place at IARC headquarters, where the Working Group carries out peer review of others' literature reviews and works toward a consensus summary evaluation. Finally, the group arrives at a final classification for each agent.

P.J. Brooks (✉)
Division of Metabolism and Health Effects, National Institute on Alcohol Abuse and Alcoholism, National Institutes of Health, Bethesda, MD, USA
e-mail: pjbrooks@mail.nih.gov

S. Zakhari et al. (eds.), *Alcohol and Cancer*, DOI 10.1007/978-1-4614-0040-0_1,
© Springer Science+Business Media, LLC 2011

The different classifications used by IARC are as follows:

Group 1: The agent is *carcinogenic to humans.*
Group 2A: The agent is *probably carcinogenic to humans.*
Group 2B: The agent is *possibly carcinogenic to humans.*
Group 3: The agent is *not classifiable as to its carcinogenicity to humans.*
Group 4: The agent is *probably not carcinogenic to humans.*

The distinction between 2A and 2B reflects the overall assessment of the strength of the available evidence.

At the conclusion of the meeting, the final classification is determined by an open vote of the Working Group members. Soon after the meeting, a summary of the findings, including the final classification, is published in *The Lancet Oncology.* Ultimately, the different group summaries, including an assessment of all of the studies that were reviewed, final summary, and final classification are published as a *Monograph.*

Classification of Alcohol as a Human Carcinogen: IARC

Prior to 2007, IARC considered the evidence for the carcinogenicity of alcohol drinking in 1998 (IARC 1998). As reported in Vol. 44, the Working Group concluded that "Alcoholic beverages are *carcinogenic to humans (Group 1)*" with the target tissues being the oral cavity, pharynx, larynx, esophagus (collectively referred to as the upper aerodigestive tract), and liver. It is worth noting in this report the use of the term alcoholic beverages, as opposed to ethanol per se. This classification left open the possibility that the carcinogenic agent(s) in alcoholic beverages was not ethanol per se but other components in alcoholic beverages. Such components could have been, for example, nitrosamines that can be found in some beers or aromatic compounds present in some distilled spirits.

Acetaldehyde, the first metabolite of ethanol, was evaluated in 1999, separately from alcohol (IARC 1999). Acetaldehyde is classified as carcinogenic to animals (Group 1), and *possibly carcinogenic to humans (Group 2B).* The Group 1 classification of acetaldehyde in animals was based in large part on studies showing that prolonged exposure of rats to acetaldehyde vapor caused tumors in the nasal epithelia (Woutersen et al. 1986).

In 2007, in response to mounting epidemiologic evidence relating alcohol drinking to different types of cancers, including breast cancer in women, IARC decided to convene another Working Group to reevaluate the carcinogenicity of alcohol and acetaldehyde. The results of this group confirmed the previous conclusions, but also made two significant changes (Baan et al. 2007; IARC 2007).

First, the group concluded that not only are alcoholic beverages carcinogenic to humans, but also that it is the ethanol in alcohol beverages that is carcinogenic to humans (Group 1) at the different sites listed above. This change was based in part on animal data showing an increased risk of cancers in experimental animals exposed to ethanol alone, as well epidemiologic evidence showing that the cancer risk from alcohol drinking is independent of the type of alcoholic beverage consumed.

Second, the group added two additional organs to the list of sites at which alcohol drinking increases the risk of cancer. These were the colorectum (colon plus rectum) and female breast. The addition of colorectal cancer and breast cancer in women, two of the most common cancers worldwide, substantially increases estimates of the numbers of cancers worldwide that are attributable to alcohol drinking.

The carcinogenicity of acetaldehyde was a highly contentious issue at the 2007 meeting. Some in the group felt strongly that the evidence for the carcinogenicity of acetaldehyde was strong and compelling, based in large part on the dramatically elevated risk of esophageal cancer in heavy drinking ALDH2-deficient individuals who are unable to metabolize acetaldehyde. As described in more detail in Chap. 5, when ALDH2-deficient individuals drink alcohol, acetaldehyde accumulates in their body, resulting in a dramatically increased risk of esophageal cancer (Yokoyama et al. 1996); see also (Brooks et al. 2009). However, other members of the group did not agree with changing the classification of acetaldehyde based on these data. Therefore, in spite of vigorous debate, it was not possible to resolve this issue in the time allotted for the Working Group meeting. As a compromise, the final summary (Baan et al. 2007) did state that "The Working Group agreed that the substantial mechanistic evidence in humans deficient in aldehyde dehydrogenase indicates that acetaldehyde derived from the metabolism of ethanol in alcoholic beverages contributes to causing malignant esophageal tumors."

More recently, in 2009, another IARC Working Group revisited the question of alcohol, acetaldehyde, and cancer. The 2009 Working Group (Secretan et al. 2009) confirmed the Group 1 classification of alcohol consumption and of ethanol in alcoholic beverages, but also concluded that acetaldehyde associated with the consumption of alcoholic beverages is carcinogenic to humans (Group 1).

Carcinogen Classification of Alcohol and Acetaldehyde in the USA

Within the USA, the National Toxicology Program (NTP) also publishes a biannual Report on Carcinogens (http://ntp.niehs.nih.gov/roc12/INDEXC5F2.HTM?objectid=035E57E7-BDD9-2D9B-AFB9D1CADC8D09C1). The NTP uses two classifications: substances known to be human carcinogens or substances reasonably anticipated to be human carcinogens. As of the most recent 12th Report on Carcinogens, alcoholic beverage consumption is "known to be a Human Carcinogen" while acetaldehyde is "reasonably anticipated to be a human carcinogen."

A summary of the different classifications of alcohol and acetaldehyde carcinogenicity is given in Table 1.1.

Table 1.1

Substance	Regulatory agency IARC	The US NTP
Ethanol	**Carcinogenic to humans**	**Not specifically evaluated**
Alcoholic beverages/alcoholic beverage consumption[a]	Carcinogenic to humans	Known to be a human carcinogen
Acetaldehyde	Carcinogenic to humans	Reasonably anticipated to be a human carcinogen

[a]IARC reviewed alcoholic beverages while the US NTP reviewed alcoholic beverage consumption

Conclusion

In view of the 2007 and 2009 IARC classifications, continued accumulation of additional epidemiologic evidence linking alcohol to cancer, and other considerations, the DMHE made the decision to convene an Extramural Advisory Board (EAB) meeting on the topic of alcohol and cancer as a guide to making decisions about future research funding.

In the chapters that follow, different mechanistic aspects of the relationship between alcohol and cancer are considered with a focus on unanswered questions and possible areas of future investigation.

References

Baan, R., K. Straif, et al. (2007). "Carcinogenicity of alcoholic beverages." Lancet Oncol **8**(4): 292–293.

Brooks, P. J., M. A. Enoch, et al. (2009). "The alcohol flushing response: an unrecognized risk factor for esophageal cancer from alcohol consumption." PLoS Med **6**(3): e50.

IARC (1998). Alcoholic Beverages. IARC Monographs on the Evaluation of Carcinogenic Risks to Humans IARC. Lyon, IARC. **44**.

IARC (1999). Re-evaluation of Some Organic Chemicals, Hydrazine and Hydrogen Peroxide IARC Monographs on the Evaluation of Carcinogenic Risks to Humans IARC. Lyon, IARC. **71**.

IARC (2007). Alcohol Consumption and Ethyl Carbamate. IARC Monographs on the Evaluation of Carcinogenic Risks to Humans IARC. Lyon, IARC. **96**. (http://monographs.iarc.fr/ENG/Monographs/vol96/index.php).

Secretan, B., K. Straif, et al. (2009). "A review of human carcinogens – Part E: tobacco, areca nut, alcohol, coal smoke, and salted fish." Lancet Oncol **10**(11): 1033–1034.

Woutersen, R. A., L. M. Appelman, et al. (1986). "Inhalation toxicity of acetaldehyde in rats. III. Carcinogenicity study." Toxicology **41**(2): 213–231.

Yokoyama, A., T. Muramatsu, et al. (1996). "Esophageal cancer and aldehyde dehydrogenase-2 genotypes in Japanese males." Cancer Epidemiol Biomarkers Prev **5**(2): 99–102.

Chapter 2
Cancer and Alcohol: An Overview of Tumorigenesis

William C. Dunty Jr.

Abbreviations

AKT	Protein kinase B
APC	Adenomatous polyposis coli
BRAF	v-raf Murine sarcoma viral oncogene homolog B1
Bcl2	B-cell lymphoma 2
CRC	Colorectal cancer
Kras	v-Ki-ras2 Kirsten rat sarcoma viral oncogene homolog
MAPK	Mitogen-activated protein kinase
PI3K	Phosphoinositide 3-kinase
P53	Tumor protein 53
Rb	Retinoblastoma protein
TGFβ	Transforming growth factor beta

Introduction

The word *cancer*, derived from the Greek term for crab (*carcinos*), was coined by the father of medicine, Hippocrates (460–370 BC), in describing the physical resemblance of malignant tumors that had spread throughout the human body. Today, we know cancer to be a collection of diseases characterized by uncontrolled growth and spread of abnormal cells (Kleinsmith 2006). Cancer is the second most common

W.C. Dunty Jr. (✉)
Division of Metabolism and Health Effects, National Institute on Alcohol Abuse and Alcoholism, National Institutes of Health, Bethesda, MD, USA
e-mail: duntyw@mail.nih.gov

S. Zakhari et al. (eds.), *Alcohol and Cancer*, DOI 10.1007/978-1-4614-0040-0_2,
© Springer Science+Business Media, LLC 2011

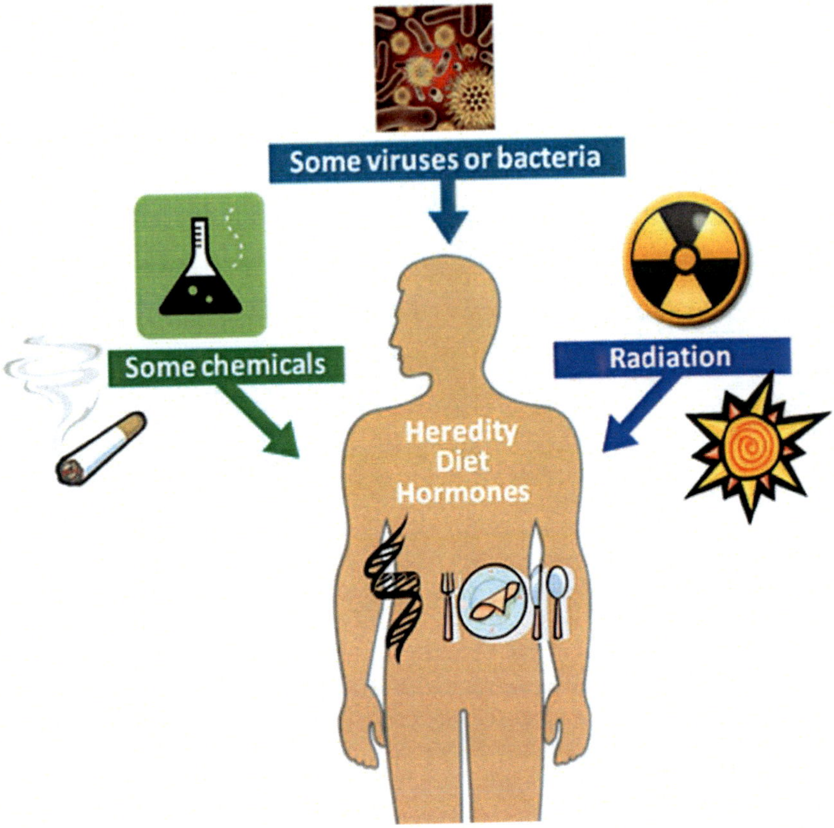

Fig. 2.1 Known causes of cancer. Modified with permission from the *Understanding Cancer Series*, National Cancer Institute (Kleinsmith et al. 2004)

cause of death, accounting for nearly one of every four deaths in the USA (American Cancer Society 2009). It encompasses more than 100 distinct diseases based on differences in their tissue of origin and the cell types involved.

The process by which a normal cell becomes malignant is referred to as *transformation*. Cellular transformation is an intricate, multistep process that typically occurs over a period of decades. Research over many years has identified several of the underlying causes of cancer (Fig. 2.1). Besides heredity, which can affect one's susceptibility to certain types of cancer, environmental and lifestyle risk factors, such as exposure to carcinogenic chemicals (e.g., those found in tobacco smoke and alcohol), radiation, infectious agents, and diet, all contribute, often in combination, to the development of cancer.

Multistep Process of Tumorigenesis

Cancer development is a multistep process by which normal cells acquire abnormal biological capabilities (Fig. 2.2) (Kleinsmith 2006). In simple terms, this neoplastic evolution begins from an initial genetic or epigenetic change in the cell. Fortunately, the cell has in place many mechanisms to repair damaged DNA, thus ensuring these are rare events. There are no outward manifestations at this stage. As the *initiated* cell proliferates, hyperplasia eventually leading to dysplasia may be histologically evident. Cancer progression describes a period after cancer has formed. During this phase, the accumulation of genetic and epigenetic abnormalities creates cells possessing increasingly aberrant traits (discussed in *Hallmarks of Cancer* section below). Such leverage provides a selective advantage to certain cells within the tumor. Repeated rounds of this clonal selection and genomic alteration generate a predominant population of cells whose cellular properties are now clearly aligned with what we recognize as *cancer*.

Cancer Genes and the Significance of Mutations

Although the main causes of cancer are quite diverse, they often lead to the common outcome of mutagenizing our genome. Currently, it is believed that mutations in at least 350 (1.6%) of the approximately 22,000 protein-coding genes in the human genome may contribute to cancer development (Futreal et al. 2004; Stratton et al. 2009). Updated lists of gene mutations causally implicated in cancer may be found at http://cgap.nci.nih.gov/cgap.html and http://www.sanger.ac.uk/genetics/CGP/Census/.

For a given human cancer, it is believed that at least four to six distinct somatic mutations are required for tumorigenesis (Hahn and Weinberg 2002). Cancer-relevant genes fall into three main classes: oncogenes, tumor-suppressor genes, and stability genes.

Oncogenes are altered genes whose protein products contribute to cancer development. They arise from normal genes (*proto-oncogenes*) which encode proteins that function as mitogenic growth factors and their corresponding receptors, cytoplasmic protein kinases, cell cycle or cell death regulators, and nuclear transcription factors. Proto-oncogenes may be converted to oncogenes by a number of mechanisms, including mutation, gene amplification, and chromosomal translocation. By these mechanisms, cancer cells produce excessive amounts or abnormal versions of these proteins, thus creating an advantageous condition for unrestrained growth. Since their discovery in the 1970s, several dozens of oncogenes have been identified in human cancer (see Chap. 6), many of which have become therapeutic targets for drug development.

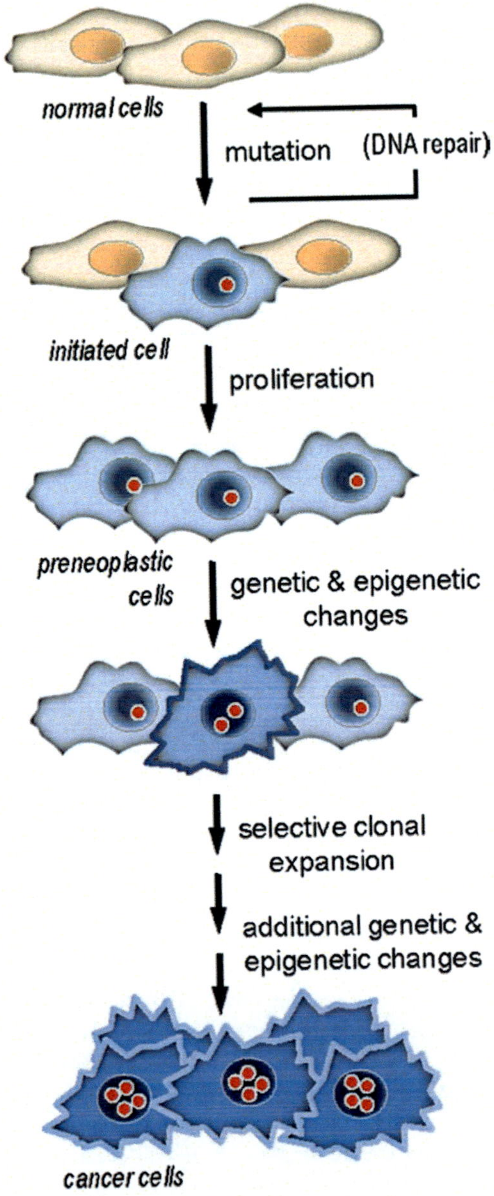

Fig. 2.2 Multistep carcinogenesis

Tumor-suppressor genes are normal genes whose absence or inactivation by mutation or epigenetic silencing may also contribute to cancer. Occasionally referred to as *anti-oncogenes*, they encode proteins which normally constrain cell growth or promote cell death. Functional loss of such genes would, therefore, allow cancer cells to evade normal growth and survival controls. In contrast to oncogenes,

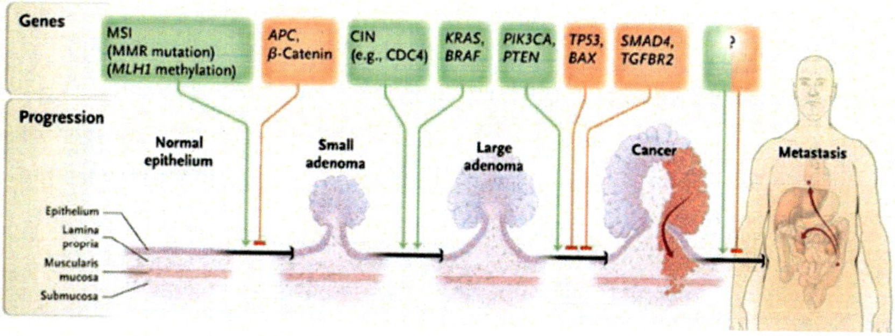

Fig. 2.3 Molecular basis of colorectal cancer. *Green* denotes oncogenic mediators that are activated while *red* represents tumor-suppressor factors that are turned off in colorectal cancer. Each successive genetic or epigenetic alteration is associated with increasingly abnormal cellular properties, all of which occur over a period of years. *Question mark* (?) denotes unknown genetic and epigenetic changes involved in metastasis. *MSI* microsatellite instability, *MMR* mismatch repair, *CIN* chromosomal instability. Adapted from *N Engl J Med,* Molecular origins of cancer: Molecular basis of colorectal cancer, Markowitz SD, Bertagnolli MM. Copyright © 2009 Massachusetts Medical Society. All rights reserved

tumor-suppressor genes generally follow the "two-hit hypothesis" first proposed by Knudson (1971) which implies that both alleles of a particular gene must be affected before an effect is manifested.

The third class of cancer genes, called *stability genes* (Vogelstein and Kinzler 2004), promotes carcinogenesis in a completely different manner when mutated. As compared to oncogenes and tumor suppressors which, when altered, drive the proliferative and survival aspects of carcinogenesis, stability genes are responsible for repairing errors made during DNA replication and those induced by carcinogen exposure. Stability genes also control chromosomal segregation and mitotic recombination processes. Inactivation of this class of cancer genes would facilitate genome-wide increases in mutation rates and chromosomal anomalies, thus indirectly contributing to cancer development.

Stepwise Model for Colorectal Cancer

The concept by which a series of mutations leads to malignancy is best illustrated by the disease of colorectal cancer (CRC). Data from a number of laboratories have contributed to a sequence of transformation from normal colonic epithelium to metastatic carcinoma driven by a stepwise accumulation of genetic and epigenetic alterations that may take decades to accrue (Fig. 2.3).

Characteristic molecular changes observed in patient-derived samples include the activation of the Wnt-signaling pathway and inactivation of the p53 and transforming growth factor beta (TGFβ) pathways by loss-of-function mutations in the tumor-suppressor genes *APC, P53 (or TP53),* and *SMAD4,* respectively (Fig. 2.3; Baker et al. 1989, 1990; Kinzler et al. 1991; Powell et al. 1992; Takagi et al. 1996; Howe et al. 1998; reviewed by Markowitz and Bertagnolli 2009). These changes are often accompanied by the oncogenic mutation of *KRAS* or *BRAF* which activates the mitogen-activated protein kinase (MAPK)-signaling pathway (Bos et al. 1987; Rajagopalan et al. 2002; reviewed by Markowitz and Bertagnolli 2009). Accumulation of these genetic and epigenetic changes correlates with increasing malignancy such that benign adenomas possess only a few of these genetic lesions, whereas aggressive tumors display most if not all of them (Fig. 2.3). It is also important to note that these molecular alterations may not always occur in the order depicted in Fig. 2.3. Taken together, our understanding of CRC serves as an excellent example **of how a defined set of genetic and epigenetic alterations may confer a sequential,** selective advantage to the cells in which they arise.

Acquired Capabilities of Cancer Cells

The Hallmarks of Cancer

Hanahan and Weinberg (2000) **proposed a simplified model of cancer development** consisting of six molecular, biochemical, and cellular traits which are shared by most, if not all, highly advanced human cancers. According to their theory, these traits or novel capabilities, referred to as the *hallmarks of cancer* (Fig. 2.4, *top half*), are acquired during tumorigenesis through both genetic and epigenetic (see Chap. 5) mechanisms. These are the following:

1. ***Self-sufficiency in growth signals.*** Normal cells require exogenous mitogenic signals prior to undergoing cell division. Cancer cells escape such a prerequisite by production of abnormal proteins that inappropriately trigger cell proliferation in the absence of environmental cues, a feat achieved primarily through the activity of oncogenes. Mechanistically, cancer cells may achieve growth factor autonomy by (a) ectopically secreting growth factors in a cell autonomous manner; (b) overexpressing growth factor receptors or possessing, by mutation, structurally altered forms which establish a hyperresponsive signaling environment; and (c) acquiring mutations in downstream intracellular components that facilitate ligand-independent signaling. Indeed, Hanahan and Weinberg (2000) have suggested that growth-signaling pathways are dysregulated in virtually all human cancers.
2. *Insensitivity to antigrowth signals.* If they are to continue to divide, cancer cells must evade a variety of inhibitory mechanisms that protect normal tissues from inappropriate growth. At the molecular level, many antiproliferative factors, such as the TGFβ family of ligands, impinge upon late G_1 phase of the cell cycle at a transition known as the restriction point. These inhibitory effects often converge on the retinoblastoma protein, Rb, a tumor-suppressor protein whose hyperphosphorylation allows passage into the S phase of the cell cycle and whose functional disruption renders cells insensitive to cell cycle control.

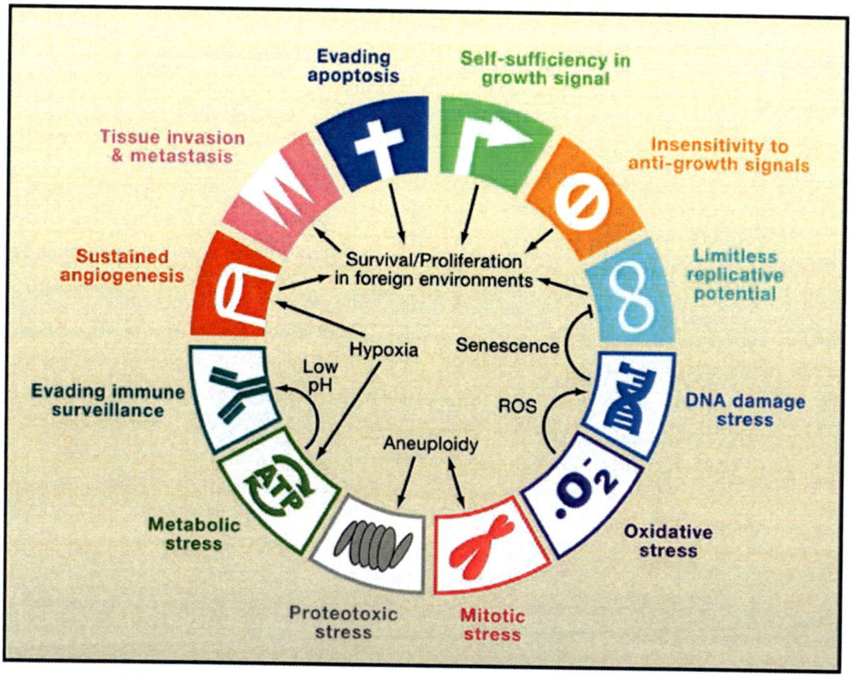

Fig. 2.4 The expanded hallmarks of cancer. In addition to the six hallmarks of cancer first proposed by Hanahan and Weinberg in 2000 (upper half, *white symbols*) and evasion of immune surveillance suggested by Kroemer and Pouyssegur (2008), Elledge and colleagues recently proposed a set of additional hallmarks that depict the stress phenotypes of cancer cells (lower half, *colored symbols*). Reprinted from *Cell*,136, Luo J, Solimini NL, and Elledge SJ, *Principles of Cancer Therapy: Oncogene and Non-oncogene Addition*, p823–836, (2009), with permission from Elsevier

3. *Evading apoptosis.* In normal tissue, a balance exists between the production of new cells by cell division and the elimination of damaged or unwanted cells by a genetic mode of cellular suicide or *apoptosis.* The intrinsic apoptotic pathway functions in response to various intracellular stresses, including DNA damage to lead to the accumulation of the p53 tumor-suppressor protein, mitochondrial release of cytochrome c, activation of caspase proteases, and ultimate cell killing. In cancer, this program of cell death is functionally silenced. Moreover, other anti-apoptotic pathways, such as survival signals mediated by PI3K and AKT protein kinases, are also enhanced in a substantial number of human tumors. The ability to evade apoptosis appears to be a hallmark of nearly all types of cancers and likely contributes to their ability to accumulate mutations and progress toward malignancy.
4. *Limitless replicative potential.* Normal cells are limited in the number of times they may divide. When this limit is reached, cells enter senescence. This replicative potential is determined by structures at the ends of chromosomes called telomeres, which are progressively lost upon completion of each cell cycle.

To avoid such chromosomal attrition which would otherwise lead to apoptosis, cancer cells have acquired mechanisms to maintain and lengthen telomeric DNA, thereby achieving the ability to replicate indefinitely. The vast majority of malignancies accomplish this feat through transcriptional activation of *telomerase*, an enzyme which promotes telomere repair and is aberrantly activated in cancer cells.

5. *Sustained angiogenesis.* Formation of a blood vasculature to nourish cancer cells is an essential step in allowing a neoplasm to expand and metastasize. Cancer cells initially lack the capacity to initiate tumor angiogenesis, the process by which new blood vessels are formed from preexisting vessels, and thus remain physically confined to their site of origin. However, during early tumorigenesis, neoplastic cells shift the balance between pro- and anti-angiogenic factors in favor of establishing an independent blood supply, thereby fueling tumor growth.
6. *Tissue invasion and metastasis.* Metastasis is the most common cause of cancer deaths from solid tumors. In order for cancers to spread, cells must dissociate from the primary tumor mass, invade the surrounding tissues, enter and travel through the lymphatic or circulatory systems, and colonize new tissues elsewhere in the body. At a mechanistic level, both invasion and metastasis utilize similar physical strategies involving (a) loss of cell–cell adhesion; (b) activation of extracellular proteases; and (c) enhanced cell motility. Among the hallmarks of human cancer, the acquisition of invasiveness and metastatic ability by cancer cells are often the very last to emerge.

   According to Hanahan and Weinberg (2000), each of these physiologic changes represents the successful breaching of an anticancer defense mechanism hardwired into normal human cells, the sum of which dictates malignant growth. Since their report was published, additional hallmarks, for which no further detail would be provided, have been proposed.
7. The ability to evade elimination by the immune system (Zitvogel et al. 2006; Kroemer and Pouyssegur 2008) and
8. The presence of an inflammatory microenvironment (Coussens and Werb 2002; Colotta et al. 2009; Mantovani 2009). The role of alcohol in enhancing inflammation and suppressing immune surveillance and its implications for cancer are discussed in detail in Chaps. 9 and 10, respectively.

   A conceptual update by Elledge and colleagues (Luo et al. 2009) expanded upon the classic hallmarks to include the "stress phenotypes of tumorigenesis" (Fig. 2.4, *lower half*). These are
9. DNA damage and replication stress;
10. Proteotoxic stress;
11. Mitotic stress;
12. Metabolic stress; and
13. Oxidative stress.

Although these cancer phenotypes may not be responsible for initiating tumorigenesis, Elledge and colleagues suggest that they represent a common set of oncogenesis-associated cellular stresses that cancer cells must endure through stress-supported pathways if they are to survive. Ultimately, cancer development is a complex interplay among these hallmarks, whether they involve traits that promote cell proliferation and survival or capabilities that mitigate cellular stresses. For example, most cancer cells rely on aerobic glycolysis, the conversion of glucose to lactate regardless of whether oxygen is present, as a means of generating ATP (Vander Heiden et al. 2009). Known as the Warburg effect, this reliance on glycolysis allows cancer cells to adapt to hypoxia and acidify their microenvironment, conditions which favor subsequent tumor invasion and suppression of immune surveillance (Fig. 2.4; Luo et al. 2009).

Molecular Bases of Cancer Hallmarks

The molecular underpinnings of these cancer hallmarks involve somatic mutations to key cancer genes that accumulate over the lifetime of the cancer patient (reviewed by Hahn and Weinberg 2002; Vogelstein and Kinzler 2004; Stratton et al. 2009). These *driver mutations* impart clonal growth advantages to cells and have been causally implicated in oncogenesis (reviewed by Stratton et al. 2009). Also present are *passenger mutations* that, due to the nature of the genetic change, fail to impart carcinogenic properties to a cell. These mutations propagate during clonal expansion, but are thought not to contribute to cancer development. A half-dozen driver mutations may be sufficient to convert normal cells to cancerous ones, though recent analyses suggest that number may be underestimated (Sjoblom et al. 2006; Beerenwinkel et al. 2007). The ability to distinguish driver from passenger mutations is a major goal of ongoing efforts cataloging somatic mutations of individual cancer genomes and provides insight into the mutational processes that drive human malignancies (Fig. 2.5; reviewed by Futreal et al. 2004; Stratton et al. 2009).

Although cancer genes are important, it is really the dysregulation of associated signaling pathways resulting from their mutation that promotes carcinogenesis. Genetic and epigenetic alterations to cancer genes lead to the derailment of homeostatic programs controlling growth, migration, and survival (see Chap. 6), and thus serve as the driving force behind the phenotypic traits of malignancy.

For example, gain-of-function mutation, copy number changes, and chromosomal rearrangements allow for the conversion of proto-oncogenes to oncogenes during cancer development (Fig. 2.5). As seen in activating mutations in members of the *RAS* family of GTPases, dysregulation and inappropriate activation of the MAPK pathway follow (see Chap. 6). Continuous mitogenic signaling independent of ligand binding represents an essential step of malignant transformation. Indeed, approximately 20–30% of all human cancers produce mutant RAS protein (Bos 1989; Medema and Bos 1993) making it the most frequently mutated oncogene in human cancers.

Loss of tumor suppressors via deletion, loss-of-function mutation, or epigenetic silencing also facilitates the acquisition of malignant phenotypes. For instance,

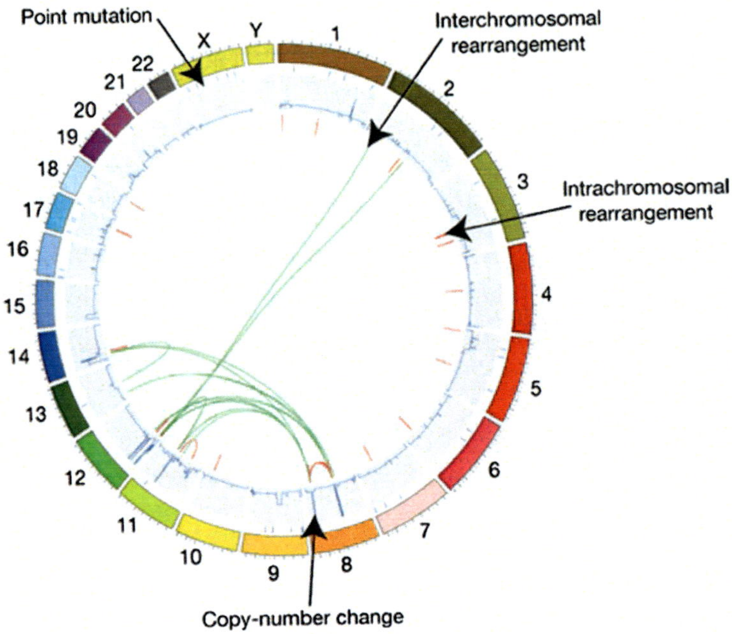

Fig. 2.5 A catalogue of somatic mutations present in a single cancer genome. Part of catalogue of somatic mutations in the small-cell lung cancer cell line NCI-H2171. Individual chromosomes are depicted on the outer circle followed by concentric tracks for point mutation, copy number, and rearrangement data relative to mapping position in the genome. *Arrows* indicate examples of the various types of somatic mutations present in this cancer genome. Reprinted by permission from Macmillan Publishers Ltd: *Nature*, Stratton et al., *The Cancer Genome*, © (2009)

somatic mutations involving the tumor-suppressor gene *p53* occur in greater than half of all tumor specimens examined, making it arguably the most commonly mutated gene in human malignancies (reviewed by Levine and Oren 2009). Loss of this tumor-suppressor protein eliminates a cell's ability to either arrest the cell cycle and repair damaged DNA following a genotoxic insult or initiate apoptosis if the DNA damage proves to be irreparable (see Chap. 6). While a detailed discussion of cancer genes and the signaling pathways they control during carcinogenesis is beyond the scope of this chapter, we refer the reader to several comprehensive reviews on the topic of the molecular circuitry of cancer cells (Hahn and Weinberg 2002; Vogelstein and Kinzler 2004; Yeang et al. 2008).

As more cancer genomes are sequenced, it is becoming clear that a large number of cancer genes function in a handful of signaling pathways (Copeland and Jenkins 2009; see Chap. 6), corroborating the hypotheses proposed by Hanahan and Weinberg nearly a decade ago. Understanding this tenant is critical for the development of target-based cancer therapeutics directed against the deregulated signaling pathways themselves rather than the individually mutated genes (Copeland and Jenkins 2009).

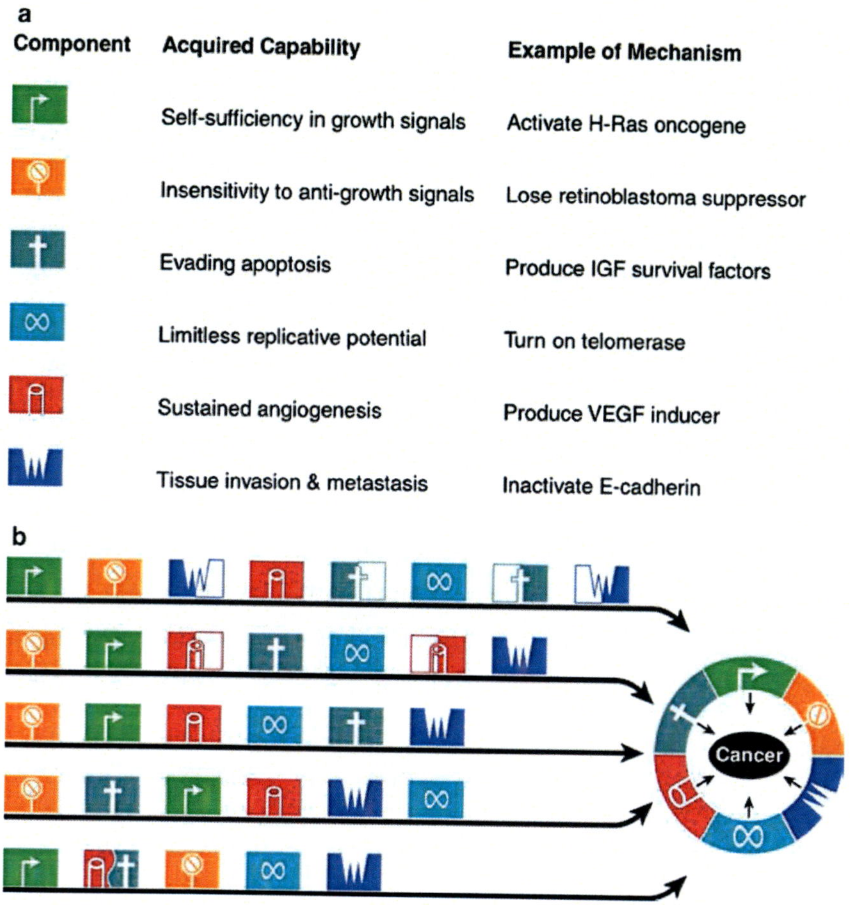

Fig. 2.6 Parallel pathways of tumorigenesis. Reprinted from *Cell*, 100 Hanahan D, and Weinberg RA, *The Hallmarks of Cancer*, p57–70, (2000), with permission from Elsevier

Conceptual Oncogenesis: Hallmarks Revised

While Hanahan and Weinberg propose that virtually all cancers acquire the same six originally proposed hallmarks (Fig. 2.6a), the timing and mechanisms governing such transformation may differ among malignancies (Fig. 2.6b). Mutations in certain oncogenes and tumor suppressors could vary sequentially, occurring early in some models of carcinogenesis while late in others. Consequently, the order in which hallmark capabilities appear during tumor progression may vary, both within and between cancer types (Fig. 2.6b).

In certain cancers, a specific genetic alteration may confer not only one, but also multiple traits simultaneously, thus lowering the number of distinct mutations required for completion of tumor progression (Fig. 2.6b). As an example, loss of the tumor-suppressor *p53* may contribute to both the anti-apoptotic and pro-angiogenic properties of a cancer cell (***as illustrated in the five-step scheme of*** Fig. 2.6b). Alternatively, a given hallmark may only be achieved through the functional cooperation of two or more genetic or epigenetic lesions, thereby increasing the total number of molecular events required for tumorigenesis. This concept is illustrated by the eight-step scheme (Fig. 2.6b) in which the novel capabilities of invading tissues and resisting apoptosis are each acquired in two distinct steps, involving separate genetic alterations.

Nonetheless, Hanahan and Weinberg (2000) propose "that independent of how the steps in these genetic pathways are arranged, the biological endpoints that are ultimately reached – the hallmark capabilities of cancer – will prove to be shared in common by all types of tumors."

Cancer and Alcohol

The mechanisms by which alcohol consumption exerts its carcinogenic effect are not fully understood but appear to occur during all stages of tumorigenesis (Fig. 2.7; reviewed by Poschl and Seitz 2004; Boffetta and Hashibe 2006; Seitz and Stickel 2007). Both animal and in vitro studies have shown that the main metabolite of alcohol, acetaldehyde, is capable of causing DNA damage that may lead to cancer

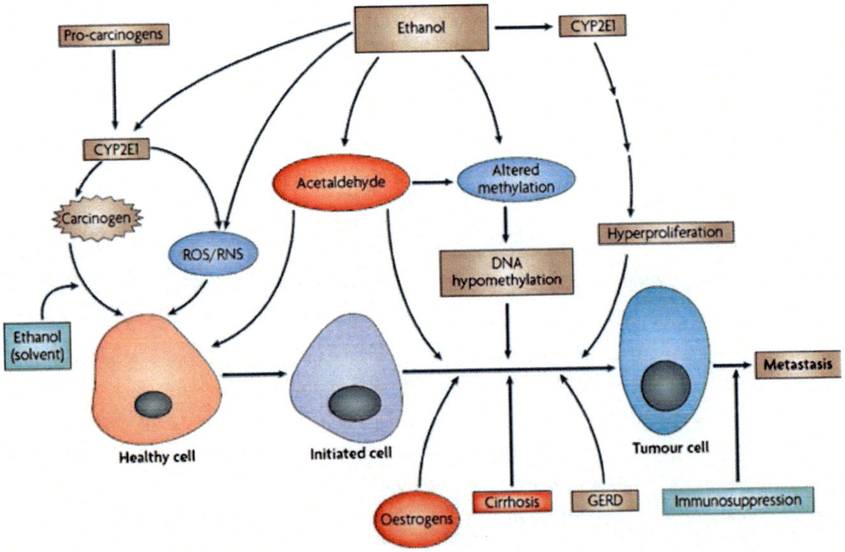

Fig. 2.7 Alcohol may promote carcinogenesis at many levels. Mechanisms with *strong evidence* are shown in *red*, with *moderate evidence* in *blue* and with *weak evidence* in *green*. Details contained within this text and cited reviews. Reprinted by permission from Macmillan Publishers Ltd: *Nat Rev Cancer*, Molecular mechanism of alcohol-mediated carcinogenesis, Seitz HK, Stickel F, © 2007

(see Chaps. 1 and 4). Alcohol metabolism or the presence of its metabolite acetaldehyde per se may *initiate* carcinogenesis by increasing the cytochrome P450 2E1 (CYP2E1)-mediated activation of various procarcinogens present in alcoholic beverages, tobacco smoke, and diets (see Chap. 4). Production of reactive oxygen species and successive lipid peroxidation may also contribute to the mutagenic effects of alcohol. During cancer *promotion* and/or *progression*, alcohol and acetaldehyde alter DNA methylation which may lead to epigenetic modifications to important cancer genes (see Chap. 5). Moreover, alcohol-associated damage to DNA and perturbations in both pro- and anti-oncogenic-signaling pathways have been observed following chronic alcohol use (see Chap. 6). Disruption in retinoic acid metabolism (see Chap. 7) and protein homeostasis (see Chap. 8) adds to the complexity of effects of alcohol on cancer development. And during cancer *progression*, alcohol consumption may contribute to inflammatory (see Chap. 9) and immunosuppressive (see Chap. 10) environments, thus allowing tumor cells to propagate and spread. Finally, the impact of alcohol on stem cells (see Chap. 11) and the role this interaction plays in alcohol-induced carcinogenesis warrants further investigation. These mechanisms and others by which alcohol contributes to oncogenesis are detailed in subsequent chapters.

Acknowledgments This chapter is based largely on information presented in ***Principles of Cancer Biology*** by Lewis Kleinsmith (2006) and from the seminal review ***The Hallmarks of Cancer*** by Douglas Hanahan and Robert Weinberg (2000).

References

American Cancer Society. 2009. Cancer Facts & Figures 2009. In. Atlanta: American Cancer Society.

Baker SJ, Fearon ER, Nigro JM, Hamilton SR, Preisinger AC, Jessup JM, vanTuinen P, Ledbetter DH, Barker DF, Nakamura Y et al. (1989) Chromosome 17 deletions and p53 gene mutations in colorectal carcinomas. Science 244:217–21.

Baker SJ, Preisinger AC, Jessup JM, Paraskeva C, Markowitz S, Willson JK, Hamilton S, Vogelstein B (1990) p53 gene mutations occur in combination with 17p allelic deletions as late events in colorectal tumorigenesis. Cancer Res 50:7717–22.

Beerenwinkel N, Antal T, Dingli D, Traulsen A, Kinzler KW, Velculescu VE, Vogelstein B, Nowak MA (2007) Genetic progression and the waiting time to cancer. PLoS Comput Biol 3:e225.

Boffetta P, Hashibe M (2006) Alcohol and cancer. Lancet Oncol 7:149–56.

Bos JL (1989) ras oncogenes in human cancer: a review. Cancer Res 49:4682–9.

Bos JL, Fearon ER, Hamilton SR, Verlaan-de Vries M, van Boom JH, van der Eb AJ, Vogelstein B (1987) Prevalence of ras gene mutations in human colorectal cancers. Nature 327:293–7.

Colotta F, Allavena P, Sica A, Garlanda C, Mantovani A (2009) Cancer-related inflammation, the seventh hallmark of cancer: links to genetic instability. Carcinogenesis 30:1073–81.

Copeland NG, Jenkins NA (2009) Deciphering the genetic landscape of cancer – from genes to pathways. Trends Genet 25:455–62.

Coussens LM, Werb Z (2002) Inflammation and cancer. Nature 420:860–7.

Futreal PA, Coin L, Marshall M, Down T, Hubbard T, Wooster R, Rahman N, Stratton MR (2004) A census of human cancer genes. Nat Rev Cancer 4:177–83.

Hahn WC, Weinberg RA (2002) Modelling the molecular circuitry of cancer. Nat Rev Cancer 2:331–41.

Hanahan D, Weinberg RA (2000) The hallmarks of cancer. Cell 100:57–70.

Howe JR, Roth S, Ringold JC, Summers RW, Jarvinen HJ, Sistonen P, Tomlinson IP, Houlston RS, Bevan S, Mitros FA et al. (1998) Mutations in the SMAD4/DPC4 gene in juvenile polyposis. Science 280:1086-8.

Kinzler KW, Nilbert MC, Su LK, Vogelstein B, Bryan TM, Levy DB, Smith KJ, Preisinger AC, Hedge P, McKechnie D et al. **(1991) Identification of FAP locus genes from chromosome 5q21.** Science 253:661–5.

Kleinsmith LD, D; Kelly J, Hollen B. 2004. Understanding Cancer and Related Topics. In: Understanding Cancer Tutorial Series: National Cancer Institute; http://www.cancer.gov/cancertopics/UnderstandingCancer.

Kleinsmith LJ (2006) *Principles of Cancer Biology*. Pearson Benjamin Cummings. San Francisco.

Knudson AG, Jr. (1971) Mutation and cancer: statistical study of retinoblastoma. Proc Natl Acad Sci U S A 68:820–3.

Kroemer G, Pouyssegur J (2008) Tumor cell metabolism: cancer's Achilles' heel. Cancer Cell 13:472–82.

Levine AJ, Oren M (2009) The first 30 years of p53: growing ever more complex. Nat Rev Cancer 9:749–58.

Luo J, Solimini NL, Elledge SJ (2009) Principles of cancer therapy: oncogene and non-oncogene addiction. Cell 136:823–37.

Mantovani A (2009) Cancer: Inflaming metastasis. Nature 457:36–7.

Markowitz SD, Bertagnolli MM (2009) Molecular origins of cancer: Molecular basis of colorectal cancer. N Engl J Med 361:2449–60.

Medema RH, Bos JL (1993) The role of p21ras in receptor tyrosine kinase signaling. Crit Rev Oncog 4:615–61.

Poschl G, Seitz HK (2004) Alcohol and cancer. Alcohol Alcohol 39:155–65.

Powell SM, Zilz N, Beazer-Barclay Y, Bryan TM, Hamilton SR, Thibodeau SN, Vogelstein B, Kinzler KW (1992) APC mutations occur early during colorectal tumorigenesis. Nature 359:235–7.

Rajagopalan H, Bardelli A, Lengauer C, Kinzler KW, Vogelstein B, Velculescu VE (2002) Tumorigenesis: RAF/RAS oncogenes and mismatch-repair status. Nature 418:934.

Seitz HK, Stickel F (2007) Molecular mechanisms of alcohol-mediated carcinogenesis. Nat Rev Cancer 7:599–612.

Sjoblom T, Jones S, Wood LD, Parsons DW, Lin J, Barber TD, Mandelker D, Leary RJ, Ptak J, Silliman N et al. (2006) The consensus coding sequences of human breast and colorectal cancers. Science 314:268–74.

Stratton MR, Campbell PJ, Futreal PA (2009) The cancer genome. Nature 458:719–24.

Takagi Y, Kohmura H, Futamura M, Kida H, Tanemura H, Shimokawa K, Saji S (1996) Somatic alterations of the DPC4 gene in human colorectal cancers in vivo. Gastroenterology 111:1369–72.

Vander Heiden MG, Cantley LC, Thompson CB (2009) Understanding the Warburg effect: the metabolic requirements of cell proliferation. Science 324:1029–33.

Vogelstein B, Kinzler KW (2004) Cancer genes and the pathways they control. Nat Med 10:789-99.

Yeang CH, McCormick F, Levine A (2008) Combinatorial patterns of somatic gene mutations in cancer. FASEB J 22:2605–22.

Zitvogel L, Tesniere A, Kroemer G (2006) Cancer despite immunosurveillance: immunoselection and immunosubversion. Nat Rev Immunol 6:715–27.

Chapter 3
Alcohol and Cancer Epidemiology

R. Thomas Gentry

Introduction

In a comprehensive worldwide assessment of cancer risk related to food and nutrition, the American Institute for Cancer Research (AICR 2007) identified alcohol consumption as a "convincing" or "probable" risk factor for esophageal, mouth, and laryngeal cancers, for liver cancer, for breast cancer in women, and for colorectal cancer especially in men. The World Health Organization's *Global Burden of Disease Project* concluded that "A total of 390,000 cases of cancer are attributable to alcohol drinking worldwide, representing 3.6% of all cancers (5.2% in men, 1.7% in women)" each year, with a corresponding annual mortality rate of 233,000, representing 3.5% of all cancer deaths (Boffetta et al. 2006). For the USA, the Alcohol-Related Disease Impact (ARDI) report indicates an annual rate of 2,464 deaths in six different alcohol-related cancer categories for the period 2001–2006 (CDC 2010).

This overview chapter serves as a summary of the impact of alcohol consumption on various cancers while highlighting evidence of the remarkably synergistic interaction between alcohol and other risk factors. The use of Alcohol-Attributable Fraction (AAF) to account for both independent and synergistic effects suggests that the magnitude of alcohol's impact on cancer may be greater than otherwise indicated. Also, the sensitization of alcohol's effect by another risk factor suggests that rates of drinking usually considered safe may in fact be hazardous *if* both factors are concurrent.

R.T. Gentry (✉)
Division of Metabolism and Health Effects, National Institute on Alcohol Abuse and Alcoholism, National Institutes of Health, Bethesda, MD, USA
e-mail: tgentry@niaaa.nih.gov

S. Zakhari et al. (eds.), *Alcohol and Cancer*, DOI 10.1007/978-1-4614-0040-0_3,
© Springer Science+Business Media, LLC 2011

Upper Aerodigestive Tract Cancers

Cancers of the pharynx, larynx, esophagus, and the oral cavity including the tongue account for about 64,500 new cases per year in the USA, or 4.4% of all new cancers and 25,790 or 4.6% of all cancer deaths (American Cancer Society 2009). As a group, these Upper Aerodigestive Tract (UADT) cancers (Fig. 3.1) are characterized by direct exposure to high (i.e., beverage) concentrations of ethanol and clear evidence of alcohol effects as exhibited by significant increases in relative risks (RR) for cancer even at moderate daily doses of 25 g/day (Corrao et al. 2004) and with relative risks in the four- to sixfold range with higher rates of alcohol consumption. But this large analysis of 156 studies covering 15 alcohol-related diseases did not report possible alcohol–tobacco interactions.

Alcohol and tobacco use interaction: Indications of alcohol–tobacco interactions on UADT cancers were noted early on (Wynder et al. 1957) and then supported by Rothman's evaluation of these data using his calculations of a synergy index (*S*, Rothman 1974, 1976). More recent studies use large meta-analyses and scaling to control for spurious associations such as heavier drinkers also being heavier smokers. The data presented in Table 3.1 (Hashibe et al. 2009) are typical of these studies (see also Ansary-Moghaddam et al. 2009) pooling over 11,000 cases and 16,000 controls to evaluate alcohol–tobacco interactive effects on UADT cancers. Note that "alcohol alone" failed to increase the odds ratio (OD) for any of the subsites or for UADT cancers as a whole. By contrast, there is a consistent synergistic effect between smoking and drinking for each of the three cancers included in the study. Using the

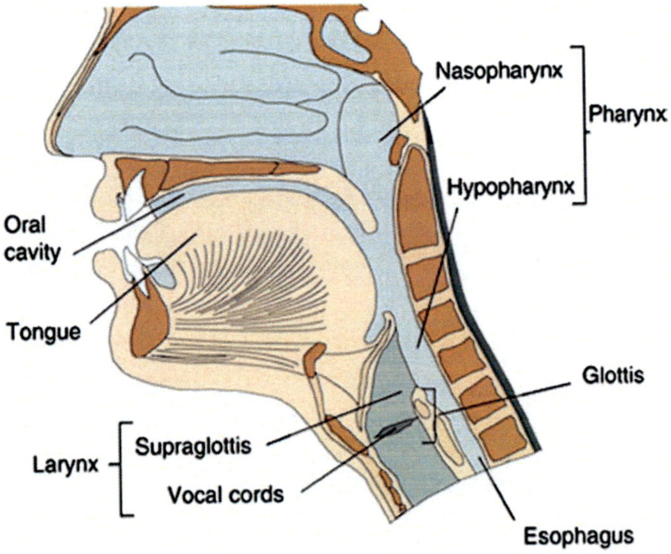

Fig. 3.1 Diagram of upper aerodigestive tract (UADT) cancer sites

Table 3.1 UADT cancers: alcohol and tobacco use on odds ratios (OR), multiplicative interaction parameters (ψ) and population attributable risks (PAR) for head and neck cancer and subsites (from Hashibe et al. 2009)

	Cases, *n* (%)	Controls, *n* (%)	OR (95% CI)	PAR (95% CI)
Head and neck cancer overall				
Alcohol alone	831 (7.4%)	1,587 (9.8%)	1.06 (0.88–1.28)	4.0 (1.5–5.3)
Tobacco alone	673 (6.0%)	3,653 (22.6%)	2.37 (1.66–3.39)	33.0 (42.6–25.9)
Tobacco and alcohol	9,146 (81.6%)	8,574 (53.1%)	5.73 (3.62–9.06)	34.9 (17.2–48.0)
Total	11,211	16,152	*ψ=2.15 (1.53–3.04)*	72.0 (61.2–79.1)
Oral cavity				
Alcohol alone	221 (7.4%)	1,587 (9.8%)	0.79 (0.60–1.04)	−1.1 (−11.4–3.7)
Tobacco alone	191 (6.4%)	3,653 (22.6%)	1.74 (1.10–2.76)	24.8 (19.6–31.1)
Tobacco and alcohol	2,354 (78.7%)	8,574 (53.1%)	4.78 (2.59–8.81)	39.9 (24.9–51.4)
Total	2,992	16,152	*ψ=3.09 (1.82–5.23)*	63.7 (44.7–74.7)
Pharynx				
Alcohol alone	247 (6.1%)	1,587 (9.8%)	1.28 (0.91–1.80)	5.6 (1.9–7.3)
Tobacco alone	289 (7.2%)	3,653 (22.6%)	1.91 (1.39–2.62)	24.3 (30.7–19.2)
Tobacco and alcohol	3,321 (82.2%)	8,574 (53.1%)	5.42 (3.21–9.16)	41.6 (25.0–53.7)
Total	4,038	16,152	*ψ=1.90 (1.41–2.56)*	71.5 (57.6–80.2)
Larynx				
Alcohol alone	284 (9.6%)	1,308 (10.0%)	1.21 (0.77–1.92)	2.9 (−0.3–4.4)
Tobacco alone	89 (3.0%)	3,041 (23.2%)	6.76 (4.58–9.96)	52.2 (77.8–36.0)
Tobacco and alcohol	2,541 (85.9%)	6,850 (52.2%)	14.22 (8.26–24.46)	33.4 (4.5–52.1)
Total	2,959	13,130	*ψ=1.62 (0.85–3.09)*	88.5 (82.1–92.4)

combined data for "Head and neck cancer overall" as an example, in the presence of tobacco use the added effect of alcohol increased the odds ratio (OR) from 2.37 to 5.73, which indicates a tripling the number of *added* cancer cases (from a 137% increase over baseline to a 473% increase over baseline). The statistical significance term $\psi > 1$ indicates a joint effect greater than expected under a multiplicative model (Hashibe et al. 2009).

Hashibe et al. (2009) go on to calculate the population attributable risk (PAR) for each condition thereby providing estimates of the impact of each risk factor, including interactions, in terms of the fraction (%) of the population affected. Again using overall data, the percentage of cancers attributable to alcohol-alone was 4.0% and to smoking-alone was 33.0%; and the portion attributable to the interaction was 34.9%, which suggests the total PAR for alcohol (also called the alcohol-attributable fraction, AAF) is 38.9%. Or looking at it another way, while the tobacco-attributable fraction is 67.9%, half of that is dependent on alcohol.

Sensitization: A study of women in Great Britain (Allen et al. 2009) designed and sufficiently powered (n = 1.28 million) to assess the effect of moderate drinking on cancer incidence revealed an additional manifestation of the smoking–alcohol interaction on UADT cancers as indicated in Table 3.2. Alcohol consumption, including the category with an intake of ≥7 units/week exhibited no impact on rates for UADT cancers *if* the women were "never smokers". If, however, women were current

Table 3.2 UADT cancers: sensitization of low doses of alcohol associated with tobacco smoking (from Allen et al. 2009)

Alcohol category (units[a]/week)	Never smokers		Current smokers	
	No. of cancers	RR (95% FCI[b])	No. of cancers	RR (95% FCI)
2 or less	165	*1.00* (0.86–1.17)	112	*2.54* (2.10–3.06)
3–6	121	*1.04* (0.87–1.25)	126	*3.57* (2.99–4.26)
7 or more	83	*0.93* (0.75–1.16)	257	*5.22* (4.60–5.92)

[a]One unit is equivalent to about 10 g alcohol
[b]Floated confidence interval

smokers then even the lowest intake category (≤2 units/week) exhibited increased risk (RR = 2.54) for UADT cancers. And women smokers consuming 3–6 units/week had a 3.57-fold increase in UADT cancers compared to nonsmokers. Since each unit = 10 g of ethanol, this means that intake less that 20 g/week, that is 1 ½ drinks *per week* (where one drink equals 14 g of ethanol, NIAAA 2007) is sufficient to more than double the risk for cancers of the upper aerodigestive tract. This magnitude of sensitization caused by smoking raises the question whether consumption of alcohol in a range otherwise deemed safe may in fact carry a significant risk if a sensitizing cofactor is also present.

Hepatocellular Carcinoma

Hepatocellular carcinoma (HCC) is said to be the fifth most common cancer worldwide and the third most common cause of cancer-related death, with an annual incidence of 564,000 new cases nearly matched by an annual mortality of 549,000 in 2000 (AICR 2007).

Global variation in HCC highlights the impact of multiple risk factors: The concentration of HCC cases in East Asia reflects the impact of infectious hepatitis, particularly HBV in China, Southeast Asia and HCV in Japan, and the combination of HBV and HCV in Mongolia (Globocan 2002; AICR 2007). Hepatitis B also prevails in much of Africa and in Haiti (Andernach et al. 2009), and other risk factors include food-borne aflatoxin exposure in sub-Saharan Africa, Southeast Asia, and China (Liu and Wu 2010), and isolated instances of dietary iron exposure (Kew and Asare 2007).

Alcohol's primary effects and synergistic interactions: Chronic heavy consumption of alcohol is a primary risk factor with significant effects on HCC depending on the quantities consumed. Table 3.3 summarizes the main results of three studies (Donato et al. 2002; Hassan et al. 2002; Yuan et al. 2004). Relatively high alcohol consumption (greater than 4 drinks per day) increased the odds ratios (ORs) to 2.6, 7.0, or 8.0 in the three studies in the absence of viral hepatitis. But a remarkably greater effect occurs when alcohol acts in concert with HBV or HCV, yielding odds ratios for HCC 48, 54, and 109-fold above baseline, respectively. This observation illustrates that the *synergistic* impact of alcohol on HCC can far outweigh its *independent*

Table 3.3 Hepatocellular carcinoma: summary of three studies evaluating the interaction between alcohol consumption and infectious hepatitis, HCV or HBV (representing +/– for HCV RNA and +/– for HBsAg)

	Low alcohol		High alcohol[a]	
	HCV– and HBV–	HCV+ or HBV+	HCV– and HBV–	HCV+ or HBV+
Donato et al. (2002)	*1.0* (ref)	*55* (30–101), *23* (12–43)[b]	*7.0* (4.5–11.1)	*109* (51–233), *49* (24–98)
Hassan et al. (2002)	*1.0* (ref)	*19.1* (4.1–89.1)	*2.4* (1.3–4.4)	*53.9* (7–415.7)
Yuan et al. (2004)	*1.0* (ref)	*8.1* (4.6–14)	*2.6* (1.3–5.1)	*48.3* (11.0–212.1)

[a]Definitions of high alcohol intake differed in each case but all approximated 4 drinks/day
[b]Donato et al. listed HCV and HBV independently

effects (i.e., effects occurring in the absence of other risk factors). Moreover, the combination of alcoholic liver disease and HCV occurs in a significant portion of patients with liver disease (Singal and Anand 2007), which suggests a frequently underestimated contribution to HCC (Mueller et al. 2009).

Alcohol and smoking interaction: While the effects of alcohol and smoking in combination on HCC suggest synergism, results are not always consistent. In a Japanese study, the RR for developing HCC was higher in those who both drank alcohol and smoked than in those who either drank or smoked (Mukaiya et al. 1998). And in another report, heavy smoking had no effect on HCC among light drinkers, but did have a significant effect among heavy drinkers (OR = 5.6; Kuper et al. 2000). Other studies found that while smoking alone increased the ORs for HCC (3.9 for men and 3.1 in women), a significant interaction with alcohol was only observed in women (OR = 2.8 for men and 13.7 for women; Hassan et al. 2008).

Global trends in hepatocellular carcinoma: In countries with the highest incidence rates of HBV such as China, recent trends are toward *decreasing* incidence of HCC largely attributable to widespread HBV vaccination and reduced aflatoxin exposure (Bosch et al. 2004). In Japan, the incidence of HCC is decreasing in younger people, although mortality rates lag behind, reflecting the acquisition of HCV several decades earlier (Tanaka et al. 2008). By contrast, several countries with historically low rates of HCC are experiencing steady increases in the annual incidence of HCC cases. These include Scotland (McDonald et al. 2008), Canada (Cancer Care Ontario 2006), France (Remontet et al. 2003), Australia (Law et al. 2000), and the USA (El-Serag et al. 2003).

Hepatocellular carcinoma epidemic in the USA: The National Cancer Institute's ongoing "*Surveillance, Epidemiology and End Results*" has documented the steadily increasing incidence rate for HCC from 1975 to 2005, with an annual percent change of +4.5%, and a threefold increase (from 1.5 to 4.9 per 100,000) over the 30-year period (Fig. 3.2; Altekruse et al. 2009).

One factor contributing to this increase in liver cancer is that it is the result of the increasing impact of viral hepatitis (mainly HCV) during the 1990s (El-Serag and Mason 2000; El-Serag et al. 2004). Even so, the majority of hepatocellular cancer

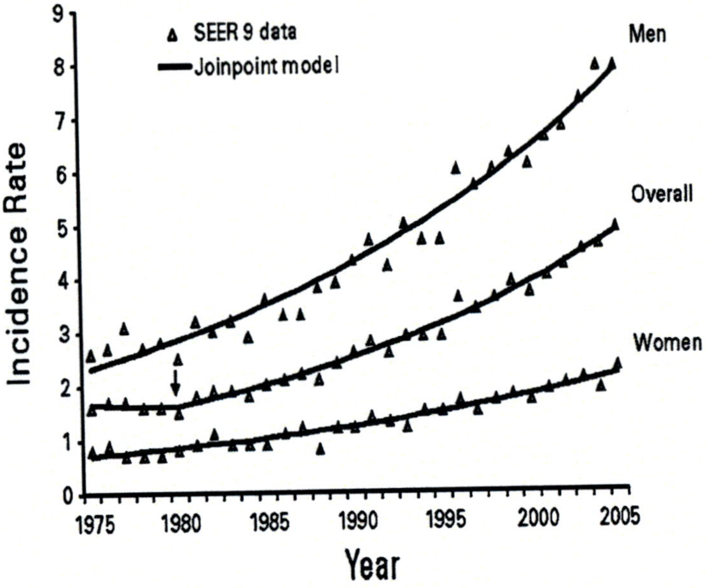

Fig. 3.2 HHC: Annual age-adjusted incidence rates per 100,000 and trends, all hepatocellular carcinoma cases and by sex, 1975–2005 (Surveillance, Epidemiology, and End Results 9, SEER9) (from Altekruse et al. 2009)

patients in the USA (55–78%) remained seronegative for both HCV and HBV (El-Serag et al. 2004; Hassan et al. 2002; Davila et al. 2004) and separate CDC data indicate that there has been a multifold *decrease* in the incidence of HBV and HCV acute hepatitis since the early 1980s (Daniels et al. 2009). Together, this suggests that other factors play a role in the rise in HCC.

The single largest identifiable risk factor among HCC patients, alcoholic liver disease (ALD), is present in about 25% of HCC patients (Davila et al. 2004), but alcohol consumption has been relatively stable (LaVallee and Yi 2010) and thus unlikely to contribute to the rising HCC rate, at least not independently. Instead, some assessments have focused attention on categories of HCC patients who were neither virus positive nor alcoholic (categories designated "non-specific cirrhosis" or "idiopathic", El-Serag et al. 2004) which together account for the majority of patients with HCC. Also referred to as "cryptogenic cirrhosis," these contributing factors of HCC are often assumed to be related to the obesity epidemic in the USA and other Western countries (Marchesini et al. 2008; Qian and Fan 2005), or more specifically to the following: diabetes, nonalcoholic fatty liver disease, dyslipidemia, and other manifestations of the metabolic syndrome (Osterreicher and Brenner 2007; Bugianesi et al. 2007; Siegel and Zhu 2009).

The linkage between obesity and the rising incidence of hepatocellular carcinoma is supported by several observations: the timing of the adult obesity epidemic and the rising incidence of HCC are approximately concurrent over the last 25 years

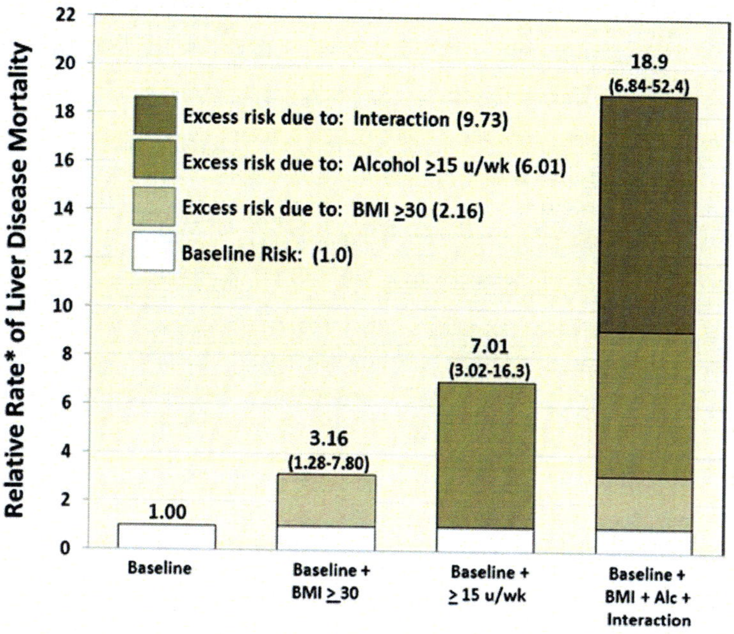

Fig. 3.3 Liver disease mortality as a function of BMI and alcohol consumption in men (data from Hart et al. 2010)
Units = 10 g ethanol.
*Relative Rate (95% CI) adjusted for age, study, social class, smoking, height, bronchitis, FEV1, angina, ischemia on electrocardiogram, and diabetes

(NCHS 2008), and the prevalence of obesity (BMI ≥ 30) in the USA is 32.2% among men and 35.5% among women (Flegal et al. 2010) is sufficient to have a large impact. However, a question arises when taking into account the male to female ratio for hepatocellular carcinoma (about 3.5:1 in Fig. 3.2). If the HCC epidemic were driven by the obesity epidemic, one would expect that men and women would be equally affected and the gender gap evident in Fig. 3.3 should be narrowing.

These observations do not eliminate obesity as an important contributor to the HCC epidemic; rather, they suggest that one or more additional cofactors play a significant role – a role that accounts for the observed gender bias. Likely candidates among risk factors include viral hepatitis B and C, and alcohol consumption. Each is a significant risk factor for HCC on its own, exhibits a greater incidence in men, and has the capacity to interact synergistically with obesity (Davila et al. 2004).

Alcohol and obesity interactions: A hospital-based, case–control study among HCC patients and controls conducted at the M. D. Anderson Cancer Center in Houston provides evidence that alcohol acts as a synergistic agent with diabetes (Hassan et al. 2002). With a background of diabetes, heavy alcohol consumption increased the risk of HCC from OR = 2.4 to 9.9 (Synergy Index, $S = 2.9$, $p < 0.02$). Consistent with other reports (Larsson and Wolk 2007), these data show that diabetes is an independent risk factor for HCC, and support the thesis that alcohol, which is consumed more by men than by women (2.67 to one, Keyes et al. 2008), could enhance the effect of obesity (in this case from RR = 2.4 to RR = 9.9) on the incidence of HCC.

Another recent study conducted in Scotland serves to illustrate the combined effects of alcohol intake and obesity on all liver disease mortality including cancer. Results indicate that even drinking 14 or fewer units per week significantly increased the relative risk to 5.30 (CI95%: 1.36–20.7, Hart et al. 2010). Since one unit is 10 g of ethanol, this is equivalent to ten drinks per week (or less that 1 ½ per day) based on NIAAA definition of 14 g per drink (NIAAA 2007). And for intake greater than 14 units (ten drinks) per week, the RRs were 3.16 in normal weight, 7.01 in overweight, and 18.9 in obese men (Fig. 3.3, data from Hart et al. 2010). Thus, these data demonstrate the capacity for obesity to amplify the effects of alcohol on HCC and to sensitize pathophysiologic mechanisms at rates of alcohol consumption usually considered safe.

Gender differences: Given that the incidence in HCC is largely driven by risk factors and the risk factors themselves occur more frequently in men than in women, the default assumption of this chapter on epidemiology is that the gender bias for HCC is secondary to the gender bias in risk factors. However, direct biological and endocrinological causes for gender differences in alcohol-induced HCC remain possible and perhaps likely. For example, male mice and ovariectomized female mice are more sensitive to diethylnitrosamine (DEN)-induced HCC than are intact females, and estradiol treatment reinstates resistance to DEN in ovariectomized females (Shimizu et al. 1998; Maeda et al. 2005).

Breast Cancer

Breast cancer was diagnosed in about 192,000 American women in 2009, accounting for 27% of all cancers and 15% of all cancer-related deaths in women (American Cancer Society 2009).

Epidemiological data reveal a near-linear relationship between alcohol intake and breast cancer risk even at very low rates of intake (Fig. 3.4). Reflecting this apparent linearity, investigators express the effect of alcohol on breast cancer as percent increase per unit of alcohol, i.e., 10 g consumed daily. A typical estimate is 7.1 ± 1.3% for each unit per day (Collaborative Group on Hormonal Factors in Breast Cancer 2002; see also Key et al. 2006). An increased relative risk of 7% per unit (or 10% per 14 g drink) may appear modest compared to values cited above, but breast cancer occurs very frequently and many women drink moderately. It is this combination that results in a large health burden, with breast cancer accounting for estimated 60% of all *alcohol-attributable* cancers in women (Boffetta et al. 2006).

An analysis of *interactions* between alcohol and other risk factors for breast cancer indicates few significant interactions even among risk factors known to exhibit independent effects. Thus, for women whose mother or sister had breast cancer there

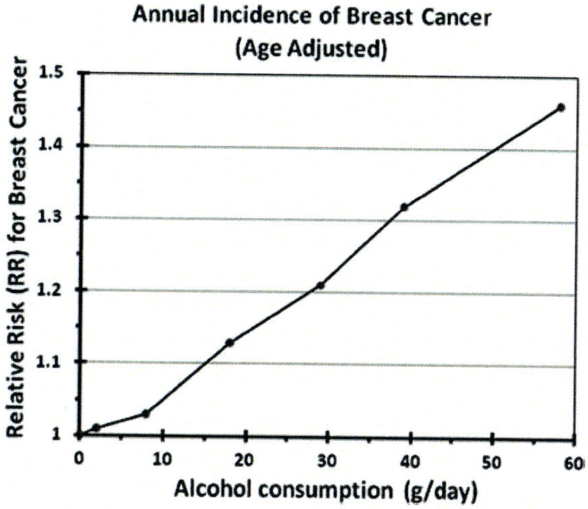

Fig. 3.4 Breast cancer: effect of alcohol consumption (g/day) on the annual incidence relative risk (RR) for breast cancer (data from Collaborative Group on Hormonal Factors in Breast Cancer 2002)

was a 12% rate increase per unit consumed. And for nonwhite women or women from developing countries, the effect of alcohol was not significant (Collaborative Group on Hormonal Factors in Breast Cancer 2002). Perhaps surprisingly, risk factors with known independent effects on breast cancer rates, such as parity, excess BMI, use of hormonal contraceptives or hormone replacement therapy did not exhibit *interactions* with alcohol (Collaborative Group on Hormonal Factors in Breast Cancer 2002). While other smaller studies have documented alcohol–HRT interactions for breast cancer; some are based on the absence of an HRT effect among women who do not drink or an alcohol effect only among "never users" of HRT (Colditz et al. 1990; Gapstur et al. 1992; Terry et al. 2006).

Recent advances have indicated that alcohol consumption is strongly related to estrogen receptor positive (ER+) breast cancers. Thus, for women with ER+ cancers, the odds ratio associated with drinking ≥13.8 g/day was 2.16 (1.68–2.76) compared to nondrinkers (Deandrea et al. 2008). Furthermore, the alcohol-associated impact on breast cancer appears to be effective in ER+ invasive lobular carcinoma, but not in ER+ invasive ductal carcinoma (Li et al. 2010).

Pancreatic Ductal Adenocarcinoma

While chronic alcohol consumption is a well-documented cause of chronic pancreatitis, alcohol's effect on pancreatic cancer (PDAC) has been inconsistent (Welsch et al. 2006). Tobacco use is the single most significant risk factor for pancreatic ductal adenocarcinoma (PDAC) (Lowenfels and Maisonneuve 2004), and the co-occurrence of drinking and smoking has made potential connection between drinking and pancreatic cancer difficult to distinguish. However, a recent case–control study found that subjects who were both heavy drinkers and heavy smokers exhibited a 4.3-fold greater risk for PDAC compared to heavy smokers who drank less than 7 drinks per week (Talamini et al. 2010). And a meta-analysis of 32 publications indicated that high rates of drinking (≥3 drinks/day) were associated with a **significantly increased relative risk for pancreatic cancer:** RR = 1.22 (1.12–1.34) (Tramacere et al. 2010).

Colorectal Cancer

Colorectal cancers (CRC) (i.e., cancer of the proximal colon, distal colon, and rectum) regularly appear on the lists of alcohol-related cancers (e.g., AICR 2007), and **various studies have identified gender differences or the differential effects of beer,** wine, or spirits (e.g., Bongaerts et al. 2008). However, reviews of this literature include both positive and negative studies (Seitz and Cho 2009). Examples of positive studies include the large NHANES follow-up study (NHEFS) that found the RR for colon cancer was 1.69 (Su and Arab 2004), and a pooled analysis of eight cohort studies indicated a RR = 1.41 for subjects drinking more than 45 g/day (Cho et al. 2004), **but with no indication of gender differences or specific beverage** effects. Finally, two recent reports came to different conclusions. While a large prospective study in Europe concluded that alcohol consumption was not associated with CRC (Park et al. 2009), a large meta-analysis of 103 cohort studies concluded the pooled RR for alcohol-associated CRC was 1.56 (1.42–1.79), which was about **twice that of other significant lifestyle factors including, diabetes, consumption of** red meat, obesity, or smoking (Huxley et al. 2009). Finally, it has been suggested that additional confounding effects for CRC may be associated with diet (Larsson et al. 2005) or the microbiome resident in the GI tract (Seitz and Cho 2009; Koivisto and Salaspuro 1998). It is anticipated that an understanding of these additional factors may help resolve apparent discrepancies in the existing literature.

Lung Cancer

Epidemiological studies consistently find strong association between tobacco smok-ing and the risk for lung cancer, but evidence for an effect of alcohol has been **elusive. Some studies found a significant effect of alcohol at doses greater than 50 g/**week (Korte et al. 2002). But other studies, each using large pooled-analyses yielded opposing results. One case showed a strong effect of alcohol in male "never smokers" with risk ratios RR = 2.53 for men drinking 5–15 g/day and RR = 6.38 for men drinking ≥15 g/day (Freudenheim et al. 2005), **while another focused specifically on life-**long nonsmokers reported "substantial evidence against the hypothesis that alcohol consumption *independently* increases lung cancer risk" (Thun et al. 2009). These results are not easily reconciled into a clear pattern. And an important caveat with all these studies is that the effects of alcohol need not be *independent* to be important, as is the case with the UADT cancers cited above.

Two indirect lines of evidence suggest that the potential interaction between alcohol and tobacco smoking on lung cancer should be reexamined. The first is that contrary to previous expectations there is now clear evidence that chronic alcohol exposure renders the lung susceptible to another stressor, such as sepsis. Characteristics of what has come to be called the "alcoholic lung" include the following: depletion of glutathione, dysfunction of the alveolar epithelium, and the consequent clinical manifestation: acute respiratory distress syndrome (ARDS) (Moss and Burnham 2003; Guidot and Hart 2005; Joshi and Guidot 2007). The second is the emerging evidence indicating a genetic susceptibility to lung cancer associated with the alcohol and acetaldehyde metabolizing enzymes already associated with UADT cancers (Segado Soriano et al. 2005; Minegishi et al. 2007; Park et al. 2010).

Prostate Cancer

The American Institute for Cancer Research report concluded that there were insufficient data to implicate alcohol as a significant contributor of prostate cancer (AICR 2007). The Alcohol-Related Disease Impact (ARDI) report indicated an annual rate of 232 deaths in the USA due to prostate cancer, which is less than one percent of the 27,000 annual total (American Cancer Society 2009). A recent review of the evidence from NCI indicated that while alcohol modestly increases the risk for nonadvanced prostate cancer, there was no association with advanced prostate cancers or mortality (Watters et al. 2010).

Stomach Cancer

The evidence for alcohol-associated stomach cancer is relatively weak. Thus, a population-based case–control study conducted in Montreal found no effect of 7+ drinks per week vs. <7 drinks/week for either all alcoholic beverages or each beverage tested individually (OR = 1.15 for all alcoholic beverages). But then, the same study found there was an effect among subjects drinking 7+ drinks weekly at the highest level of total exposure, i.e., >180 drink-years (Benedetti et al. 2009). Negative results have also been noted in India (Sumathi et al. 2009). On the contrary, ALDH2*2 is associated with increased susceptibility to gastric cancer (Yokoyama et al. 1998).

Thyroid Cancer (Alcohol Lowers the Risk)

Recent US data indicate that thyroid cancer is diagnosed in about 22,000 individuals each year with a relative low mortality rate of about 1,600 (ACS Table, 2009). Thyroid cancer is unusual in several ways: First, it is one of the few cancers with a significantly higher incidence rate (2.7-fold) in women than in men (i.e., other than breast and female reproductive system cancers, ACS Table, 2009). Second, very few risk factors have been identified for thyroid cancer, and those that have been identified are uncharacteristic of other cancers (iodine deficiency and childhood exposure to ionizing radiation, Dal Maso et al. 2009). Finally, the risk for thyroid cancer is *decreased* with alcohol consumption especially in women (Nagano et al. 2007; Mack et al. 2003). In the Million Women Study, alcohol reduced the incidence of thyroid cancer by nearly 50% (RR = 0.54, $p < 0.005$; Allen et al. 2009). The National Cancer Institute's NIH-AARP study confirmed a protective effect due to alcohol (RR = 0.57, $p < 0.01$) with two or more drinks per day and also indicated that beer was more effective than wine or distilled spirits (Meinhold et al. 2009). Finally, thyroid cancer may not be unique, since several sources including the Million Women Study also found decreased incidence of non-Hodgkin lymphoma (RR = 0.77, $p = 0.001$) and renal cell carcinoma (RR = 0.66, $p = 0.03$) associated with alcohol consumption.

Estimating Alcohol's Impact on Cancer Mortality in the USA

As a means for estimating alcohol's total impact on cancer mortality in the USA, Table 3.4 uses two sets of published data: alcohol-attributable fraction (AAF) as determined in Canada (Rehm et al. 2006) and the American Cancer Society (2009) table for 2009. Note that the AAF data approximate those in Table 3.1 (Hashibe et al. 2009), which explicitly takes into account tobacco–alcohol interactions on UADT cancers. The fifth and sixth columns of Table 3.4 are calculated for males and females, which are then summed and compared to the ARDI data cited in the Introduction. The total alcohol-attributable cancer deaths per year are calculated to

Table 3.4 Estimation of alcohol-attributable annual cancer mortality (from Rehm et al. 2006; American Cancer Society 2009; CDC 2010)

Malignant neoplasms listed by Rehm et al. (2006)	Rehm et al. (2006) AAF% deaths		Am Cancer Soc table estimated deaths		AAF% × estimated deaths		Alc. Attr. deaths	ARDI deaths
	Male	Female	Male	Female	Male	Female	Total M + F	Total M + F
Mouth and oropharynx cancers	32.7%	18.5%	5,240	2,360	1,713	437	2,150	376
Esophageal cancer	37.7%	24.2%	11,490	3,040	4,332	736	5,067	478
Laryngeal cancer	42.8%	31.0%	2,900	760	1,241	236	1,477	237
Liver cancer	31.7%	22.0%	12,090	6,070	3,833	1,335	5,168	786
Breast cancer	–	6.4%	440	40,170	–	2,571	2,571	355
Other neoplasms	8.7%	5.1%	–	–	–	–	–	–
Prostate cancer	–	–	27,360	–	–	–	–	232
Totals	30.5%	9.1%	59,520	52,400	11,119	5,314	16,433	2,464

be 16,433, which is much greater than the number (2,464) provided in the ARDI report (CDC 2010) and does not include prostate cancer or "other neoplasms" for which there were missing data cells. This sixfold difference raises the question whether an incomplete accounting of alcohol's synergistic effects may have led to underestimations of alcohol's total impact on cancer deaths in the USA.

Summary

From the overview presented here, it is clear that alcohol consumption is a major risk factor for cancers of the pharynx, larynx, esophagus, and other UADT tissues directly impacted by alcohol during drinking, and for cancer of the liver where alcohol is metabolized. Drinking is also a significant risk factor for breast cancer in women especially in developed countries. Among men, alcohol is a significant risk factor for CRC and for nonadvanced prostate cancer.

Epidemiological evidence emphasizes the observation that while alcohol is an independent risk factor for cancer, it also interacts with other major risk factors including viral hepatitis B and C, smoking and obesity, and that these interactions are typically synergistic.

Synergism can be manifested in several ways, including the following: (1) by a rate of cancer incidence significantly greater than the sum of each of the risk factors alone and (2) by sensitization to low doses of alcohol that would otherwise be considered safe, as in the case of smoking and alcohol on UADT cancers.

There is consistent evidence that alcohol-related cancers occur in about three men for every one woman (other than breast cancer, of course). One of the reasons for this difference probably is the gender bias in the risk factors that contribute to cancer. This is true for alcohol consumption, for HBV and HCV, and for smoking (albeit increasingly less so), but not for obesity. Also, it is likely that biological factor, including the effects of steroid hormones, contributes to the sex differences in cancer rates.

Finally, the epidemiological assessment of recent trends in the incidence of hepatocellular carcinoma indicates decreasing rates in parts of the world where incidence is highest, and increasing rates in developed countries. It is suggested that the increasing trends in HCC could result from the growing impact of obesity interacting with the gender-biased risk factors: alcohol consumption, HCV, and HBV.

References

AICR: American Institute for Cancer Research Diet and Cancer Report, Chapter 7 (2007) http://www.dietandcancerreport.org/downloads/chapters/chapter_07.pdf.

Allen NE, Beral V, Casabonne D, Kan SW, Reeves GK, Brown A, Green J (2009) Million Women Study Collaborators. Moderate alcohol intake and cancer incidence in women. J Natl Cancer Inst 101:296–305.

Altekruse SF, McGlynn AK, Reichman ME (2009) Hepatocellular Carcinoma Incidence, Mortality, and Survival Trends in the United States From 1975 to 2005. J Clin Oncology 27: 1485–1491.

American Cancer Society (2009) Cancer Facts & Figures for 2009. http://www.cancer.org/acs/groups/content/@nho/documents/document/500809webpdf.pdf.
Andernach IE, Nolte C, Pape JW, Muller CP (2009) Slave trade and hepatitis B virus genotypes and subgenotypes in Haiti and Africa. Emerg Infect Dis. 15:1222–8.
Ansary-Moghaddam A, Huxley RR, Lam TH, Woodward M (2009) The risk of upper aero digestive tract cancer associated with smoking, with and without concurrent alcohol consumption. Mt Sinai J Med. 76:392–403.
Benedetti A, Parent ME, Siemiatycki J (2009) Lifetime consumption of alcoholic beverages and risk of 13 types of cancer in men: results from a case-control study in Montreal. Cancer Detect Prev 32:352–62.
Boffetta P, Hashibe M, La Vecchia C, Zatonski W, Rehm J (2006) The burden of cancer attributable to alcohol drinking. Int J Cancer 119:884–7.
Bongaerts BW, van den Brandt PA, Goldbohm RA, de Goeij AF, Weijenberg MP (2008) Alcohol **consumption, type of alcoholic beverage and risk of colorectal cancer at specific subsites. Int J** Cancer 123:2411–7.
Bosch FX, Ribes J, Díaz M, Cléries R (2004) Primary liver cancer: worldwide incidence and trends. Gastroenterology 127:S5-S16.
Bugianesi E, Vanni E, Marchesini G (2007) NASH and the risk of cirrhosis and hepatocellular carcinoma in type 2 diabetes. Curr Diab Rep 7:175–80.
Cancer Care Ontario (2006) Cancer Fact: Increase in liver and intrahepatic bile duct cancer rates in Ontario August 2006. http://www.cancercare.on.ca/cms/one.aspx?pageId=9621.
CDC (2010) Alcohol-Attributable Deaths Report, Average for United States 2001–2005 https://apps.nccd.cdc.gov/ardi/Homepage.aspx.
Cho E, Smith-Warner SA, Ritz J, van den Brandt PA, Colditz GA, Folsom AR, Freudenheim JL, Giovannucci E, Goldbohm RA, Graham S, et al. (2004) Alcohol intake and colorectal cancer: a pooled analysis of 8 cohort studies. Ann Intern Med. 140:603–13.
Collaborative Group on Hormonal Factors in Breast Cancer (2002) Alcohol, tobacco and breast cancer – collaborative reanalysis of individual data from 53 epidemiological studies, including 58,515 women with breast cancer and 95,067 women without the disease. Br J Cancer 87(11):1234–45.
Colditz GA, Stampfer MJ, Willett WC, Hennekens CH, Rosner B, Speizer FE (1990) Prospective study of estrogen replacement therapy and risk of breast cancer in postmenopausal women. JAMA 264(20):2648–2653.
Corrao G, Bagnardi V, Zambon A, La Vecchia C (2004) A meta-analysis of alcohol consumption and the risk of 15 diseases. Prev Med 38:613–9.
Dal Maso L, Bosetti C, La Vecchia C, Franceschi S (2009) Risk factors for thyroid cancer: an epidemiological review focused on nutritional factors. Cancer Causes Control. 20:75–86.
Daniels D, Grytdal S, Wasley A (2009) Surveillance for Acute Viral Hepatitis – United States, 2007. Morbidity and Mortality Weekly Report 58: No. SS-3. http://www.cdc.gov/mmwr/pdf/ss/ss5803.pdf.
Davila JA, Morgan RO, Shaib Y, McGlynn KA, El-Serag HB (2004) Hepatitis C infection and the increasing incidence of hepatocellular carcinoma: a population-based study. Gastroenterology 127:1372–80.
Deandrea S, Talamini R, Foschi R, Montella M, Dal Maso L, Falcini F, La Vecchia C, Franceschi S, Negri E **(2008) Alcohol and breast cancer risk defined by estrogen and progesterone receptor** status: a case-control study. Cancer Epidemiol Biomarkers Prev 17(8):2025–8.
Donato F, Tagger A,. Gelatti U, Parrinello G, Boffetta P et al. (2002) Alcohol and hepatocellular carcinoma: The effect of lifetime Intake and hepatitis virus infections in men and women. Amer J Epidemiol 155: 323–331.
El-Serag HB, Tran T, Everhart JE (2004) Diabetes increases the risk of chronic liver disease and hepatocellular carcinoma. Gastroenterology 126:460–8.
El-Serag HB, Davila JA, Petersen NJ, McGlynn KA (2003) The continuing increase in the incidence of hepatocellular carcinoma in the United States: an update. Ann Intern Med 139: 817–823.
El-Serag HB, Mason AC. (2000) Risk factors for the rising rates of primary liver cancer in the United States. Arch Intern Med. 160(21):3227–30.

Flegal KM, Carroll MD, Ogden CL, Curtin LR (2010) Prevalence and trends in obesity among US adults, 1999–2008. JAMA 303:235–41.
Freudenheim JL, Ritz J, Smith-Warner SA, Albanes D, Bandera EV, van den Brandt PA, Colditz G, Feskanich D, Goldbohm RA, Harnack L, et al. (2005) Alcohol consumption and risk of lung cancer: a pooled analysis of cohort studies. Am J Clin Nutr 82: 657–67.
Gapstur SM, Potter JD, Sellers TA, Folsom AR (1992) Increased risk of breast cancer with alcohol consumption in postmenopausal women. Am J Epidemiol. 136(10):1221–1231.
Globocan (2002) International Agency for Research on Cancer (IARC) http://www-dep.iarc.fr.
Guidot DM, Hart CM (2005) Alcohol abuse and acute lung injury: epidemiology and pathophysiology of a recently recognized association. J Investig Med 53(5):235–45.
Hart CL, Morrison DS, Batty GD, Mitchell RJ, Davey Smith G. (2010) Effect of body mass index and alcohol consumption on liver disease: analysis of data from two prospective cohort studies. BMJ 340:c1240.
Hashibe M, Brennan P, Chuang SC, Boccia S, Castellsague X, Chen C, Curado MP, Dal Maso L, Daudt AW, Fabianova E, et al. (2009) Interaction between tobacco and alcohol use and the risk of head and neck cancer: pooled analysis in the International Head and Neck Cancer Epidemiology Consortium. Cancer Epidemiol Biomarkers Prev 18:541–50.
Hassan MM, Spitz MR, Thomas MB, El-Deeb AS, Glover KY, Nguyen NT, Chan W, Kaseb A, Curley SA, Vauthey JN, Ellis LM, Abdalla E, Lozano RD, Patt YZ, Brown TD, Abbruzzese JL, Li D (2008) Effect of different types of smoking and synergism with hepatitis C virus on risk of hepatocellular carcinoma in American men and women: case-control study. Int J Cancer 123(8):1883–91.
Hassan MM, Hwang LY, Hatten CJ, Swaim M, Li D, Abbruzzese JL, Beasley P, Patt YZ (2002) Risk factors for hepatocellular carcinoma: synergism of alcohol with viral hepatitis and diabetes mellitus. Hepatology 36: 1206–13.
Huxley RR, Ansary-Moghaddam A, Clifton P, Czernichow S, Parr CL, Woodward M (2009) The impact of dietary and lifestyle risk factors on risk of colorectal cancer: A quantitative overview of the epidemiological evidence. Int J Cancer 125:171–180.
Kew MC, Asare GA (2007) Dietary iron overload in the African and hepatocellular carcinoma. Liver Int 27:735–41.
Key J, Hodgson S, Omar RZ, Jensen TK, Thompson SG, Boobis AR, Davies DS, Elliott P (2006) Meta-analysis of studies of alcohol and breast cancer with consideration of the methodological issues. Cancer Causes Control. 17:759–770.
Keyes KM, Grant BF, Hasin DS (2008) Evidence for a closing gender gap in alcohol use, abuse, and dependence in the United States population. Drug Alcohol Depend 93:21–9.
Koivisto T, Salaspuro M (1998) Acetaldehyde alters proliferation, differentiation and adhesion properties of human colon adenocarcinoma cell line Caco-2. Carcinogenesis 19:2031–6.
Korte JE, Brennan P, Henley SJ, Boffetta P (2002) Dose-specific meta-analysis and sensitivity analysis of the relation between alcohol consumption and lung cancer risk. Am J Epidemiol 155:496–506.
Kuper H, Tzonou A, Kaklamani E, Hsieh CC, Lagiou P, Adami HO, Trichopoulos D, Stuver SO (2000) Tobacco smoking, alcohol consumption and their interaction in the causation of hepatocellular carcinoma. Int J Cancer 85(4):498–502.
Joshi PC, Guidot DM (2007) The alcoholic lung: epidemiology, pathophysiology, and potential therapies. Am J Physiol Lung Cell Mol Physiol. 292(4):L813–23.
Larsson SC, Wolk A (2007) Overweight, obesity and risk of liver cancer: a meta-analysis of cohort studies. Br J Cancer 97:1005–8.
Larsson SC, Giovannucci E, Wolk A (2005) Vitamin B6 intake, alcohol consumption, and colorectal cancer: a longitudinal population-based cohort of women. Gastroenterology 128:1830–7.
LaVallee RA, Yi H (2010) NIAAA Surveillance Report #90: Apparent per capita alcohol consumption: National, state and regional trends 1977–2008. http://pubs.niaaa.nih.gov/publications/Surveillance90/tab1_08.htm.
Law MG, Roberts SK, Dore GJ, Kaldor JM. (2000) Primary hepatocellular carcinoma in Australia, 1978–1997: increasing incidence and mortality. Med J Aust 173: 403–405.

Li CI, Chlebowski RT, Freiberg M, Johnson KC, Kuller L, Lane D, Lessin L, O'Sullivan MJ, Wactawski-Wende J, Yasmeen S, Prentice R (2010) Alcohol Consumption and Risk of Postmenopausal Breast Cancer by Subtype: The Women's Health Initiative Observational Study. J Natl Cancer Inst 102:1422–1431.

Liu Y, Wu F (2010) Global Burden of Aflatoxin-Induced Hepatocellular Carcinoma: A Risk Assessment. Environ Health Perspect. 118(6):818–824.

Lowenfels AB, Maisonneuve P (2004) Epidemiology and prevention of pancreatic cancer. Jpn J Clin Oncol 34:238–44.

Mack WJ, Preston-Martin S, Dal Maso L, Galanti R, Xiang M, Franceschi S, Hallquist A, Jin F, Kolonel L, La Vecchia C, Levi F, Linos A, Lund E, McTiernan A, Mabuchi K, Negri E, Wingren G, Ron E (2003) A pooled analysis of case-control studies of thyroid cancer: cigarette smoking and consumption of alcohol, coffee, and tea. Cancer Causes Control 14:773–85.

Maeda S, Kamata H, Luo JL, Leffert H, Karin M (2005) IKKbeta couples hepatocyte death to cytokine-driven compensatory proliferation that promotes chemical hepatocarcinogenesis. Cell 121:977–90.

Marchesini G, Moscatiello S, Di Domizio S, Forlani G (2008) Obesity-associated liver disease. J Clin Endocrinol Metab 93:S74-80.

McDonald SA, Hutchinson SJ, Bird SM, Robertson C, Mills PR, Dillon JF, Goldberg DJ (2008) A record-linkage study of the development of hepatocellular carcinoma in persons with hepatitis C infection in Scotland. Br J Cancer 99:805–10.

Meinhold CL, Park Y, Stolzenberg-Solomon RZ, Hollenbeck AR, Schatzkin A, Berrington de Gonzalez A (2009) Alcohol intake and risk of thyroid cancer in the NIH-AARP Diet and Health Study. Br J Cancer 101:1630–4.

Minegishi Y, Tsukino H, Muto M, Goto K, Gemma A, Tsugane S, Kudoh S, Nishiwaki Y, Esumi H (2007) Susceptibility to lung cancer and genetic polymorphisms in the alcohol metabolite-related enzymes alcohol dehydrogenase 3, aldehyde dehydrogenase 2, and cytochrome P450 2E1 in the Japanese population. Cancer 110:353–62.

Moss M, Burnham EL (2003) Chronic alcohol abuse, acute respiratory distress syndrome, and multiple organ dysfunction. Crit Care Med 31(4 Suppl):S207-12.

Mueller S, Millonig G, Seitz HK (2009) Alcoholic liver disease and hepatitis C: a frequently underestimated combination. World J Gastroenterol 15(28):3462–71.

Mukaiya M, Nishi M, Miyake H, Hirata K (1998) Chronic liver diseases for the risk of hepatocellular carcinoma: a case-control study in Japan. Etiologic association of alcohol consumption, cigarette smoking and the development of chronic liver diseases. Hepatogastroenterology 45:2328–32.

Nagano J, Mabuchi K, Yoshimoto Y, Hayashi Y, Tsuda N, Land C, Kodama K (2007) A case-control study in Hiroshima and Nagasaki examining non-radiation risk factors for thyroid cancer. J Epidemiol 17:76–85.

NCHS (2008) CDC: National Center for Health Statistics: Prevalence of overweight, obesity and extreme obesity among adults: United States, trends 1976–80 through 2005–2006. http://www.cdc.gov/nchs/data/hestat/overweight/overweight_adult.pdf.

NIAAA (2007) Rethinking Drinking: Alcohol and your Health http://pubs.niaaa.nih.gov/publications/rethinkingdrinking/rethinking_drinking.pdf.

Osterreicher CH, Brenner DA (2007) The genetics of nonalcoholic fatty liver disease. Ann Hepatol 6:83–8.

Park JY, Matsuo K, Suzuki T, Ito H, Hosono S, Kawase T, Watanabe M, Oze I, Hida T, Yatabe Y, Mitsudomi T, Takezaki T, Tajima K, Tanaka H (2010) Impact of smoking on lung cancer risk is stronger in those with the homozygous aldehyde dehydrogenase 2 null allele in a Japanese population. Carcinogenesis 31:660–5.

Park JY, Mitrou PN, Dahm CC, Luben RN, Wareham NJ, Khaw KT, Rodwell SA (2009) Baseline alcohol consumption, type of alcoholic beverage and risk of colorectal cancer in the European Prospective Investigation into Cancer and Nutrition-Norfolk study. Cancer Epidemiol 33:347–54.

Qian Y, Fan JG (2005) Obesity, fatty liver and liver cancer. Hepatobiliary Pancreat Dis Int 4:173–7.

Rehm J, Patra J, Popova S (2006) Alcohol-attributable mortality and potential years of life lost in Canada 2001: implications for prevention and policy. Addiction, 101: 373–384.
Remontet L, Esteve J, Bouvier AM et al. (2003) Cancer incidence and mortality in France over the period 1978-2000. Rev Epidemiol Sante Publique; 51(Pt 1): 3–30.
Rothman KJ (1974) Synergy and antagonism in cause effect relationships Am J Epidemiol 99:385–388.
Rothman KJ (1976) The estimation of synergy or antagonism. Am J Epidmiol 103:506–511.
Segado Soriano A, Santiago Dorrego C, Bañares Cañizares R, Alvarez Fernández E, Bandrés Moya F, Gómez-Gallego F (2005) Genetic susceptibility to the development of acute alcoholic hepatitis: role of genetic mutations in dehydrogenase alcohol, aldehyde dehydrogenase and cytochrome P450 2E1. Rev Clin Esp 205:528–32.
Seitz HK, Cho CH (2009) Contribution of alcohol and tobacco use in gastrointestinal cancer development. Methods Mol Biol 472:217–41.
Shimizu I, Yasuda M, Mizobuchi Y, Ma Y-R, Liu F, Shiba M, Horie T, Ito S (1998) Suppressive effect of oestradiol on chemical hepatocarcinogenesis in rats. Gut 42:112–119.
Siegel AB, Zhu AX (2009) Metabolic syndrome and hepatocellular carcinoma: two growing epidemics with a potential link. Cancer 115:5651–61.
Singal AK, Anand BS (2007) Mechanisms of synergy between alcohol and hepatitis C virus. Clin Gastroenterol 41(8):761–72.
Su LJ, Arab L (2004) Alcohol consumption and risk of colon cancer: evidence from the national health and nutrition examination survey I epidemiologic follow-up study. Nutr Cancer 50:111–9.
Sumathi B, Ramalingam S, Navaneethan U, Jayanthi V (2009) Risk factors for gastric cancer in South India. Singapore Med J 50:147–51.
Talamini R, Polesel J, Gallus S, Dal Maso L, Zucchetto A, Negri E, Bosetti C, Lucenteforte E, Boz G, Franceschi S, Serraino D, La Vecchia C (2010) Tobacco smoking, alcohol consumption and pancreatic cancer risk: a case-control study in Italy. Eur J Cancer 46:370–6.
Tanaka H, Imai Y, Hiramatsu N, Ito Y, Imanaka K, Oshita M, Hijioka T, Katayama K, Yabuuchi I, Yoshihara H, Inoue A, Kato M, Takehara T, Tamura S, Kasahara A, Hayashi N, Tsukuma H (2008) Declining incidence of hepatocellular carcinoma in Osaka, Japan, from 1990 to 2003. Ann Intern Med 148:820–6.
Terry MB, Zhang FF, Kabat G, Britton JA, Teitelbaum SL, Neugut AI, Gammon MD (2006) Lifetime alcohol intake and breast cancer risk. Ann Epidemiol 16(3):230–40.
Thun MJ, Hannan LM, DeLancey JO (2009) Alcohol consumption not associated with lung cancer mortality in lifelong nonsmokers. Cancer Epidemiol Biomarkers Prev 18:2269–72.
Tramacere I, Scotti L, Jenab M, Bagnardi V, Bellocco R, Rota M, Corrao G, Bravi F, Boffetta P, La Vecchia C (2010) Alcohol drinking and pancreatic cancer risk: a meta-analysis of the dose-risk relation. Int J Cancer 126:1474–86.
Watters JL, Park Y, Hollenbeck A, Schatzkin A, Albanes D (2010) Alcoholic beverages and prostate cancer in a prospective US cohort study. Am J Epidemiol 172(7):773–80
Welsch T, Kleeff J, Seitz HK, Büchler P, Friess H, Büchler MW (2006) Update on pancreatic cancer and alcohol-associated risk. J Gastroenterol Hepatol 21 Suppl 3:S69-75.
Wynder EE, Bross LI, Feldman R (1957) A study of etiological factors in cancer of the mouth. Cancer 10: 1300–23.
Yokoyama A, Muramatsu T, Ohmori T, Yokoyama T, Okuyama K, Takahashi H, Hasegawa Y, Higuchi S, Maruyama K, Shirakura K, Ishii H (1998) Alcohol-related cancers and aldehyde dehydrogenase-2 in Japanese alcoholics. Carcinogenesis 19:1383–7.
Yuan JM, Govindarajan S, Arakawa K, Yu MC (2004) Synergism of alcohol, diabetes, and viral hepatitis on the risk of hepatocellular carcinoma in blacks and whites in the U.S. Cancer. 2004 101(5):1009–17.

Chapter 4
Alcohol Metabolism and Its Implications for Cancer

Gary J. Murray, Philip J. Brooks, and Samir Zakhari

Abbreviations

ADH	Alcohol dehydrogenase
ALDH	Aldehyde dehydrogenase
BAL	Blood alcohol level
BHMT	Betaine homocysteine methyltransferase
CβS	Cystathionine β-synthase
CrPdG	Crotonaldehyde-derived N^2-propanodeoxyguanosine adduct
CtBP	C-terminal-binding protein
CTH	Cystathionine hydrolase
CYP2E1	Cytochrome P450-2E1
DNMT	DNA methyl transferase
GSH	Glutathione
hMLH1	Human MutL homolog 1, colon cancer
HNE	4-hydroxynonenal
JNK	JUN N-terminal kinase
MAT	Methionine adenosyltransferase
MDA	Malondialdehyde
MEOS	Microsomal ethanol-oxidizing system
MS	Methionine synthase
MTHFR	5,10 Methylenetetrahydrofolate reductase
N^2-Et-dG	N^2-Ethyl-2-deoxyguanosine
N^2-Etl-dG	N^2-Ethylidene-2-deoxyguanosine
NFκB	Nuclear factor kappa-light-chain-enhancer of activated B cells
MAP kinase	Mitogen-activated protein kinase
RA	Retinoic acid

S. Zakhari (✉)
Division of Metabolism and Health Effects, National Institute on Alcohol Abuse and Alcoholism, National Institutes of Health, Bethesda, MD, USA
e-mail: szakhari@mail.nih.gov

S. Zakhari et al. (eds.), *Alcohol and Cancer*, DOI 10.1007/978-1-4614-0040-0_4,
© Springer Science+Business Media, LLC 2011

RNS	Reactive nitrogen species
ROS	Reactive oxygen species
SAH	*S*-adenosylhomocysteine
SAM	*S*-adenosylmethionine
SHMT	Serine hydroxymethyltransferase
SIR	Silent information regulator
SRC	Src tyrosine kinase
THF	Tetrahydrofolate
UADT	Upper aero-digestive tract

Introduction

As described in Chap. 1, alcohol has been classified as carcinogenic to humans at several sites in the body by the International Agency for Research on Cancer (Secretan et al. 2009). These include the upper aero-digestive tract (UADT), liver, colon/rectum, and female breast. Numerous mechanisms have been proposed for these multiple carcinogenic effects (Zakhari 2006). In this chapter, we discuss some of the diverse mechanisms involving alcohol metabolism or alcohol-induced changes in metabolic pathways (Fig. 4.1) that may lead to cancer. These include formation of acetaldehyde, changes in the NADH/NAD$^+$ ratio, increases in oxidative stress, induction of cytochrome P450-2E1 (CYP2E1), procarcinogen activation, changes in folate and methionine metabolism, and effects on retinoid metabolism.

Metabolism of Ethanol to Acetaldehyde

Ethanol is converted to acetaldehyde by the action of both endogenous and exogenous (microbial) alcohol dehydrogenases (ADHs) and by CYP2E1 (Zakhari 2006, Fig. 4.2). Aldehyde dehydrogenase (ALDH) converts the acetaldehyde formed to acetate (reviewed in Edenberg 2007). Although CYP2E1 can also convert alcohol to acetaldehyde, under many conditions the amount of acetaldehyde generated is relatively minor compared to the contribution from ADHs. However, after induction following ethanol consumption (Salaspuro and Lieber 1978), CYP2E1 is of increasing importance to this process and thus may be more relevant to alcohol-related cancer via other mechanisms, as is discussed in more detail below.

Metabolism of Ethanol to Acetaldehyde by Alcohol Dehydrogenase

Pioneering work on the metabolism of ethanol identified multiple isoenzymes and characterized the enzyme kinetics for each (reviewed in Hurley et al. 2002). Understanding ethanol metabolism is not trivial, complicated by the presence of

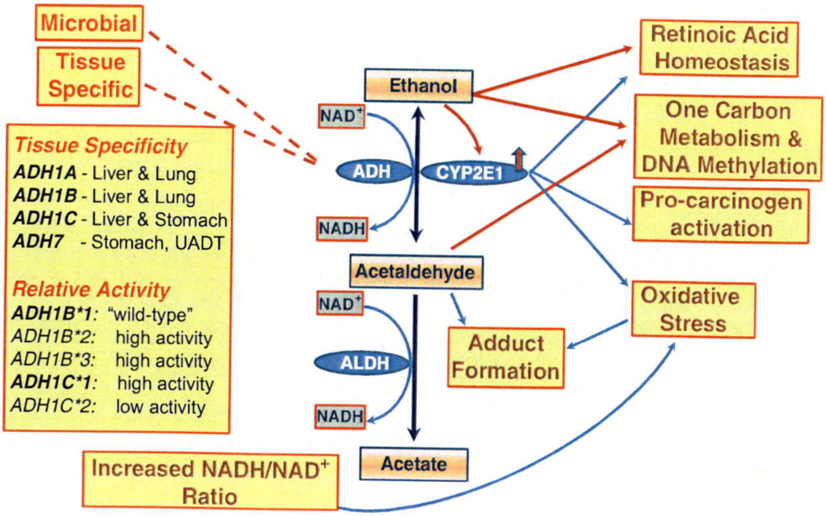

Fig. 4.1 Ethanol metabolism and its role in carcinogenesis. (1) Ethanol is metabolized to acetaldehyde mainly by ADH and CYP2E1, and is further oxidized to acetate by ALDH. ADH-mediated ethanol metabolism results in the generation of NADH and acetaldehyde. (2) CYP2E1 is inducible by chronic ethanol ingestion and leads to the production of acetaldehyde and reactive oxygen species (ROS) and also to an increased activation of various environmental procarcinogens. CYP2E1 also decreases tissue levels of retinol and retinoic acid. (3) NADH is reoxidized to NAD^+ in the mitochondria, which may further increase the generation of ROS. (4) Acetaldehyde can bind to DNA, forming stable adducts. ROS results in lipid peroxidation and lipid peroxidation products that also bind to DNA forming exocyclic DNA adducts

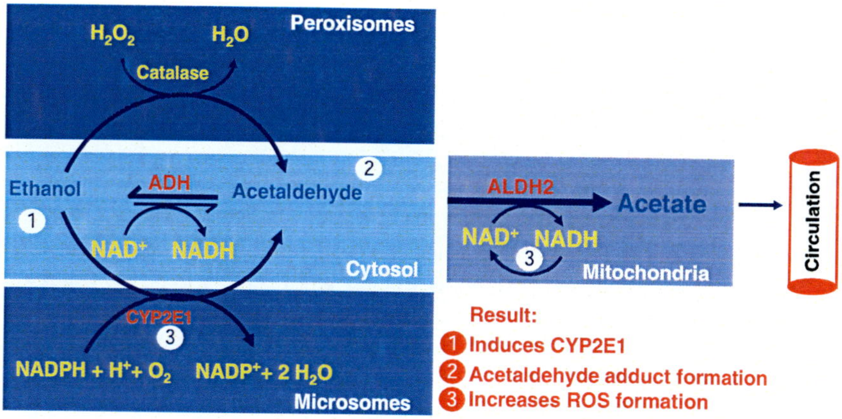

Fig. 4.2 Subcellular compartmentation of ethanol metabolism. Ethanol is metabolized to acetaldehyde by cytosolic ADH, micromal CYP2E1, and to a lesser extent by peroxisomal catalase. Acetaldehyde is oxidized to acetate by ALDH primarily in the mitochondrion

Table 4.1 Isozymes of alcohol and acetaldehyde metabolism

Official gene name[a]	Amino acid differences between alleles	Protein name	K_m for ethanol (mM)	k_{cat} turnover (min^{-1})	% contribution in liver (at 22 mM ethanol)	Organ and subcellular distribution
ADH1A		α	4.0	30	8.1[b]	Liver (cytosol)
*ADH1B*1*	Arg48, Arg370	β_1	0.05	4	21.8[b]	Liver, lung (cytosol)
*ADH1B*2*	His48, Arg370	β_2	0.9	350		Liver, lung (cytosol)
*ADH1B*3*	Arg48, Cys370	β_3	40	300		Liver, lung (cytosol)
*ADH1C*1*	Arg272, Ile350	γ_1	1.0	90	41.5[b]	Liver, stomach (cytosol)
*ADH1C*2*	Gln272, Val350	γ_2	0.6	40		
*ADH1C*3*	Thr 352	–	–	–		
ADH4		π	30	20	28.6[b]	
ADH5		χ	>1,000	100	<1	
ADH6		*ADH6*	?	?	<1	
ADH7		σ	30	1,800	<1[c]	Stomach, UADT, and other tissues

[a] Quantitative expression levels have been reported for some of the liver forms of ADH, but data are limited for other tissues

[b] Percentage contribution is calculated as an example only from data obtained for liver from an individual with the ADH1B*1 genotype

[c] ADH7 is not present in liver and would, thus, not be expected to contribute to liver alcohol oxidation (Hurley et al. 2002)

multiple isoenzymes, variable tissue-specific expression, and multiple genetic backgrounds. In humans, there are seven ADH isoenzymes and each has unique enzyme kinetic properties (K_m and k_{cat}) demonstrating tissue-specific variability in distribution and expression patterns. Four genes of the ADH family, coding for class I (ADH1A, ADH1B, and ADH1C) and class II (ADH4) enzymes, are significantly involved in the liver metabolism of ethanol (Han et al. 1998; Yin et al. 1999; Peters et al. 2005).

Extrahepatic oxidation of ethanol also occurs through the action of exogenous (microbial) or endogenous (human) ADHs. Among these is ADH7, a class IV enzyme that is found in all tissues and has a high K_m (low affinity for ethanol) but compensates with an extraordinarily high k_{cat}, resulting in an enzyme predicted to contribute significantly to ethanol metabolism at higher concentrations as may be found in the UADT following alcohol ingestion. Thus, metabolism of ethanol in the UADT which includes the oral mucosa, esophagus, and stomach may involve a combination of human isoenzymes, e.g., ADH1C and ADH7, both of which have been found in these tissues, in addition to microbial ADH enzymes.

Table 4.1 shows the various ADH isoenzymes, their individual K_m and k_{cat} values, and organ distribution (Hurley et al. 2002). Although it is tempting to use this type of data for predicting the role of specific enzyme isoforms in the metabolism of ethanol and associated risk for tissue damage, these data are only a rough guide and must be used in conjunction with information on the concentrations for each of the individual isoforms as determined by expression patterns. ADH isoforms vary considerably in the capacity to oxidize ethanol. ADH1B*2 and ADH1B*3 are "fast" relative to ADH1B*1 (Bosron and Li 1986). ADH1B*3, found primarily in individuals with Black ancestry, exhibits a high k_{cat}; however, the high K_m limits the rate of oxidation of ethanol except at very high blood alcohol levels. Under normal conditions of "social drinking," this enzyme is not saturated with substrate and thus the rate of production of acetaldehyde is not as dramatically increased as in the case of ADH1B*2. Individuals of Asian ethnicity might be expected to oxidize ethanol to acetaldehyde more rapidly due to the very high k_{cat} in combination with a low K_m. Asians have a much higher incidence for the ADH1B*2 allele [85% of the Japanese population expresses an "atypical" ADH, later identified as ADH1B*2, compared with only 20% in Caucasians (Stamatoyannopoulos et al. 1975; Ikuta et al. 1988)].

Cytochrome P450 Enzymes

In the liver, in addition to cytosolic ADH, the microsomal ethanol-oxidizing system (MEOS) contributes up to 30% to the metabolism of alcohol particularly after chronic ethanol intake. The MEOS resides primarily in the endoplasmic reticulum and includes the cytochrome P450 isozymes, CYP2E1, 1A2, and 3A4. CYP2E1 is induced by chronic ethanol consumption and although it has a moderately high K_m for ethanol of 8–10 mM (compared with the K_m of 0.05–40 mM for hepatic ADH), it is physiologically relevant especially in metabolizing ethanol at elevated alcohol concentration or in extrahepatic tissues, where ADH activity is low (for review, see Caro and Cederbaum 2004). CYP2E1 is induced by alcohol use and a variety of other conditions, including diabetes, obesity, fasting, and liver disease. As is discussed below, these enzymes have a prominent role to play in the generation of reactive oxygen species (ROS) and in the conversion of procarcinogens to carcinogens, as discussed below.

Microbial Alcohol Metabolism

Oral Cavity

Bacteria in the oral cavity and esophagus or in the colon are capable of readily converting ethanol to acetaldehyde, but have limited ability to further metabolize it to acetate. This may result in elevations in acetaldehyde in the saliva that can be 10–100 times higher than that found in the blood (Homann et al. 1997). Concentrations between 50 and 150 μM were detected in the saliva of normal individuals after ingestion of a moderate dose of ethanol (0.5 g per kg body weight) and much higher in individuals lacking ALDH2 activity. Moreover, use of an antiseptic mouthwash prior to alcohol use significantly reduced salivary acetaldehyde further demonstrating the important role of oral microbes in the production of acetaldehyde from ethanol. Coincidental heavy alcohol drinking, chronic smoking, and poor oral hygiene in drinkers who smoke result in the modification of the oral flora to contain an overabundance of aerobic bacteria and yeasts with an increased capacity to generate acetaldehyde from ethanol (Homann et al. 2000, 2001; Salaspuro and Salaspuro 2004).

Sidebar 1: Genes for Alcohol Metabolism

ADH1B: The functionally important polymorphic sites for *ADH1B* are thought to be Arg48 and Arg370. The **1* allele is considered the wild-type haplotype. Substitution of Arg48 with His constitutes the **2* allele, and Cys at position 370 constitutes the **3* allele.

*ADH1C*1* codes for Ile350 and Arg272: Substitution with Val (Ile350Val) and Gln (Arg272Gln) constitutes the *ADH1C*2* allele. The *ADH1B**2, *ADH1B**3, and *ADH1C*1* alleles each results in enzymes capable of faster metabolism of ethanol.

*ADH1B*2* and *ADH1B*3* increase ethanol oxidation by 40 and 90 times, respectively, compared with *ADH1B*1* (Bosron et al. 1983; Neumark et al. 2004), and *ADH1C*1* increases ethanol oxidation by about 2.5 times compared with *ADH1C**2.

*ALDH2*1* codes for a sequence containing Glu487: The *ALDH2*2* allele substitutes Lys for Glu (Glu487Lys) and is inactive. Homozygotes for *ALDH2*2* are unable to oxidize acetaldehyde, and heterozygote carriers do so inefficiently (Novoradovsky et al. 1995; Seitz et al. 2004; Seitz and Becker 2007). Also, since the ALDH2 isoenzyme is a tetramer, only one of every 16 ALDH2 enzymes is fully functional in heterozygous individuals (Weiner et al. 2001).

Interactions with Smoking

Another key observation is that smoking alters the microbial composition of the oral cavity in a manner that increases acetaldehyde production from alcohol (Homann et al. 2000, 2001; Salaspuro and Salaspuro 2004). An alcohol challenge to smokers without coincident smoking during the challenge showed twice the in vivo salivary acetaldehyde concentrations than in nonsmokers. Active smoking during the same challenge resulted in seven times higher salivary acetaldehyde levels due to high acetaldehyde concentrations in cigarette smoke. Morita reviewed the epidemiology for esophageal cancer risk in smokers and drinkers and noted that these well-established independent risk factors for esophageal cancer act synergistically and are not simply additive (Morita et al. 2010; Baan et al. 2007).

Alcohol alone increases the risk by approximately twofold, but when both heavy drinking and heavy smoking occur together the odds ratios increase 50-fold. Any or all of the following events may contribute to this synergy: local generation of high levels of acetaldehyde from ethanol and tobacco smoke; poor oral hygiene; solvent action of alcohol permitting transport to the esophageal mucosa of carcinogenic substances, including benzo[a]pyrene (Kuratsune et al. 1965); activation of CYP2E1; and subsequent activation of nitrosamines in tobacco smoke into active carcinogens (Seitz and Stickel 2007). The role of CYP2E1 is discussed in more detail below.

Microbial Ethanol Metabolism in the Colon

In the lower GI tract, coliforms and other intestinal bacteria possess ADHs with a low K_m for alcohol that are capable of oxidizing the moderate amounts of ethanol ingested during social drinking and generating significant levels of acetaldehyde within the colon (Jokelainen et al. 1996; Nosova et al. 1997). In germ-free rats, acetaldehyde levels in the colon were low compared to conventional rats. Similarly, treatment of rats with the antibiotic Ciprofloxacin decreased the ethanol elimination rate coincident with decreased intestinal aerobic and facultative anaerobic bacteria, fecal ADH activity, and acetaldehyde production.

Acetaldehyde Metabolism

Acetaldehyde is also classified as carcinogenic to humans (Secretan et al. 2009); therefore, understanding the different enzymatic mechanisms by which ethanol is converted to acetaldehyde is of particular importance to understanding alcohol-related carcinogenesis. The human ADH and ALDH genes are polymorphic, and studies of alcohol-related cancers in individuals with different forms of ADH and ALDH provide the most compelling evidence for the role of acetaldehyde in mediating the carcinogenic effects of ethanol (Yokoyama et al. 2002; Boccia et al. 2009; Toh et al. 2010).

The risk for tissue damage and potential for carcinogenicity due to acetaldehyde depend on the exposure time and concentration, which are determined by the net rate of production and removal of this highly reactive and potentially toxic metabolite. Acetaldehyde, produced by enzymatic oxidation of ethanol or from other sources in diet or in cigarette smoke, is normally quickly eliminated by conversion to acetate by ALDH. Importantly however, genetic variants of ALDH exist in human populations and result in decreased rates of removal of acetaldehyde with associated physiological sequelae (Smith 1986; Yoshida et al. 1991; Agarwal and Goedde 1992). Multiple human ALDH genes code for enzymes that catalyze the oxidation of acetaldehyde produced from ethanol metabolism to produce acetate and NADH, each varying in kinetics, preferred substrates, and tissue and subcellular localization. The low K_m forms (3–50 μM), ALDH1 and ALDH2, are of interest to the present discussion; the high K_m forms (5–83 mM), ALDH3 and ALDH4, are not relevant to the metabolism of acetaldehyde at physiological concentrations (Zakhari 2006). ALDH1 is a cytosolic enzyme that is found in various tissues, including liver, stomach, and brain, and that possesses a high affinity for retinal and plays a vital role in the oxidation of both all-*trans*- and 9-*cis*-retinal. ALDH2, found in the mitochondrial matrix of a smaller subset of tissue types with the highest level in the liver, appears to be the most important contributor to the oxidation of acetaldehyde.

Total alcohol consumption, drinking habits, tobacco smoking, and choice of diet may all contribute to the acetaldehyde burden (Salaspuro 2003b, 2007). Risk varies among individuals and in various organs within a single individual due to organ-specific enzyme expression, contributions to metabolism by microflora, or as a result of environmental or hormonal influences on expression. Ingested alcohol distributes rapidly among tissues of the body, eventually attaining approximately uniform concentration throughout the body; however, during transit from the oral cavity through the esophagus and gut, transient local exposure to alcohol or alcohol metabolites may vary considerably due to the variation in enzyme expression or microflora within a single individual or in different individuals. Concentrations of alcohol or acetaldehyde may greatly exceed the blood levels normally found after drinking and may also contribute to the pathology of alcohol-induced cancers.

The Inactive ALDH2 Allele and Alcohol-Related Cancer

Like the *ADH* genes, *ALDH2* is polymorphic. The most well-studied *ALDH2* polymorphism is the ALDH2 K487 variant (ALDH2*2), which is found almost exclusively in individuals of East Asian (Japanese, Chinese, Korean) descent. Individuals who are homozygous for the *ALDH2*2* allele have no detectable ALDH2 activity. Therefore, when these individuals consume even small amounts of alcohol (such as one glass of beer), acetaldehyde accumulates in the body causing severe adverse reactions, including increased heart rate, nausea, headache, and facial flushing. These adverse effects strongly discourage alcohol drinking, and as a result *ALDH2*2* homozygotes are protected against developing alcoholism. Since *ALDH2*2* homozygotes drink very little alcohol, which is a risk factor for esophageal cancer, they are at a significantly reduced risk for this disease.

When ALDH2 heterozygotes drink alcohol, they also experience aversive effects, though not to the same extent as homozygotes. In contrast to *ALDH2*2* homozygotes, ALDH2*2/*1 heterozygotes have very low, but detectable, levels of ALDH2 activity. ALDH2 exists as a tetrameric enzyme exhibiting "half-of-the-sites" reactivity, i.e., two active sites per tetramer. Also, the presence of one mutant (inactive) subunit inactivates the dimer pair resulting in much less than half the activity of the ALDH2*1 enzyme (Weiner et al. 2001). Some ALDH2 heterozygotes can become

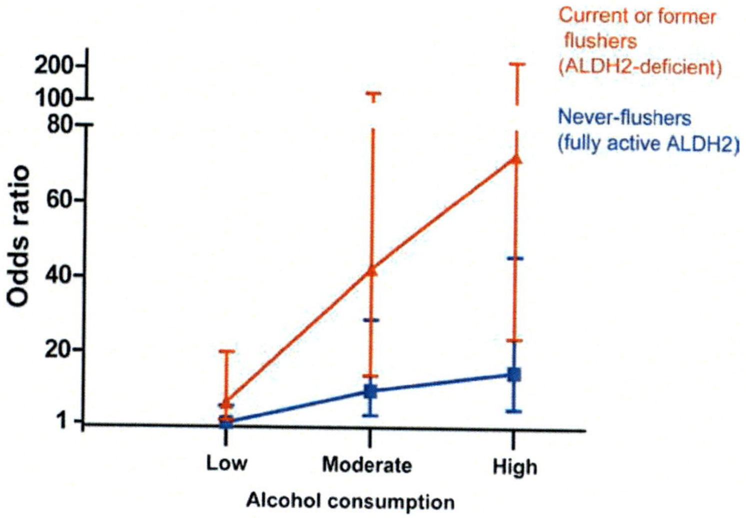

Fig. 4.3 Increased risk of esophageal cancer in ALDH2-deficient individuals

tolerant to the aversive effects and become heavy drinkers. In such individuals, the risk of squamous cell carcinoma of the esophagus rises dramatically such that at each level of consumption, the risk of cancer is increased by five- to sixfold compared to individuals with fully active ALDH2 (Fig. 4.3) (Brooks et al. 2009).

The time and concentration of exposure to acetaldehyde are dependent on the source or route of administration, the rate of acetaldehyde generation, and the local capacity to detoxify the acetaldehyde present. In normal individuals (*ALDH2*1/*1*), the plasma concentration of acetaldehyde is generally less than 5 μM, whereas in individuals homozygous for the defective enzyme, i.e., *ALDH2*2/*2*, acetaldehyde levels may be 60–100 μM, resulting in a 10- to 380-fold increased risk for UADT cancers. After consumption of alcohol, the inability of the oral mucosa and salivary glands to remove acetaldehyde results in markedly elevated concentrations of acetaldehyde in the saliva. Asian drinkers with a low-activity ADH isoenzyme may still experience significant acetaldehyde exposure time and increased risk for UADT cancer, presumably as a result of metabolism of ethanol by oral microbes and slow removal of the acetaldehyde formed.

Effect of Binge Drinking

The balance between generation and removal of acetaldehyde depends on individual genetic background but may also be overwhelmed by occasional binge drinking, where a blood alcohol level (BAL) in excess of the legal limit for intoxication of 22 mM is frequently found. Measurement of tissue biopsy specimens has shown that at concentrations of alcohol from 33 mM up to 500 mM the rate of formation of acetaldehyde is relatively constant at 600–800 nmol/min/g tissue, whereas at 200 μM acetaldehyde, the rate of removal is only 30 nmol/min/g tissue (Yin et al. 1993). The net effect generates significant local acetaldehyde accumulation without factoring in any possible contributions from microbial alcohol metabolism or other sources of acetaldehyde.

Changes in Alcohol Metabolism in Tumors

Jelski and colleagues have documented alterations in ethanol metabolism in cancerous tissues. For example, the activity of esophageal class IV ADH was shown to be doubled in cases of esophageal cancer, squamous cell carcinoma, and adenocarcinomas compared with normal esophageal tissues (Jelski et al. 2007b). Tissue-specific increases in ADH activity were observed in colorectal cancer (class I ADH) (Jelski et al. 2004), in pancreatic cancer (class III ADH) (Jelski et al. 2007a), and in gastric cancer (class IV ADH) (Jelski et al. 2007b). In breast cancer, however, the activity of class I ADH is significantly lower in cancer cells than that in healthy tissues (Jelski et al. 2006).

Physiological Acetaldehyde Concentrations

Levels of acetaldehyde in the blood have previously been a source of controversy due to the fact that many early measurements failed to correct for acetaldehyde formation during sample preparation. More recently, using methods which avoid this artifact, acetaldehyde levels in males with fully active ALDH2 are low or undetectable after drinking (Eriksson 2007). In contrast, low levels of acetaldehyde are detectable in females following alcohol drinking depending upon steroid hormone levels, which may have relevance for alcohol-related breast cancer risk. Acetaldehyde concentrations in the saliva and gut can be much higher than in the blood. Concentrations in human saliva after an intoxicating load of ethanol (BAL = 44 mM) may be as high as 450 μM depending upon ALDH2 genotype and other factors. As noted above, acetaldehyde concentration in the colon of rats fed an alcohol diet has been reported to be as high as 2.7 mM (Visapaa et al. 1998).

The Role of Acetaldehyde in Alcohol-Related Cancer

The acetaldehyde hypothesis: If acetaldehyde is a principal component of the alcohol-induced carcinogenic process, then increased acetaldehyde levels will increase the risk of head and neck cancer. Increased generation of acetaldehyde, as may result from possession of the fast-metabolizing alleles of ADH (*ADH1B*2*, *ADH1B*3*, and *ADH1C*1*) alone or in combination with slow metabolism of acetaldehyde due to

Table 4.2 Epidemiological studies

Population	Cancer type	Genotype	Result	References
European	Various	*ADH1B*	No association	Risch et al. (2003), Lilla et al. (2005)
Asian	UADT	*ADH1B*1 (slow)*	Increased risk	Yokoyama and Omori (2003), Druesne-Pecollo et al. (2009)
European	Various	*ADH1B*2 (fast)*	Protective	Hashibe et al. (2006)
Caucasians	Head and neck	*ADH1C*1 (fast)*	Increased risk	Visapaa et al. (2004), Homann et al. (2006)
European	Head and neck	*ADH1C*	No association	Brennan et al. (2004)
European	Head and neck	*ADH1C*2 (slow)*	Increased risk	Salaspuro (2003a), Hashibe et al. (2006)
Caucasian	Head and neck	*ADH1C*2 (slow)*	Increased risk	Schwartz et al. (2001), Peters et al. (2005)

the presence of the null allele for ALDH (ALDH2*2), might be predicted to lead to significantly higher concentrations of acetaldehyde and thus a greater relative risk of developing some forms of cancer. This prediction has posed some difficulty, especially in some older epidemiological studies (Table 4.2) (Boffetta and Hashibe 2006).

Conflicting Epidemiological Data

Conflicting data have appeared in the literature relating mutations in ADH to carcinogenesis (Table 4.2). However, more recent data with respect to cancer risk in the UADT appears to be more consistent with the acetaldehyde hypothesis. All studies in Asian populations have consistently associated the *ADH1B*1* allele (rare in Asians) with an increased risk of esophageal cancer (Yokoyama and Omori 2003; Druesne-Pecollo et al. 2009). However, in some studies in European populations, *ADH1B* was not associated with alcohol-related cancer (Risch et al. 2003; Lilla et al. 2005), whereas later studies in Europeans found a protective effect of *ADH1B*2* (faster alcohol oxidation) for UADT cancer (Hashibe et al. 2006). In some reports, Caucasian heavy drinkers with high-activity ADH1C*1 have a significantly increased risk for head and neck cancers in association with elevated levels of acetaldehyde in saliva after alcohol consumption (Visapaa et al. 2004; Homann et al. 2006). In reports published in 2004, the *ADH1C* genotype was not associated with the risk of head and neck cancer in populations of European origin (Brennan et al. 2004), but in later studies a moderately increased risk for individuals carrying the "slow"-allele *ADH1C*2* was reported (Salaspuro 2003b; Hashibe et al. 2006). Two additional studies have reported a significantly increased risk for head and neck cancer associated with the low-activity *ADH1C*2* genotype in heavy drinkers (Schwartz et al. 2001; Peters et al. 2005). Reduced alcohol metabolism as a result of a variant (low activity) *ADH7* allele also results in a pronounced protective effect (Hashibe et al. 2008). The class IV enzyme ADH7, mentioned earlier, is of interest in UADT cancers despite the apparently high K_m, since this isoform has a very high k_{cat}, is found in the tissues of the UADT, and may be exposed to high concentrations of ethanol up to 0.5–1 M during drinking.

On the surface, the results showing an association between lower ADH1B activity (*ADH1B*1*) and increased cancer risk are paradoxical; however, the decrease in the liver enzyme may have no effect on the enzymes expressed locally in the UADT or may reduce the rate of liver metabolism leaving higher concentrations of alcohol to be removed by other systems. The most recent results showing association of cancer risk with "faster" metabolism due to the presence of the ADH1C*1 allele are more consistent with a model that attributes the greater risk in this instance to the enzyme capable of generating higher (local) concentrations of acetaldehyde and are independent of enzyme activity in the liver. The observed tissue-specific expression of ADH1C in the UADT (Liao et al. 1991; Moreno et al. 1994) supports an increased risk of cancer associated with increased metabolism. Since the primary ADH activity in UADT arises from *ADH1C* and *ADH7*, variations in these enzymes may explain variable risk for cancer. The absence of effect of the *ADH1B* genotype may also be explained by the absence of expression of this gene in the UADT.

The primary difficulty with the acetaldehyde hypothesis is that it oversimplifies the metabolism of alcohol. It fails to recognize differences in localized expression patterns for various ADH isoforms and the complexity in the etiology of various cancers. Recognizing the tissue specificity of the metabolic enzymes involved requires a limitation to the hypothesis as follows: acetaldehyde is an important factor in the generation of cancers of the UADT, but may play a relatively minor role in liver or breast cancer where any number of additional factors, such as generation of ROS, procarcinogen activation, epigenetic modifications, alteration of retinoid homeostasis, changes in cell signaling, or changes in hormone expression, may take preeminence.

As noted above, alcohol drinking increases the risk of cancer at several sites in the body. Below, we review the evidence for acetaldehyde in alcohol-related cancer at different sites.

Squamous Cell Carcinoma of the Esophagus

The most compelling evidence for a role for acetaldehyde in alcohol-related carcinogenesis comes from epidemiological studies from Asian individuals with ALDH2 deficiency. A series of studies by Yokoyama and colleagues have shown that individuals who lack ALDH2 activity due to the K487 ALDH2 variant have a dramatically increased risk of esophageal cancer from alcohol consumption. In the absence of alcohol consumption, no increased risk was observed, indicating that the risk is due to the formation of acetaldehyde from ethanol metabolism. At all levels of alcohol consumption studied, ALDH2-deficient individuals have about a five- to six-fold increase in the risk of squamous cell cancer of the esophagus compared to individuals with fully active ALDH2. In these studies, the groups have been matched for alcohol consumption, smoking, and consumption of fruits and vegetables. It is notable here that ALDH2-deficient individuals drink less alcohol than those with fully active ALDH2, due to the aversive affects they experience from alcohol consumption, yet still have elevated risks of esophageal cancer. The data from ALDH2 individuals provided the primary basis for the classification of acetaldehyde generated as a consequence of alcohol consumption as a group 1 carcinogen (Secretan et al. 2009).

Other UADT Sites

In addition to the esophagus, the presence of inactive ALDH2 appears to be consistently linked to an increased risk of oral, pharyngeal, laryngeal, lung, and colon cancer. Yokoyama (Yokoyama et al. 1998) reported that the presence of the *ALDH2*2* allele significantly increased the odds ratios for oropharyngolaryngeal (11.14), stomach (3.49), colon (3.35), lung (8.20), and esophageal cancer concomitant with oropharyngolaryngeal and/or stomach cancer (54.20), but not for liver or other cancers (after adjustment for age, daily alcohol consumption, and amount of cigarette smoking). Also, ALDH2 deficiency among Asian heavy drinkers and high-activity ADH among Caucasians drinking over 30 g alcohol/day have also been shown to be associated with an enhanced incidence of colorectal cancers (Yokoyama et al. 1998; Homann et al. 2009).

Breast Cancer

There is also some evidence supporting a role for acetaldehyde in alcohol-related breast cancer. Two studies (Freudenheim et al. 1999; Terry et al. 2006) have linked the ADH1C*1 allele to alcohol-related breast cancer while one study (Hines et al. 2000) did not observe this effect. However, as has been discussed (Seitz and Stickel 2007), the negative study included women who consumed relatively low levels of alcohol. Therefore, it is possible that the high-activity ADH1C*1 allele increases alcohol-related breast cancer risk in women, but only if they consume sufficiently high levels of ethanol.

Liver Cancer

Finally, it is notable that while the liver is the major site of ethanol metabolism to acetaldehyde, there is no evidence supporting a role for acetaldehyde in alcohol-related liver cancer. Although the liver is the major site of acetaldehyde metabolism by ALDH2, there is also no evidence for increased alcohol-related liver cancer in ALDH2-deficient individuals (Yokoyama et al. 1998). It is highly likely that acetaldehyde-DNA adducts are increased in the liver of ALDH2-deficient alcoholics, since studies in ALDH2-deficient mice given chronic ethanol show a dramatic increase in N^2-Et-dG adducts compared to wild-type mice.

This apparent dissociation between acetaldehyde-DNA adduct formation and liver carcinogenesis may reflect the fact that cells in the liver are largely quiescent, providing time for DNA repair. In contrast, other alcohol-related cancer sites contain stratified epithelia with basal cells that are constantly dividing.

Conclusion

Studies of alcohol-related esophageal cancer in ALDH2-deficient individuals have provided compelling evidence in support of a role for acetaldehyde in squamous cell cancer of the esophagus. Other epidemiologic studies also support a role for acetaldehyde in alcohol-related UADT cancers in Asian populations. In non-Asian populations, some genetic epidemiologic studies support a role for acetaldehyde in alcohol-related cancer, whereas others do not support such a role. Reports of association of cancer with differentially active ADH variants must be interpreted in the light of the above discussion of localized enzyme expression. In future studies, additional information on acetaldehyde levels within specific target tissues will be valuable in assessing the role of acetaldehyde.

In Asian populations, the presence or absence of the inactive ALDH2*2 allele dominates the risk factors for cancer of the UADT as a result of alcohol consumption. However, in other populations, there is also evidence for a role for acetaldehyde in alcohol-related cancers, though there are conflicting findings as well.

Mechanisms of Acetaldehyde Carcinogenicity

Acetaldehyde-DNA Adduct Formation

Acetaldehyde from ethanol metabolism leads to adduct formation with both DNA and proteins. In terms of carcinogenesis, the DNA adducts are of primary relevance. The immediate reaction of acetaldehyde with DNA is a Schiff base adduct, N^2-Ethylidene-2-deoxyguanosine (N^2-Etl-dG). Studies of N^2-Ethyl-2-deoxyguanosine (N^2-Et-dG), a reduced version of this adduct, have indicated that this adduct has limited mutagenicity and genotoxicity. However, physiological concentrations of acetaldehyde and polyamines, such as spermidine, have also been shown to generate crotonaldehyde in vitro (Theruvathu et al. 2005) which may subsequently form the DNA adduct alpha-methyl-gamma hydroxypropano-deoxyguanosine, also known as Crotonaldehyde-derived N^2-propanodeoxyguanosine adduct (CrPdG) (Fig. 4.4).

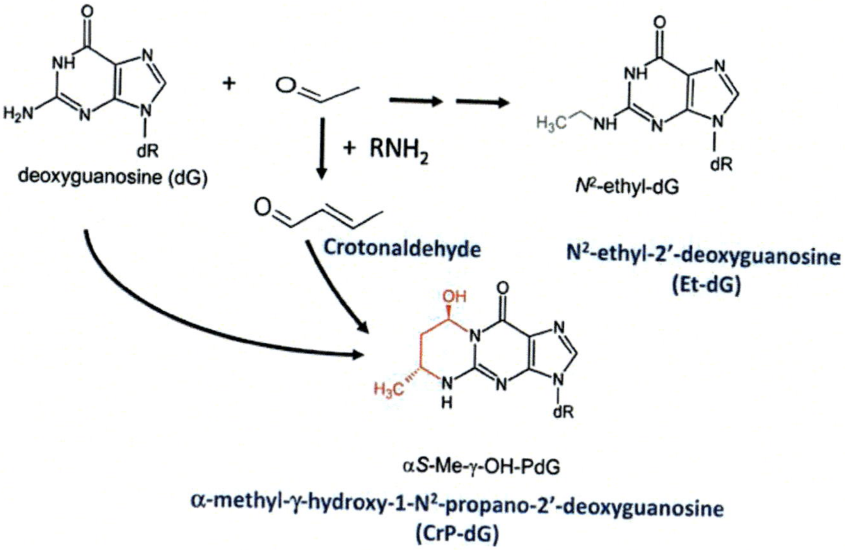

Fig. 4.4 DNA adduct formation

Although the need to first generate crotonaldehyde from acetaldehyde followed by formation of adducts results in a much lower abundance for CrPdG than for N^2Etl-dG; the former is more mutagenic and genotoxic due to the capacity of these adducts to interconvert into a ring-opened form containing an aldehyde moiety. Via the aldehyde, this form of the adduct can react with proteins (most likely histones) to form DNA–protein cross-links and with guanosine residues on the opposite strand of DNA to form DNA interstrand cross-links. Consistent with such effects, exposure of human cells to acetaldehyde triggers a DNA damage response involving the Fanconi anemia–BRCA network, which is known to be activated by chemicals that induce DNA interstrand cross-links (Marietta et al. 2009).

Importantly, there is in vivo evidence supporting the physiologic relevance of these adducts. Matsuda and colleagues (Matsuda et al. 2006) showed that the levels of N^2-Et-dG as well as those of the CrPdG adducts are elevated in white blood cell DNA from ALDH2-deficient alcoholics compared to those with fully active ALDH2. Both groups were matched for smoking and other demographic variables, and as expected those with ALDH2 deficiency activity drank slightly less than those with fully active ALDH2, yet still had higher levels of adducts, supporting a role for ALDH2 in protecting against acetaldehyde-related DNA damage in humans.

Hyperregeneration

In addition to genotoxic effects, acetaldehyde may contribute to carcinogenesis by other mechanisms. Studies by Seitz and colleagues (reviewed in Seitz and Stickel 2007) showed that chronic acetaldehyde results in a hyperregenerative phenomenon in several sites in the gastrointestinal tract. One aspect of this hyperregeneration is increased levels of ornithine decarboxylase, the rate-limiting enzyme for polyamine biosynthesis (Simanowski et al. 1995). In this manner, acetaldehyde causes increases in cell division and increased polyamine levels which in turn facilitate the formation of the more genotoxic CrPdG adducts (Theruvathu et al. 2005). More cell division increases the chance for mutations as cells replicate DNA-containing mutagenic adducts.

CYP2E1, ROS, and Oxidative Stress

CYP2E1 and Oxidative Stress

As mentioned above, CYP2E1 is induced by alcohol use, plays an important role in ethanol metabolism in the liver, and is responsible for the generation of ROS and the conversion of procarcinogens to carcinogens. Ethanol increases CYP2E1 levels by stabilizing the CYP2E1 protein (Buhler et al. 1991; Seitz and Stickel 2007). This increase in CYP2E1 enzyme, together with the alteration of the $NADH/NAD^+$ balance, results in production of ROS, including hydroxyl (•OH), superoxide anion (•O_2), hydrogen peroxide (H_2O_2), and hydroxyethyl radicals (CH_3C•HOH) and generation of numerous lipid peroxidation products. Chronic alcohol exposure also causes increase in reactive nitrogen species (RNS) by inducing nitric oxide synthase, thus increasing nitric oxide production and generating highly reactive peroxynitrite ($ONOO^-$) (Frank et al. 2004; Wang et al. 2009). ROS and RNS are thought to play an important role in carcinogenesis as a result of oxidative stress, including oxidative injury, inflammation, and lipid peroxidation. Detrimental effects (Schetter et al. 2010) include the activation of the immune system through the release of TNF-α with subsequent tissue damage and scar formation and interaction with lipids, proteins, and DNA. Increases in these reactive species lead to protein and DNA adduct formation, DNA strand breaks, point mutations, and aberrant DNA cross-linking (Wright et al. 1999; Koch et al. 2004). More than 20 different types of base alterations have been characterized, including 8-hydroxy-2′-guanosine and thymine glycols (Albano et al. 1996; Dupont et al. 1998). Additionally, elevated ROS or RNS can increase angiogenesis and transcriptional activation of proto-oncogenes (Suh et al. 1999) and increase the metastatic potential of tumors (Ren et al. 2009). Such posttranslational modification of proteins can render them autoantigenic contributing to the proinflammatory process (Thiele et al. 2004).

Redox Balance

Both acute and chronic alcohol consumption can disturb the normal balance that exists between ROS and antioxidants in the cells. Normally, despite the constant generation of ROS, mitochondria remain functional due to an antioxidant defense system that starts with manganese-dependent superoxide dismutase that converts the $^{\bullet}O_2$ to H_2O_2. Reduction of the peroxide to H_2O by mitochondrial glutathione (GSH) is able to prevent protein and lipid peroxidation. Induction of oxidative stress by ethanol is a multifactorial process attributed to an increase in the $NADH/NAD^+$ ratio, acetaldehyde formation, CYP2E1 induction, hypoxia, cytokine signaling, mitochondrial damage, LPS activation of Kupffer cells, reduction in antioxidants particularly GSH, and the conversion of xanthine dehydrogenase to xanthine oxidase. The mechanisms of depletion in mitochondrial GSH as a consequence of chronic alcohol consumption are discussed further as part of the methionine cycle discussion.

Oxidative Stress in Carcinogenesis

In support for a role of ethanol-induced oxidative stress in carcinogenesis, studies have shown that chemically induced carcinogenesis or ethanol-associated mucosal hyperregeneration was counteracted by the concomitant administration of radical scavengers, such as α-tocopherol (Eskelson et al. 1993). Replenishment of GSH by administering the GSH precursor *S*-adenosylmethionine (SAM) or through the use of other antioxidants attenuated alcohol-induced liver damage (Wu and Cederbaum 2003).

Several studies of CYP2E1 polymorphisms provide support for the hypothesis that alcohol-induced changes in basal activity of CYP2E1 may result in increased risk for cancer. Several polymorphisms in CYP2E1 (*Rsa*I, *Dra*I, and *Taq*I) result in elevated CYP2E1 activity compared with the wild-type allele, and each results in increased risk of cancer. The c1 allele of *Rsa*I has higher enzyme activity than the c2 allele and is associated with higher incidence of esophageal cancer in Chinese populations (Lin et al. 1998; Niu et al. 2010) and liver cancer in smokers (Munaka et al. 2003). The *Dra*I variant has been reported to be associated with elevated risk of lung cancer in Mexican American smokers (Wu et al. 1998).

Adduct Formation

Ethanol may be converted to the hydroxyethyl radical in the presence of ROS and generate adducts with DNA. ROS also promote lipid peroxidation leading to the generation of malondialdehyde (MDA) and 4-hydroxynonenal (HNE) among others (Table 4.3). Oxidation of lipids induces the formation of aldehydes and lipid peroxidation products (Table 4.3 and Fig. 4.5) that when present in low concentrations may act as signaling transducers of ROS-mediated metabolic reactions, and thus may also modulate several cell functions, including gene expression and cell proliferation (Uchida 2003). At higher concentrations, the same lipid-derived products are considerably more damaging because of their ability to form toxic adducts with proteins, DNA, and phospholipids that lead to the propagation and amplification of oxidative stress (Blair 2001) and result in a variety of possible oncogenic events. DNA adducts generated by interaction with lipid peroxidation products result in the

Table 4.3 Ethanol metabolites and adducts generated during ethanol metabolism (modified from Niemela 1999)

Compound	Abbreviation	References
Acetaldehyde	AA	Nomura and Lieber (1981), Yokoyama et al. (1995)
Malondialdehyde	MDA	French et al. (1993), Niemela et al. (1994)
4-Hydroxynonenal	HNE	Kamimura et al. (1992)
Malondialdehyde–acetaldehyde hybrid	MAA	Tuma et al. (1996)
Hydroxyethyl radical	HER	Moncada et al. (1994)
Crotonaldehyde	Cr	Brooks and Theruvathu (2005)

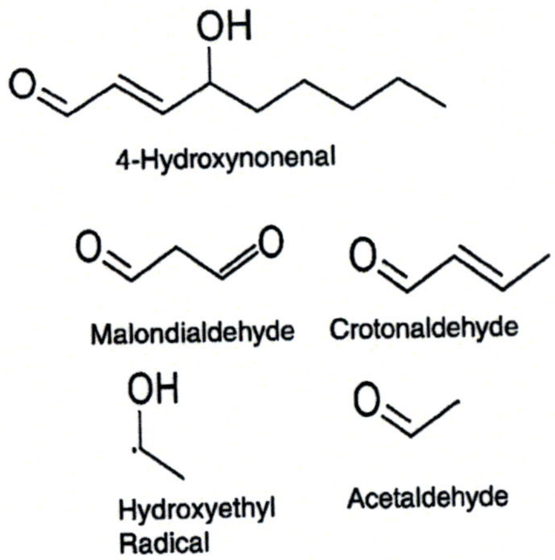

Fig. 4.5 Free radicals, lipid peroxidation products, and reactive aldehydes

generation of miscoding etheno- and propano-modified DNA bases (Fig. 4.4) that have been shown to correlate with the presence of persistent inflammation and may provide essential biomarkers for monitoring and diagnosis of precancerous tissue.

MDA is a highly reactive dialdehyde originating in part from nonenzymatic lipid peroxidation of a variety of unsaturated fatty acids. Formation of hybrid adducts containing both acetaldehyde and MDA in livers of ethanol-fed rats (Tuma et al. 1996) may generate the stable immunogenic MDA–acetaldehyde adduct in vivo. The free radical-mediated oxidation of long-chain polyunsaturated fatty acids leads to the production of HNE, which can react with the sulfhydryl groups of proteins (Esterbauer et al. 1991; Stadtman 1992). HNE generated as a consequence of ROS production may also react with DNA bases to form highly mutagenic adducts with deoxyadenosine and deoxycytidine (Hu et al. 2002), thus altering *TP53* (which encodes p53), upregulating COX-2 expression, and further amplifying the problem by inducing an enhanced production of ROS. The net effect is to give cells some growth advantage and make cells more resistant to apoptosis. Adducts have been demonstrated at the fatty liver stage of alcoholic liver disease (ALD) and increase in frequency in advanced ALD (Frank et al. 2004). Oxidative DNA damage in chronic pancreatitis caused by alcohol abuse was found to result from lipid peroxidation together with depletion of GSH (Braganza 1983). Promutagenic DNA lesions, together with oxidative DNA damage, cause an increased mutation load promoting malignancy. ROS-induced DNA damage, including single- or double-stranded DNA breaks, nucleotide modifications, DNA intrastrand adducts, and protein cross-links, may result in either arrest or induction of transcription, induction of signal transduction pathways, replication errors, and genomic instability, all processes associated with carcinogenesis (Marnett 2000; Valko et al. 2006).

Recent studies by Seitz and colleagues have provided compelling evidence linking elevated levels of CYP2E1 to increased levels of mutagenic DNA damage. Millonig et al. showed that in nontumor-containing biopsies from esophageal cancer patients, samples from alcohol drinkers had elevated levels of CYP2E1, as well as elevated numbers of cells staining for the mutagenic DNA adducts etheno-dA and etheno-dC (Millonig et al. 2009). Adduct levels were particularly high in individuals who were both smokers and alcohol drinkers. Similarly, in samples from patients with alcoholic liver disease, levels of etheno adducts correlate with CYP2E1 levels (Wang et al. 2009). In this same study, elevated levels of etheno adducts were observed following incubation of HepG2 cells expressing CYP2E1 with ethanol, and this effect could be blocked by the CYP2E1 inhibitor chlormethiazole (Wang et al. 2009) directly linking ethanol metabolism by CYP2E1 to increased levels of etheno adducts. The most likely mechanism for this effect involves the formation of ROS leading to elevated lipid peroxide levels.

Changes in NADH/NAD$^+$ Levels and Gene Activation

Ethanol oxidation both by ADH and ALDH consumes NAD$^+$ and produces NADH, resulting in a significant increase in the hepatic NADH/NAD$^+$ ratio in both the cytosol and mitochondria (Cunningham 1986; Bailey and Cunningham 1998). This creates an imbalance in the cellular redox potential, affecting a broad range of important cellular reactions. The energy equivalents of the NADH generated by conversion of ethanol to acetaldehyde are transported into the mitochondria primarily by the malate–aspartate shuttle, which in combination with the NADH produced by ALDH significantly increases the availability of NADH to the electron transport chain in the mitochondria. Changes in the NADH/NAD$^+$ ratio also influence gene expression through changes in activity of NAD$^+$-dependent enzymes that influence transcription. For example, under conditions of caloric restriction, high NAD$^+$ levels may activate certain genes (Imai et al. 2000) that have been shown to extend the lifespan in a wide variety of organisms and reduce the incidence of age-related diseases, such as diabetes, cancer, immune deficiencies, and cardiovascular disorders (Bordone and Guarente 2005).

Examples include the C-terminal-binding protein (CtBP) and the silent information regulator (SIR), among others. CtBP is an NAD^+-dependent D2-hydroxyacid dehydrogenase which mediates transcriptional repression (Kumar et al. 2002). As such, NAD^+ can be seen as a modulator of gene expression and thus, when alcohol induces a decrease in available NAD^+, these genes may be expressed at higher levels. At the same time, in the absence of adequate supply of NAD^+, the NAD^+-dependent histone deacetylase activity of SIR is reduced, resulting in a decrease in gene silencing, suppression of DNA recombination, and silencing of the clock/NPAS2 gene that is involved in the regulation of the circadian clock. Important SIR substrates include histones and the transcription factor p53 (Vaziri et al. 2001; Smith et al. 2002). A number of other critical cellular proteins also respond to changes in redox state, including AP1 transcription factor, NFkB transcription factor, human insulin receptor kinase, protein tyrosine phosphatases, SRC family kinases, JNK and p38 MAP kinase-signaling pathways, and angiogenesis signaling (see Chap. 6).

Conversion of Procarcinogens to Carcinogens

Another mechanism by which alcohol may increase cancer risk through the induction of CYP2E1 is by changing the metabolism of certain procarcinogens. CYP2E1 can enzymatically activate numerous procarcinogens found in tobacco smoke or in the environment, notably including nitrosamines and polycyclic hydrocarbons (Seitz et al. 1998). This mechanism may in part explain the apparent synergistic effect of drinking and smoking on cancer risk. Conversion of procarcinogens by CYP2E1 occurs even at low concentrations and has been demonstrated using the microsomes from a variety of tissues, including the liver, lungs, intestines, and esophagus. Each of these organs represents important portals of entry for xenobiotics, tobacco smoke, and dietary carcinogens. Ultimately, the significance of this mechanism for alcohol-related carcinogenesis depends upon the amount of procarcinogens.

Folate Cycle: Global Hypomethylation, Focal Hypermethylation, and Epigenetics

Methylation of CpG islands in the promoter region is a general mechanism of gene silencing and, thus, may reduce the risk of cancer due to oncogenes. Hypomethylation may result in increased expression of a variety of genes and may, therefore, increase risk. For example, hypomethylation of certain oncogenes, such as c-myc and c-N-ras, may lead to dedifferentiation and proliferation (Wainfan et al. 1989; Shen et al. 1998). On the other hand, hypermethylation of tumor-suppressor genes can result in decreased gene transcription of p53 and HIC-1 (Kanai et al. 1999), and thus both global hypomethylation and regional hypermethylation are associated with an increase in the risk for cancer (Davis and Uthus 2004).

Several dietary factors, such as vitamins (B6, B12), folate (B9), methionine, choline, and zinc, can modulate DNA methylation and cancer susceptibility through

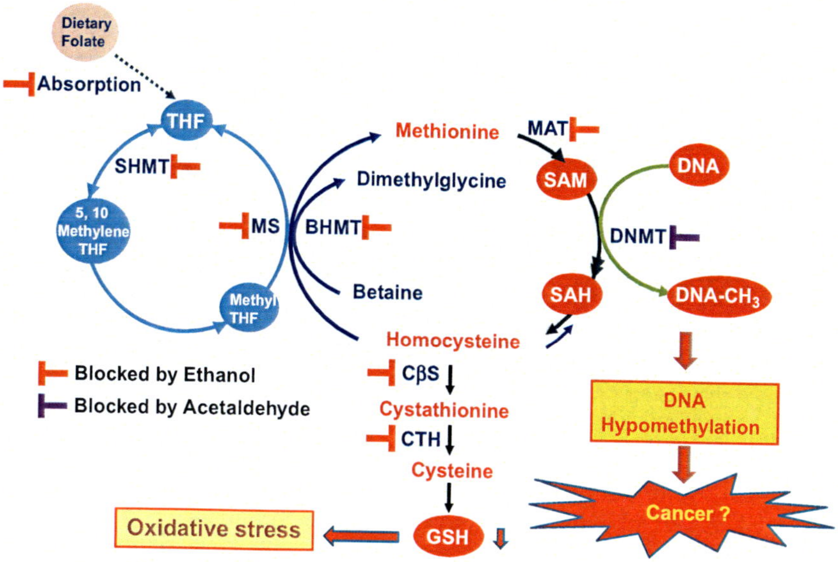

Fig. 4.6 Ethanol and one-carbon metabolism. Ethanol and acetaldehyde block multiple steps in the generation of methyl transfer intermediates. (1) Inhibits absorption of dietary folic acid in the gut and decreased urinary reabsorption. (2) Interrupts methyl group generation from serine by interaction with pyridoxal-5′phosphate. (3) Inhibits methionine synthase. (4) Inhibits BHMT interfering with methyl group transfer from betaine to homocysteine. (5) Inhibits MAT blocking the synthesis of SAM. (6) Disrupts transsulfuration of homocysteine by inactivation of CβS. (7) Inhibits CTH blocking formation of cysteine needed for the generation of glutathione. (8) Acetaldehyde and SAH act independently to block DNA methyl transfers

their involvement in one-carbon metabolism. The folate and the methionine cycles act in concert to control the supply of methyl groups and, thus, exert a strong influence on the methylation of DNA. Chronic alcohol consumption blocks absorption of dietary folate and also blocks multiple points in the folate and methionine cycles, resulting in increased plasma homocysteine level, decreased level of SAM, and folate deficiency (Seitz and Stickel 2007; Bleich and Hillemacher 2009) (Fig. 4.6).

Excessive alcohol consumption interferes with the bioavailability and metabolism of folate (Mason and Choi 2005) and prevents the formation of 5,10-methylenetetrahydrofolate by serine hydroxymethyl transferase (SHMT). Ethanol also blocks the enzyme methionine synthase (MS), which is responsible for the methyl transfer from methyl-tetrahydrofolate (THF) to homocysteine and formation of methionine. Conversion of methionine to SAM is also blocked by ethanol, thus preventing the formation of the donor molecule for the subsequent methyl transfer to DNA. SAM is important for transmethylation, transsulfuration, and polyamine synthesis, processes that are critical for intracellular functions including nucleic acid synthesis and DNA methylation. Decreases in SAM and folate (Cravo et al. 1996) and elevations in homocysteine (de la Vega et al. 2001) in liver or serum samples after alcohol consumption have been reported. The reduction in SAM and concurrent increase in *S*-adenosylhomocysteine (SAH) (a potent inhibitor of numerous methyl transferases) lead to a decrease in DNA methylation.

Despite the increased levels of homocysteine as a result of the block of methionine synthase, alcohol blockade of the enzymes, cystathionine β-synthase and cystathionine hydrolase, results in decreased levels of glutathione and leads to increased oxidative stress. Decreased generation of GSH is combined with decreased transport of GSH into the mitochondria from the cytosol. The depletion of GSH, which is the main intracellular free radical scavenger, exacerbates the disequilibrium between formation of ROS and the antioxidant defense system.

Direct inhibition of MS by ethanol results in a clinical condition that cannot be corrected by mere folate supplementation; however, some studies indicate that high dietary folate intake or adequate circulating levels of folate may reduce breast cancer risk, especially among women with higher alcohol intake (Negri et al. 2000; Sellers et al. 2001; Zhang 2004). The effect of folate intake on breast cancer risk is more evident among subjects with the *MTHFR 677TT* genotype (Shrubsole et al. 2004) or in association with a family history of breast cancer (Sellers et al. 2004). Moreover, in animal models, folate supplementation has a protective effect against mitochondrial DNA deletions induced after cancer chemotherapy (Branda et al. 2002) and reduces the DNA strand breaks in the *p53* gene (Kim et al. 2000). In addition, chronic alcohol consumption induces hypomethylation in genomic DNA, but not in *p53* gene (Choi et al. 1999), resulting in the upregulation of oncogenes and downregulation of tumor-suppressor genes.

Ethanol blockade of the folate and methionine cycles results in a general state of hypomethylation; however, focal hypermethylation is still possible. For example,

Sidebar 2: Methyl Group Transfers and Pancreatic Cancer

A compelling case for the effect of alcohol consumption on pancreatic cancer risk has been made by (Suzuki et al. 2008) in a case-control study examining the effect of alcohol on pancreatic cancer in conjunction with polymorphisms in four enzymes that are essential for one-carbon metabolism. None of the polymorphisms in the enzymes, methylene-tetrahydrofolate reductase (MTHFR C677T), methionine synthase (MTR A2756G), methionine synthase reductase (MTRR A66G), and thymidylate synthase (TS) variable number of tandem repeat, showed any significant effect on pancreatic cancer risk by genotype alone; however, in stratified analysis, the effect of alcohol consumption on pancreatic cancer was observed in individuals with the MTHFR 667 CC, MTR 2756 AA, or MTRR 66 G allele. OR (95% CI) of pancreatic cancer for heavy drinkers compared with never drinkers was 4.50 (1.44–14.05) in the MTHFR 667 CC genotype, 2.65 (1.17–6.00) in the MTR 2756 AA genotype, and 3.35 (1.34–8.36) in the MTRR 66 G allele carriers. These results suggest strongly that the folate-related enzyme polymorphisms that reduce normal function are further stressed by alcohol use, strengthening the association between drinking habit and pancreatic cancer risk.

smoking and alcohol consumption were associated with a higher risk for gastric cancer with hypermethylation of the gene promoter for hMLH1, a mismatch repair enzyme responsible for maintaining the fidelity of the genome during cellular proliferation (Nan et al. 2005). A more detailed discussion of epigenetics is presented in Chap. 5.

Retinol and Impairment of Other Metabolic Processes

Chronic ethanol consumption and alcohol metabolism also may influence various other metabolic pathways, thereby contributing to metabolic disorders frequently found in alcoholics, such as fatty liver and excessive levels of lipids in the blood (i.e., hyperlipidemia), accumulation of lactic acid in body fluids (i.e., lactic acidosis), excessive production of chemical compounds known as ketones in the body (i.e., ketosis), and elevated levels of uric acid in the blood (i.e., hyperuricemia).

Other metabolic derangements associated with ethanol metabolism result from the fact that ADH and ALDH show specificity not only for ethanol, but also for other compounds. For example, ADH and ALDH oxidize retinol (i.e., vitamin A1) to retinal and, subsequently, retinoic acid, which plays an important role in growth and differentiation (Fig. 4.7). Ethanol competes for the active sites of ADH and ALDH, thus inhibiting retinol metabolism. These interactions may have serious implications for fetal development, stem cell differentiation, maintenance of differentiated tissue function, and the normal structure and function of stellate cells in the liver (Crabb et al. 2001; Liu and Gudas 2002). Long-term alcohol intake results in impaired nutritional status of retinoic acid by either inhibiting its biosynthesis and/or enhancing its catabolism (Liu and Gudas 2002), interfering with retinoic acid signaling and altering "cross talk" with the MAP kinases, including JNK, ERK, and p38-signaling cascade, which plays an essential role in cellular proliferation, apoptosis, stress, inflammatory response, and carcinogenesis. Rats receiving chronic

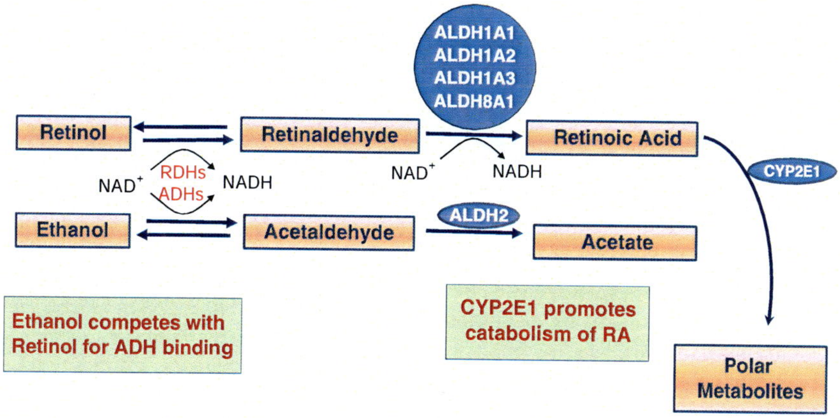

Fig. 4.7 Retinoic acid homeostasis

ethanol treatment exhibited significant elevations in cell nuclear antigen-positive hepatocytes and a number of proliferative factors in hepatocytes, including hepatic c-Jun protein, cyclin D1 protein, and increased activator protein 1 (AP-1) DNA binding, all of which could be restored to normal levels by RA supplementation suggesting a role for preventing or reversing certain types of ethanol-induced liver injury (Chung et al. 2001). Induction of CYP2E1 also plays a major role in the degradation of RA, thus providing an additional mechanism by which chronic and excessive ethanol intake may increase risk for both hepatic and extrahepatic cell proliferation and carcinogenesis (Liu et al. 2001). These important metabolic pathways are discussed in greater detail in Chaps. 6, 7, and 9.

Chronic alcohol consumption also is associated with disturbances in the metabolism of sulfur-containing amino acids, leading to increased levels of the amino acids glutamate, aspartate, and homocysteine in alcoholic patients. These increases may have serious adverse effects. For example, homocysteine increases and modulates certain nerve-signaling processes, particularly during alcohol withdrawal, and increases in homocysteine levels may possibly contribute to the atrophy observed in brain tissue of alcohol abusers (Bleich and Kornhuber 2003). In addition to ethanol, CYP2E1 metabolizes numerous other compounds, including propranolol, acetaminophen, warfarin, and diazepam. Metabolism of these and other xenobiotics should be considered as potentially negative side effects of chronic alcohol use; however, the connection to carcinogenesis may be tenuous.

Conclusions and New Directions

In this chapter, we reviewed the potential role of alcohol metabolism in alcohol-related carcinogenesis. With the exception of squamous cell cancer of the esophagus, where the evidence for a role for acetaldehyde is compelling, it is unclear which of the above mechanisms is most important in causing alcohol-related cancers at other sites in the body. The multiple possibilities outlined above may each contribute in different tissues under various environmental exposures and in differing genetic backgrounds. Generation of DNA adducts, induction of CYP2E1 by chronic ethanol use resulting in increases in ROS and lipid peroxidation products, and the conversion of procarcinogens present in diet and tobacco smoke to their ultimate carcinogens (Cederbaum 1991, 1998) may each play a role in different tissues. Underlying all may be the effect exerted by alcohol on the folate and methionine metabolic pathways, thus altering the methylation of DNA and resulting in epigenetic changes with potentially negative impact. If left unrepaired, DNA lesions can initiate carcinogenesis, generate carcinogens, or influence signaling pathways with attendant negative consequences. Finally, alcohol may exert direct and indirect effects on retinoid metabolism through its influence on the action of ADH and ALDH.

Studies are needed to clarify the suspected link between the generation of acetaldehyde, the formation of DNA adducts, and the development of cancer. Another area of interest is the apparent paradox between ADH activity and cancer development in some tissues. Animal models in which ADH levels can be manipulated in specific target tissues could be useful here. Measurement of external sources of acetaldehyde and the synergistic effects of smoking and alcohol consumption may provide further clues to the link between alcohol and cancer. Promising drugs to inhibit CYP2E1 or to eliminate the microbial contribution to acetaldehyde burden should be further evaluated. At present, no satisfying explanation exists for the apparent link between moderate alcohol consumption and the risk of breast cancer, though there is suggestive evidence for a role for estrogens. Identification of the molecular and cellular mechanisms by which alcohol disrupts normal cell cycle controls may shed additional light on this area.

References

Agarwal DP, Goedde HW. 1992. Pharmacogenetics of alcohol metabolism and alcoholism. Pharmacogenetics 2:48–62.
Albano E, Clot P, Morimoto M, Tomasi A, Ingelman-Sundberg M, French SW. 1996. Role of cytochrome P4502E1-dependent formation of hydroxyethyl free radical in the development of liver damage in rats intragastrically fed with ethanol. Hepatology 23:155–163.
Baan R, Straif K, Grosse Y, Secretan B, El Ghissassi F, Bouvard V, Altieri A, Cogliano V. 2007. Carcinogenicity of alcoholic beverages. Lancet Oncol 8:292–293.
Bailey SM, Cunningham CC. 1998. Acute and chronic ethanol increases reactive oxygen species generation and decreases viability in fresh, isolated rat hepatocytes. Hepatology 28:1318–1326.
Blair IA. 2001. Lipid hydroperoxide-mediated DNA damage. Exp Gerontol 36:1473–1481.
Bleich S, Hillemacher T. 2009. Homocysteine, alcoholism and its molecular networks. Pharmacopsychiatry 42 Suppl 1:S102–109.
Bleich S, Kornhuber J. 2003. Relationship between plasma homocysteine levels and brain atrophy in healthy elderly individuals. Neurology 60:1220; author reply 1220.
Boccia S, Hashibe M, Galli P, De Feo E, Asakage T, Hashimoto T, Hiraki A, Katoh T, Nomura T, Yokoyama A, van Duijn CM, Ricciardi G, Boffetta P. 2009. Aldehyde dehydrogenase 2 and head and neck cancer: a meta-analysis implementing a Mendelian randomization approach. Cancer Epidemiol Biomarkers Prev 18:248–254.
Boffetta P, Hashibe M. 2006. Alcohol and cancer. Lancet Oncol 7:149–156.
Bordone L, Guarente L. 2005. Calorie restriction, SIRT1 and metabolism: understanding longevity. Nat Rev Mol Cell Biol 6:298–305.
Bosron WF, Crabb DW, Li TK. 1983. Relationship between kinetics of liver alcohol dehydrogenase and alcohol metabolism. Pharmacol Biochem Behav 18 Suppl 1:223–227.
Bosron WF, Li TK. 1986. Genetic polymorphism of human liver alcohol and aldehyde dehydrogenases, and their relationship to alcohol metabolism and alcoholism. Hepatology 6:502–510.
Braganza JM. 1983. Pancreatic disease: a casualty of hepatic "detoxification"? Lancet 2:1000–1003.
Branda RF, Brooks EM, Chen Z, Naud SJ, Nicklas JA. 2002. Dietary modulation of mitochondrial DNA deletions and copy number after chemotherapy in rats. Mutat Res 501:29–36.
Brennan P, Lewis S, Hashibe M, Bell DA, Boffetta P, Bouchardy C, Caporaso N, Chen C, Coutelle C, Diehl SR, Hayes RB, Olshan AF, Schwartz SM, Sturgis EM, Wei Q, Zavras AI, Benhamou S. 2004. Pooled analysis of alcohol dehydrogenase genotypes and head and neck cancer: a HuGE review. Am J Epidemiol 159:1–16.
Brooks PJ, Enoch MA, Goldman D, Li TK, Yokoyama A. 2009. The alcohol flushing response: an unrecognized risk factor for esophageal cancer from alcohol consumption. PLoS Med 6:e50.
Brooks PJ, Theruvathu JA. 2005. DNA adducts from acetaldehyde: implications for alcohol-related carcinogenesis. Alcohol 35:187–193.

Buhler R, Lindros KO, von Boguslawsky K, Karkkainen P, Makinen J, Ingelman-Sundberg M. 1991. Perivenous expression of ethanol-inducible cytochrome P450 IIE1 in livers from alcoholics and chronically ethanol-fed rats. Alcohol Alcohol Suppl 1:311–315.

Caro AA, Cederbaum AI. 2004. Oxidative stress, toxicology, and pharmacology of CYP2E1. Annu Rev Pharmacol Toxicol 44:27–42.

Cederbaum AI. 1991. Microsomal generation of reactive oxygen species and their possible role in alcohol hepatotoxicity. Alcohol Alcohol Suppl 1:291–296.

Cederbaum AI. 1998. Ethanol-related cytotoxicity catalyzed by CYP2E1-dependent generation of reactive oxygen intermediates in transduced HepG2 cells. Biofactors 8(1–2):93–96.

Cravo ML, Gloria LM et al. 1996. Hyperhomocysteinemia in chronic alcoholism: correlation with folate, vitamin B-12, and vitamin B-6 status. Am J Clin Nutr 63(2):220–224.

Choi SW, Stickel F, Baik HW, Kim YI, Seitz HK, Mason JB. 1999. Chronic alcohol consumption induces genomic but not p53-specific DNA hypomethylation in rat colon. J Nutr 129:1945–1950.

Chung J, Liu C, Smith DE, Seitz HK, Russell RM, Wang XD. 2001. Restoration of retinoic acid concentration suppresses ethanol-enhanced c-Jun expression and hepatocyte proliferation in rat liver. Carcinogenesis 22:1213–1219.

Crabb DW, Pinairs J, Hasanadka R, Fang M, Leo MA, Lieber CS, Tsukamoto H, Motomura K, Miyahara T, Ohata M, Bosron W, Sanghani S, Kedishvili N, Shiraishi H, Yokoyama H, Miyagi M, Ishii H, Bergheim I, Menzl I, Parlesak A, Bode C. 2001. Alcohol and retinoids. Alcohol Clin Exp Res 25:207S–217S.

Cunningham CC. 1986. Use of nuclear magnetic resonance spectroscopy to study the effects of ethanol consumption on liver metabolism and pathology. Alcohol Clin Exp Res 10:246–250.

Davis CD, Uthus EO. 2004. DNA methylation, cancer susceptibility, and nutrient interactions. Exp Biol Med (Maywood) 229:988–995.

de la Vega MJ, Santolaria F et al. 2001. High prevalence of hyperhomocysteinemia in chronic alcoholism: the importance of the thermolabile form of the enzyme methylenetetrahydrofolate reductase (MTHFR). Alcohol 25(2):59–67.

Druesne-Pecollo N, Tehard B, Mallet Y, Gerber M, Norat T, Hercberg S, Latino-Martel P. 2009. Alcohol and genetic polymorphisms: effect on risk of alcohol-related cancer. Lancet Oncol 10:173–180.

Dupont I, Lucas D, Clot P, Menez C, Albano E. 1998. Cytochrome P4502E1 inducibility and hydroxyethyl radical formation among alcoholics. J Hepatol 28:564–571.

Edenberg HJ. 2007. The genetics of alcohol metabolism: role of alcohol dehydrogenase and aldehyde dehydrogenase variants. Alcohol Res Health 30:5–13.

Eriksson CJ. 2007. Measurement of acetaldehyde: what levels occur naturally and in response to alcohol? Novartis Found Symp 285:247–255; discussion 256–260.

Eskelson CD, Odeleye OE, Watson RR, Earnest DL, Mufti SI. 1993. Modulation of cancer growth by vitamin E and alcohol. Alcohol Alcohol 28:117–125.

Esterbauer H, Schaur RJ, Zollner H. 1991. Chemistry and biochemistry of 4-hydroxynonenal, malonaldehyde and related aldehydes. Free Radic Biol Med 11:81–128.

Frank A, Seitz HK et al. 2004. Immunohistochemical detection of 1,N6-ethenodeoxyadenosine in nuclei of human liver affected by diseases predisposing to hepato-carcinogenesis. Carcinogenesis 25(6):1027–1031.

French SW, Wong K, Jui L, Albano E, Hagbjork AL, Ingelman-Sundberg M. 1993. Effect of ethanol on cytochrome P450 2E1 (CYP2E1), lipid peroxidation, and serum protein adduct formation in relation to liver pathology pathogenesis. Exp Mol Pathol 58:61–75.

Freudenheim JL, Ambrosone CB, Moysich KB, Vena JE, Graham S, Marshall JR, Muti P, Laughlin R, Nemoto T, Harty LC, Crits GA, Chan AW, Shields PG. 1999. Alcohol dehydrogenase 3 genotype modification of the association of alcohol consumption with breast cancer risk. Cancer Causes Control 10:369–377.

Han CL, Liao CS, Wu CW, Hwong CL, Lee AR, Yin SJ. 1998. Contribution to first-pass metabolism of ethanol and inhibition by ethanol for retinol oxidation in human alcohol dehydrogenase family – implications for etiology of fetal alcohol syndrome and alcohol-related diseases. Eur J Biochem 254:25–31.

Hashibe M, Boffetta P, Zaridze D, Shangina O, Szeszenia-Dabrowska N, Mates D, Janout V, Fabianova E, Bencko V, Moullan N, Chabrier A, Hung R, Hall J, Canzian F, Brennan P. 2006. Evidence for an important role of alcohol- and aldehyde-metabolizing genes in cancers of the upper aerodigestive tract. Cancer Epidemiol Biomarkers Prev 15:696–703.

Hashibe M, McKay JD, Curado MP, Oliveira JC, Koifman S, Koifman R, Zaridze D, Shangina O, Wunsch-Filho V, Eluf-Neto J, Levi JE, Matos E, Lagiou P, Lagiou A, Benhamou S, Bouchardy C, Szeszenia-Dabrowska N, Menezes A, Dall'Agnol MM, Merletti F, Richiardi L, Fernandez L, Lence J, Talamini R, Barzan L, Mates D, Mates IN, Kjaerheim K, Macfarlane GJ, Macfarlane TV, Simonato L, Canova C, Holcatova I, Agudo A, Castellsague X, Lowry R, Janout V, Kollarova H, Conway DI, McKinney PA, Znaor A, Fabianova E, Bencko V, Lissowska J, Chabrier A, Hung RJ, Gaborieau V, Boffetta P, Brennan P. 2008. Multiple ADH genes are associated with upper aerodigestive cancers. Nat Genet 40:707–709.

Hines LM, Hankinson SE, Smith-Warner SA, Spiegelman D, Kelsey KT, Colditz GA, Willett WC, Hunter DJ. 2000. A prospective study of the effect of alcohol consumption and ADH3 genotype on plasma steroid hormone levels and breast cancer risk. Cancer Epidemiol Biomarkers Prev 9:1099–1105.

Homann N, Karkkainen P, Koivisto T, Nosova T, Jokelainen K, Salaspuro M. 1997. Effects of acetaldehyde on cell regeneration and differentiation of the upper gastrointestinal tract mucosa. J Natl Cancer Inst 89:1692–1697.

Homann N, Konig IR, Marks M, Benesova M, Stickel F, Millonig G, Mueller S, Seitz HK. 2009. Alcohol and colorectal cancer: the role of alcohol dehydrogenase 1C polymorphism. Alcohol Clin Exp Res 33:551–556.

Homann N, Stickel F, Konig IR, Jacobs A, Junghanns K, Benesova M, Schuppan D, Himsel S, Zuber-Jerger I, Hellerbrand C, Ludwig D, Caselmann WH, Seitz HK. 2006. Alcohol dehydrogenase 1C*1 allele is a genetic marker for alcohol-associated cancer in heavy drinkers. Int J Cancer 118:1998–2002.

Homann N, Tillonen J, Meurman JH, Rintamaki H, Lindqvist C, Rautio M, Jousimies-Somer H, Salaspuro M. 2000. Increased salivary acetaldehyde levels in heavy drinkers and smokers: a microbiological approach to oral cavity cancer. Carcinogenesis 21:663–668.

Homann N, Tillonen J, Rintamaki H, Salaspuro M, Lindqvist C, Meurman JH. 2001. Poor dental status increases acetaldehyde production from ethanol in saliva: a possible link to increased oral cancer risk among heavy drinkers. Oral Oncol 37:153–158.

Hu W, Feng Z, Eveleigh J, Iyer G, Pan J, Amin S, Chung FL, Tang MS. 2002. The major lipid peroxidation product, trans-4-hydroxy-2-nonenal, preferentially forms DNA adducts at codon 249 of human p53 gene, a unique mutational hotspot in hepatocellular carcinoma. Carcinogenesis 23:1781–1789.

Hurley TD, Edenberg, H.J., Li, T.K. 2002. Pharmacogenomics of Alcoholism. In: Pharmacogenomics: The Search for Individualized Therapies. Weinheim, Germany: Wiley-VCH. pp 417–441.

Ikuta T, Shibuya A, Yoshida A. 1988. Direct determination of usual (Caucasian-type) and atypical (Oriental-type) alleles of the class I human alcohol dehydrogenase-2 locus. Biochem Genet 26:519–525.

Imai S, Johnson FB et al. 2000. SIR2: an NAD-dependent histone deacetylase that connects chromatin silencing, metabolism, and aging. Cold Spring Harb Symp Quant Biol 65:297–302.

Jelski W, Chrostek L, Markiewicz W, Szmitkowski M. 2006. Activity of alcohol dehydrogenase (ADH) isoenzymes and aldehyde dehydrogenase (ALDH) in the sera of patients with breast cancer. J Clin Lab Anal 20:105–108.

Jelski W, Chrostek L, Szmitkowski M. 2007a. The activity of class I, II, III, and IV of alcohol dehydrogenase isoenzymes and aldehyde dehydrogenase in pancreatic cancer. Pancreas 35: 142–146.

Jelski W, Chrostek L, Szmitkowski M. 2007b. The activity of class I, III, and IV of alcohol dehydrogenase isoenzymes and aldehyde dehydrogenase in gastric cancer. Dig Dis Sci 52:531–535.

Jelski W, Zalewski B, Chrostek L, Szmitkowski M. 2004. The activity of class I, II, III, and IV alcohol dehydrogenase isoenzymes and aldehyde dehydrogenase in colorectal cancer. Dig Dis Sci 49:977–981.

Jokelainen K, Heikkonen E, Roine R, Lehtonen H, Salaspuro M. 1996. Increased acetaldehyde production by mouthwashings from patients with oral cavity, laryngeal, or pharyngeal cancer. Alcohol Clin Exp Res 20:1206–1210.

Kamimura S, Gaal K, Britton RS, Bacon BR, Triadafilopoulos G, Tsukamoto H. 1992. Increased 4-hydroxynonenal levels in experimental alcoholic liver disease: association of lipid peroxidation with liver fibrogenesis. Hepatology 16:448–453.

Kanai Y, Hui AM, Sun L, Ushijima S, Sakamoto M, Tsuda H, Hirohashi S. 1999. DNA hypermethylation at the D17S5 locus and reduced HIC-1 mRNA expression are associated with hepatocarcinogenesis. Hepatology 29:703–709.

Kim YI, Shirwadkar S, Choi SW, Puchyr M, Wang Y, Mason JB. 2000. Effects of dietary folate on DNA strand breaks within mutation-prone exons of the p53 gene in rat colon. Gastroenterology 119:151–161.

Koch OR, Pani G, Borrello S, Colavitti R, Cravero A, Farre S, Galeotti T. 2004. Oxidative stress and antioxidant defenses in ethanol-induced cell injury. Mol Aspects Med 25:191–198.

Kumar V, Carlson JE, Ohgi KA, Edwards TA, Rose DW, Escalante CR, Rosenfeld MG, Aggarwal AK. 2002. Transcription corepressor CtBP is an NAD(+)-regulated dehydrogenase. Mol Cell 10:857–869.

Kuratsune M, Kohchi S, Horie A. 1965. Carcinogenesis in the Esophagus. I. Penetration of Benzo(a) Pyrene and Other Hydrocarbons into the Esophageal Mucosa. Gann 56:177–187.

Liao CS, Lin JS, Chang CP, Chao TJ, Chao YC, Cheng TC, Wu CW, Yin SJ. 1991. Stomach and duodenal alcohol and aldehyde dehydrogenase isozymes in Chinese. Proc Natl Sci Counc Repub China B 15:92–96.

Lilla C, Koehler T, Kropp S, Wang-Gohrke S, Chang-Claude J. 2005. Alcohol dehydrogenase 1B (ADH1B) genotype, alcohol consumption and breast cancer risk by age 50 years in a German case-control study. Br J Cancer 92:2039–2041.

Lin DX, Tang YM, Peng Q, Lu SX, Ambrosone CB, Kadlubar FF. 1998. Susceptibility to esophageal cancer and genetic polymorphisms in glutathione S-transferases T1, P1, and M1 and cytochrome P450 2E1. Cancer Epidemiol Biomarkers Prev 7:1013–1018.

Liu L, Gudas LJ. 2002. Retinoic acid induces expression of the interleukin-1beta gene in cultured normal human mammary epithelial cells and in human breast carcinoma lines. J Cell Physiol 193:244–252.

Liu S, Park JY et al. 2001. Elucidation of CYP2E1 5' regulatory RsaI/PstI allelic variants and their role in risk for oral cancer. Oral Oncol 37(5):437–445.

Marietta C, Thompson LH et al. 2009. Acetaldehyde stimulates FANCD2 monoubiquitination, H2AX phosphorylation, and BRCA1 phosphorylation in human cells in vitro: implications for alcohol-related carcinogenesis. Mutat Res 664(1–2):77–83.

Marnett LJ. 2000. Oxyradicals and DNA damage. Carcinogenesis 21:361–370.

Mason JB, Choi SW. 2005. Effects of alcohol on folate metabolism: implications for carcinogenesis. Alcohol 35(3):235–241.

Matsuda T, Yabushita H, Kanaly RA, Shibutani S, Yokoyama A. 2006. Increased DNA damage in ALDH2-deficient alcoholics. Chem Res Toxicol 19:1374–1378.

Millonig G, Hegedusch S, Becker L, Seitz HK, Schuppan D, Mueller S. 2009. Hypoxia-inducible factor 1 alpha under rapid enzymatic hypoxia: cells sense decrements of oxygen but not hypoxia per se. Free Radic Biol Med 46:182–191.

Moncada C, Torres V, Varghese G, Albano E, Israel Y. 1994. Ethanol-derived immunoreactive species formed by free radical mechanisms. Mol Pharmacol 46:786–791.

Moreno A, Pares A, Ortiz J, Enriquez J, Pares X. 1994. Alcohol dehydrogenase from human stomach: variability in normal mucosa and effect of age, gender, ADH3 phenotype and gastric region. Alcohol Alcohol 29:663–671.

Morita M, Kumashiro R, Kubo N, Nakashima Y, Yoshida R, Yoshinaga K, Saeki H, Emi Y, Kakeji Y, Sakaguchi Y, Toh Y, Maehara Y. 2010. Alcohol drinking, cigarette smoking, and the development of squamous cell carcinoma of the esophagus: epidemiology, clinical findings, and prevention. Int J Clin Oncol 15:126–134.

Munaka M, Kohshi K, Kawamoto T, Takasawa S, Nagata N, Itoh H, Oda S, Katoh T. 2003. Genetic polymorphisms of tobacco- and alcohol-related metabolizing enzymes and the risk of hepatocellular carcinoma. J Cancer Res Clin Oncol 129:355–360.

Nan HM, Song YJ, Yun HY, Park JS, Kim H. 2005. Effects of dietary intake and genetic factors on hypermethylation of the hMLH1 gene promoter in gastric cancer. World J Gastroenterol 11:3834–3841.

Negri E, La Vecchia C, Franceschi S. 2000. Re: dietary folate consumption and breast cancer risk. J Natl Cancer Inst 92:1270–1271.

Neumark YD, Friedlander Y, Durst R, Leitersdorf E, Jaffe D, Ramchandani VA, O'Connor S, Carr LG, Li TK. 2004. Alcohol dehydrogenase polymorphisms influence alcohol-elimination rates in a male Jewish population. Alcohol Clin Exp Res 28:10–14.

Niemela O, Parkkila S, Yla-Herttuala S, Halsted C, Witztum JL, Lanca A, Israel Y. 1994. Covalent protein adducts in the liver as a result of ethanol metabolism and lipid peroxidation. Lab Invest 70:537–546.

Niemela O. 1999. Aldehyde-protein adducts in the liver as a result of ethanol-induced oxidative stress. Front Biosci 4:D506–513.

Niu Y, Yuan H, Leng W, Pang Y, Gu N, Chen N. 2010. CYP2E1 Rsa I/Pst I polymorphism and esophageal cancer risk: a meta-analysis based on 1,088 cases and 2,238 controls. Med Oncol.

Nomura F, Lieber CS. 1981. Binding of acetaldehyde to rat liver microsomes: enhancement after chronic alcohol consumption. Biochem Biophys Res Commun 100:131–137.

Nosova T, Jousimies-Somer H, Kaihovaara P, Jokelainen K, Heine R, Salaspuro M. 1997. Characteristics of alcohol dehydrogenases of certain aerobic bacteria representing human colonic flora. Alcohol Clin Exp Res 21:489–494.

Novoradovsky A, Tsai SJ, Goldfarb L, Peterson R, Long JC, Goldman D. 1995. Mitochondrial aldehyde dehydrogenase polymorphism in Asian and American Indian populations: detection of new ALDH2 alleles. Alcohol Clin Exp Res 19:1105–1110.

Peters ES, McClean MD, Liu M, Eisen EA, Mueller N, Kelsey KT. 2005. The ADH1C polymorphism modifies the risk of squamous cell carcinoma of the head and neck associated with alcohol and tobacco use. Cancer Epidemiol Biomarkers Prev 14:476–482.

Ren JL, Pan JS, Lu YP, Sun P, Han J. 2009. Inflammatory signaling and cellular senescence. Cell Signal 21:378–383.

Risch A, Ramroth H, Raedts V, Rajaee-Behbahani N, Schmezer P, Bartsch H, Becher H, Dietz A. 2003. Laryngeal cancer risk in Caucasians is associated with alcohol and tobacco consumption but not modified by genetic polymorphisms in class I alcohol dehydrogenases ADH1B and ADH1C, and glutathione-S-transferases GSTM1 and GSTT1. Pharmacogenetics 13: 225–230.

Salaspuro M. 2007. Interrelationship between alcohol, smoking, acetaldehyde and cancer. Novartis Found Symp 285:80–89; discussion 89–96, 198–199.

Salaspuro MP. 2003a. Acetaldehyde, microbes, and cancer of the digestive tract. Crit Rev Clin Lab Sci 40:183–208.

Salaspuro MP. 2003b. Alcohol consumption and cancer of the gastrointestinal tract. Best Pract Res Clin Gastroenterol 17:679–694.

Salaspuro MP, Lieber CS. 1978. Non-uniformity of blood ethanol elimination: its exaggeration after chronic consumption. Ann Clin Res 10:294–297.

Salaspuro V, Salaspuro M. 2004. Synergistic effect of alcohol drinking and smoking on in vivo acetaldehyde concentration in saliva. Int J Cancer 111:480–483.

Schetter AJ, Heegaard NH, Harris CC. 2010. Inflammation and cancer: interweaving microRNA, free radical, cytokine and p53 pathways. Carcinogenesis 31:37–49.

Schwartz SM, Doody DR, Fitzgibbons ED, Ricks S, Porter PL, Chen C. 2001. Oral squamous cell cancer risk in relation to alcohol consumption and alcohol dehydrogenase-3 genotypes. Cancer Epidemiol Biomarkers Prev 10:1137–1144.

Secretan B, Straif K, Baan R, Grosse Y, El Ghissassi F, Bouvard V, Benbrahim-Tallaa L, Guha N, Freeman C, Galichet L, Cogliano V. 2009. A review of human carcinogens – Part E: tobacco, areca nut, alcohol, coal smoke, and salted fish. Lancet Oncol 10:1033–1034.

Seitz HK, Becker P. 2007. Alcohol metabolism and cancer risk. Alcohol Res Health 30:38–41, 44–37.

Seitz HK, Stickel F. 2007. Molecular mechanisms of alcohol-mediated carcinogenesis. Nat Rev Cancer 7:599–612.

Seitz HK, Stickel F, Homann N. 2004. Pathogenetic mechanisms of upper aerodigestive tract cancer in alcoholics. Int J Cancer 108:483–487.

Seitz HK, Poschl G et al. 1998. Alcohol and cancer. Recent Dev Alcohol 14:67–95.

Sellers TA, Grabrick DM et al. 2004. Does folate intake decrease risk of postmenopausal breast cancer among women with a family history? Cancer Causes Control 15(2):113–120.

Sellers TA, Kushi LH, Cerhan JR, Vierkant RA, Gapstur SM, Vachon CM, Olson JE, Therneau TM, Folsom AR. 2001. Dietary folate intake, alcohol, and risk of breast cancer in a prospective study of postmenopausal women. Epidemiology 12:420–428.

Shen L, Fang J, Qiu D, Zhang T, Yang J, Chen S, Xiao S. 1998. Correlation between DNA methylation and pathological changes in human hepatocellular carcinoma. Hepatogastroenterology 45:1753–1759.

Shrubsole MJ, Gao YT, Cai Q, Shu XO, Dai Q, Hebert JR, Jin F, Zheng W. 2004. MTHFR polymorphisms, dietary folate intake, and breast cancer risk: results from the Shanghai Breast Cancer Study. Cancer Epidemiol Biomarkers Prev 13:190–196.

Simanowski UA, Stickel F, Maier H, Gartner U, Seitz HK. 1995. Effect of alcohol on gastrointestinal cell regeneration as a possible mechanism in alcohol-associated carcinogenesis. Alcohol 12:111–115.

Smith M. 1986. Genetics of human alcohol and aldehyde dehydrogenases. Adv Hum Genet 15:249–290.

Smith JS, Avalos J et al. 2002. SIR2 family of NAD(+)-dependent protein deacetylases. Methods Enzymol 353:282–300.

Stadtman ER. 1992. Protein oxidation and aging. Science 257:1220–1224.

Stamatoyannopoulos G, Chen SH, Fukui M. 1975. Liver alcohol dehydrogenase in Japanese: high population frequency of atypical form and its possible role in alcohol sensitivity. Am J Hum Genet 27:789–796.

Suh YA, Arnold RS, Lassegue B, Shi J, Xu X, Sorescu D, Chung AB, Griendling KK, Lambeth JD. 1999. Cell transformation by the superoxide-generating oxidase Mox1. Nature 401:79–82.

Suzuki T, Matsuo K, Sawaki A, Mizuno N, Hiraki A, Kawase T, Watanabe M, Nakamura T, Yamao K, Tajima K, Tanaka H. 2008. Alcohol drinking and one-carbon metabolism-related gene polymorphisms on pancreatic cancer risk. Cancer Epidemiol Biomarkers Prev 17:2742–2747.

Terry MB, Gammon MD, Zhang FF, Knight JA, Wang Q, Britton JA, Teitelbaum SL, Neugut AI, Santella RM. 2006. ADH3 genotype, alcohol intake and breast cancer risk. Carcinogenesis 27:840–847.

Theruvathu JA, Jaruga P, Nath RG, Dizdaroglu M, Brooks PJ. 2005. Polyamines stimulate the formation of mutagenic 1,N2-propanodeoxyguanosine adducts from acetaldehyde. Nucleic Acids Res 33:3513–3520.

Thiele GM, Duryee MJ, Willis MS, Sorrell MF, Freeman TL, Tuma DJ, Klassen LW. 2004. Malondialdehyde-acetaldehyde (MAA) modified proteins induce pro-inflammatory and pro-fibrotic responses by liver endothelial cells. Comp Hepatol 3 Suppl 1:S25.

Toh Y, Oki E, Ohgaki K, Sakamoto Y, Ito S, Egashira A, Saeki H, Kakeji Y, Morita M, Sakaguchi Y, Okamura T, Maehara Y. 2010. Alcohol drinking, cigarette smoking, and the development of squamous cell carcinoma of the esophagus: molecular mechanisms of carcinogenesis. Int J Clin Oncol.

Tuma DJ, Thiele GM, Xu D, Klassen LW, Sorrell MF. 1996. Acetaldehyde and malondialdehyde react together to generate distinct protein adducts in the liver during long-term ethanol administration. Hepatology 23:872–880.

Uchida K. 2003. 4-Hydroxy-2-nonenal: a product and mediator of oxidative stress. Prog Lipid Res 42:318–343.

Valko M, Rhodes CJ, Moncol J, Izakovic M, Mazur M. 2006. Free radicals, metals and antioxidants in oxidative stress-induced cancer. Chem Biol Interact 160:1–40.

Vaziri H, Dessain SK et al. 2001. hSIR2(SIRT1) functions as an NAD-dependent p53 deacetylase. Cell 107(2):149–159.

Visapaa JP, Gotte K, Benesova M, Li J, Homann N, Conradt C, Inoue H, Tisch M, Horrmann K, Vakevainen S, Salaspuro M, Seitz HK. 2004. Increased cancer risk in heavy drinkers with the alcohol dehydrogenase 1C*1 allele, possibly due to salivary acetaldehyde. Gut 53:871–876.
Visapaa JP, Jokelainen K, Nosova T, Salaspuro M. 1998. Inhibition of intracolonic acetaldehyde production and alcoholic fermentation in rats by ciprofloxacin. Alcohol Clin Exp Res 22:1161–1164.
Wainfan E, Dizik M, Stender M, Christman JK. 1989. Rapid appearance of hypomethylated DNA in livers of rats fed cancer-promoting, methyl-deficient diets. Cancer Res 49:4094–4097.
Wang Y, Millonig G, Nair J, Patsenker E, Stickel F, Mueller S, Bartsch H, Seitz HK. 2009. Ethanol-induced cytochrome P4502E1 causes carcinogenic etheno-DNA lesions in alcoholic liver disease. Hepatology 50:453–461.
Weiner H, Wei B, Zhou J. 2001. Subunit communication in tetrameric class 2 human liver aldehyde dehydrogenase as the basis for half-of-the-site reactivity and the dominance of the oriental subunit in a heterotetramer. Chem Biol Interact 130–132:47–56.
Wright RM, McManaman JL, Repine JE. 1999. Alcohol-induced breast cancer: a proposed mechanism. Free Radic Biol Med 26:348–354.
Wu D, Cederbaum AI. 2003. Alcohol, oxidative stress, and free radical damage. Alcohol Res Health 27:277–284.
Wu X, Amos CI, Kemp BL, Shi H, Jiang H, Wan Y, Spitz MR. 1998. Cytochrome P450 2E1 DraI polymorphisms in lung cancer in minority populations. Cancer Epidemiol Biomarkers Prev 7:13–18.
Yin SJ, Chou FJ, Chao SF, Tsai SF, Liao CS, Wang SL, Wu CW, Lee SC. 1993. Alcohol and aldehyde dehydrogenases in human esophagus: comparison with the stomach enzyme activities. Alcohol Clin Exp Res 17:376–381.
Yin SJ, Han CL, Lee AI, Wu CW. 1999. Human alcohol dehydrogenase family. Functional classification, ethanol/retinol metabolism, and medical implications. Adv Exp Med Biol 463:265–274.
Yokoyama A, Muramatsu T, Ohmori T, Yokoyama T, Okuyama K, Takahashi H, Hasegawa Y, Higuchi S, Maruyama K, Shirakura K, Ishii H. 1998. Alcohol-related cancers and aldehyde dehydrogenase-2 in Japanese alcoholics. Carcinogenesis 19:1383–1387.
Yokoyama A, Omori T. 2003. Genetic polymorphisms of alcohol and aldehyde dehydrogenases and risk for esophageal and head and neck cancers. Jpn J Clin Oncol 33:111–121.
Yokoyama A, Watanabe H, Fukuda H, Haneda T, Kato H, Yokoyama T, Muramatsu T, Igaki H, Tachimori Y. 2002. Multiple cancers associated with esophageal and oropharyngolaryngeal squamous cell carcinoma and the aldehyde dehydrogenase-2 genotype in male Japanese drinkers. Cancer Epidemiol Biomarkers Prev 11:895–900.
Yokoyama H, Nagata S, Moriya S, Kato S, Ito T, Kamegaya K, Ishii H. 1995. Hepatic fibrosis produced in guinea pigs by chronic ethanol administration and immunization with acetaldehyde adducts. Hepatology 21:1438–1442.
Yoshida A, Hsu LC, Yasunami M. 1991. Genetics of human alcohol-metabolizing enzymes. Prog Nucleic Acid Res Mol Biol 40:255–287.
Zakhari S. 2006. Overview: how is alcohol metabolized by the body? Alcohol Res Health 29:245–254.
Zhang SM. 2004. Role of vitamins in the risk, prevention, and treatment of breast cancer. Curr Opin Obstet Gynecol 16:19–25.

Chapter 5
Epigenetics, Alcohol, and Cancer

Dale Hereld and Q. Max Guo

Abbreviations

CpG	Cytosine-guanine dinucleotide
DNMT	DNA methyl transferase
ER	Endoplasmic reticulum
GSH	Glutathione
GST	Glutathione *S*-transferase
HAT	Histone acetyltransferase
HCC	Hepatocellular carcinoma
HDAC	Histone deacetylase
HERP	Homocysteine-induced endoplasmic reticulum protein
HMT	Histone methyltranferase
HNSCC	Head and neck squamous cell carcinoma
JAK	Janus kinase
MAP kinase	Mitogen-activated protein kinase
MAT	Methionine adenosyltransferase
miRNA	microRNA
MTHFR	Methylene tetrahydrofolate reductase
NAD and NADH	Oxidized and reduced nicotinamide adenine dinucleotide, respectively
ncRNA	Nonprotein-coding RNA
PLP	Pyridoxal-5′ phosphate
RISC	RNA-induced silencing complex
RITS	RNA-induced transcriptional silencing
SAH	*S*-adenosyl-homocysteine

D. Hereld (✉)
Division of Metabolism and Health Effects, National Institute on Alcohol Abuse and Alcoholism, National Institutes of Health, Bethesda, MD, USA
e-mail: hereldd@mail.nih.gov

S. Zakhari et al. (eds.), *Alcohol and Cancer*, DOI 10.1007/978-1-4614-0040-0_5,
© Springer Science+Business Media, LLC 2011

SAM (or SAMe)	*S*-adenosylmethionine
STAT	Signal transducer and activator of transcription
TGS	Transcriptional gene silencing
THF	Tetrahydrofolate
UTRs	Untranslated regions

Introduction

Chronic or excessive alcohol consumption often leads to various medical disorders, including liver cirrhosis, pancreatitis, cardiomyopathy, fetal abnormalities, brain damage, and various cancers. To effectively prevent or treat these disorders, a better understanding of their underlying mechanisms is pivotal. Alcohol and its metabolites alter cellular functions through changes at the levels of DNA, RNA, protein, and metabolites, resulting in pathophysiological changes. Although the amount of RNA, protein, or metabolites is determined by dynamic processes of synthesis and degradation with many regulators involved, it is initially predominantly determined by the activity of the genes involved. Two major mechanisms of gene regulation involve genetic and epigenetic controls of gene expression. In the past half century, research and technological innovations have led to a remarkable progress in understanding the genetic controls of gene activities. However, only in recent years, epigenetic controls of gene expression drew immense interest, especially in the biomedical fields of cancer and ageing. To date, research efforts to understand effects of alcohol on regulation of gene activity have been primarily focused on genetic factors. The mechanisms of epigenetic modifications in alcohol-induced organ damage, including cancers, have only started to be tackled in the past few years.

Epigenetics refers to the study of heritable changes in gene function that occur without altering DNA sequences. These epigenetic changes can be either inherited mitotically from cell to cell or meiotically from generation to generation. Increasing evidence has demonstrated that epigenetic modifications play an important role in gene activity and chromosomal stability through covalent modification of genomic DNA and histones, and RNA-mediated silencing. Thus, epigenetic modifications introduce another layer of complexity to the regulation of gene expression. For example, genetically identical monozygotic twins could have different susceptibility to Beckwith–Wiedemann syndrome, a rare disease with about 850-fold increased risk for developing Wilms' tumor and other malignancies. The increased risk results from a DNA methylation defect during early embryogenesis in the promoter region of CNQ1OT1 gene (Weksberg et al. 2002). A recent study reported that while locus-specific and global differences of DNA methylation and histone acetylation in young monozygotic twins are almost indistinguishable, these epigenetic differences increase dramatically as the twin pairs age (Fraga et al. 2005a). Consistent with these increased epigenetic differences, the differences in gene

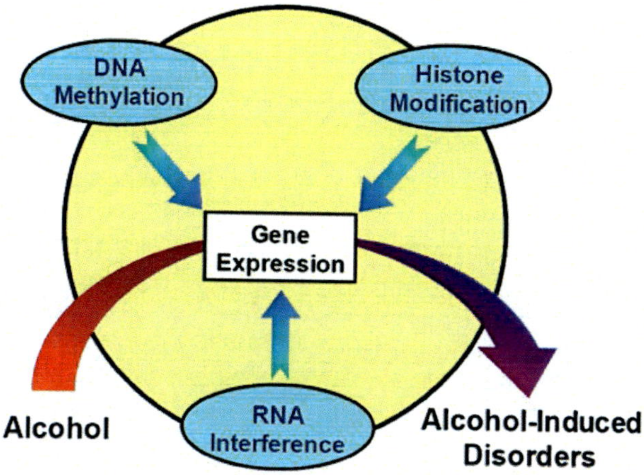

Fig. 5.1 DNA methylation, histone modification, and RNA-associated gene silencing regulate gene expression and are involved in actions of alcohol

expression in 50-year-old twin pairs are four times greater than those of 3-year-old twin pairs (Fraga et al. 2005a). These epigenetic differences reflect mostly the impact of different environmental exposure over time. The effects of various environmental factors, such as pup licking and grooming, smoking, and diet on epigenetic regulations, have been widely documented (reviewed by Zhang and Meaney 2010). However, inheritance (gene imprinting) and environment are not the sole sources of epigenetic differences. Monozygotic twins or cloned animals with identical genomes can display subtle or dramatic phenotypic differences even when placed in the same environment. For example, monozygotic twins can be readily distinguished through close examination of their fingerprints. The first cloned cat displayed different coat patterns and personality from her genetic mother (Shin et al. 2002). It appears that these phenotypic variations are inevitable because of the stochastic nature of biological processes in a given cell or an organism. The variability in epigenetic regulation of gene expression also contributes a large part to this stochastic nature of biology.

Epigenetic regulation of gene expression primarily involves three systems: DNA methylation, histone modification, and RNA-mediated gene silencing. Studies have shown that alcohol affects all three systems, thus modulating the expression of many genes either directly or indirectly (Fig. 5.1). In turn, these alcohol-induced changes in gene expression may affect various biochemical and signaling pathways influencing the function of cells and organs, leading to diseases or beneficial effects (for moderate alcohol intake). Understanding alcohol-induced epigenetic regulation will provide mechanistic insights, diagnostic biomarkers, and therapeutic targets for alcohol-related cancers.

DNA Methylation

DNA Methylation and Cancer

DNA methylation occurs on the CpG dinucleotides by transferring a methyl group from *S*-adenosylmethionine (SAMe) onto the cytosine residue, which protrudes into the major groove of the DNA (Fig. 5.2 and Sidebar 1). DNA methylation can be maintained during DNA replication by DNA methyl transferases (DNMTs), which transfer the methyl groups to the hemimethylated DNA (Iacobuzio-Donahue 2009). DNA methylation can also occur after DNA replication by de novo DNMTs. In mammals, three functional DNMTs (DNMT1, 3a, and 3b) have been identified, of which DNMT3a and DNMT3b are responsible for the de novo DNA methylation (Edwards and Ferguson-Smith 2007). In general, methylation of CpG islands represses gene expression by changing the chromatin structure or by interfering with the binding of some transcription factors to the promoter. DNA methylation has been shown to play a critical role in many cellular and biological processes, including X-chromosome inactivation, cancer, ageing, addiction, development, and the maintenance and differentiation of stem cells (reviewed by Zhang and Meaney 2010).

An important biological phenomenon involving epigenetic modification is called genomic imprinting, in which the gene is only expressed from either paternally or maternally inherited chromosomes. Approximately 70 imprinted genes have been found so far, but it is estimated that as many as 1% of human genes are imprinted. While some of these genes are imprinted individually, approximately 80% of them are found in clusters in the genome (Edwards and Ferguson-Smith 2007; Bartolomei 2009). In the imprinted genes, DNA methylation patterns, thus gene expression state, differ between the maternally and paternally inherited alleles. Imprinting of some genes has been found to be linked to human cancers. For example, loss of imprinting in IGF2 gene has been shown in both mice and humans to be associated with increased cancer risk in intestine, colon, and prostate (Cui et al. 2003; Sakatani et al. 2005; Bjornsson et al. 2007). In addition to imprinted genes, methylation of nonimprinted genes also plays an important role in cancers (Sharma et al. 2010). Tumorigenesis involves both hypomethylation and hypermethylation. Since methylation of DNA is closely associated with gene silencing, hypomethylation of

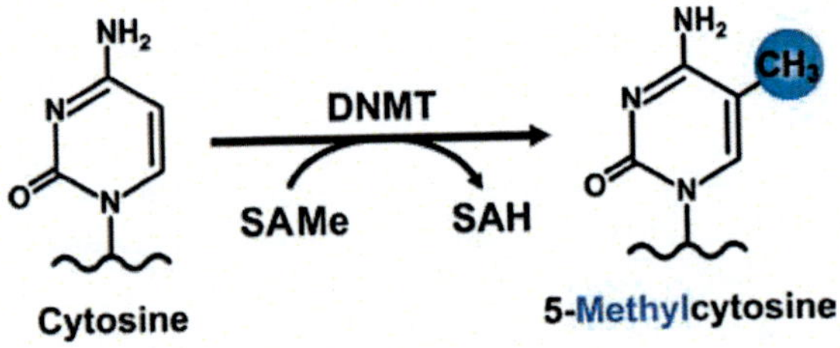

Fig. 5.2 DNA methylation. *DNMT* DNA methyl transferase, *Me* methyl, *SAH S*-adenosylhomocysteine, *SAMe S*-adenosylmethionine. *Wavy lines* symbolize the phospho-deoxyribose backbone of DNA

Sidebar 1: CpG Island

CpG is a cytosine-guanine dinucleotide connected by a phosphodiester bond. The "p" in CpG is used to distinguish this linear nucleotide sequence from the G:C base pair in DNA. Regions of chromosome containing a high frequency of CpG sites are called CpG islands. The CpG islands are defined as having greater than 55% of (G+C) content with a CpG dinucleotide ratio of greater than 0.60 in a stretch of DNA greater than 500 bp. Given the GC frequency, the number of CpG dinucleotides appears to be vastly underrepresented in genomes. For example, with 42% GC content, human genome is expected to have 4.41% (21×21%) CpG dinucleotides. The actual frequency of CpG dinucleotides is only 1% in human genome. This phenomenon, known as CG suppression, is proposed to be due to an increased vulnerability of methylcytosines to transition mutation in CpG dinucleotides during evolution. Through spontaneous deamination, the methylcytosines tend to turn into thymines, thus be selected out over time. Despite being underrepresented, CpG dinucleotides are common in promoter regions. About 70% of promoters have a high CpG content in human genome. In the mammalian genome, 80% of CpG dinucleotides are estimated to be methylated. The unmethylated CpG dinucleotides are largely located in CpG islands of promoter regions of actively expressed genes. The hypermethylation of CpG islands in tumor-suppressor genes can silence their expression, as found in a number of human cancers. The hypomethylation of CpG islands in the promoters of oncogenes can also lead to their overexpression, contributing to cancer development.

oncogenes could result in their activation. On the other hand, hypermethylation of tumor-suppressor genes can cause their silencing and contribute to cancer initiation and progression. Extrinsic factors, including insufficiencies in dietary methionine/choline, folate, zinc, and other micronutrient, as well as excessive alcohol intake, can cause hypomethylation or hypermethylation. Sufficient evidence has been accumulated that alterations caused by environmental factors could lead to changes in gene expression and increased risk to cancers (Iacobuzio-Donahue 2009; Zhang and Meaney 2010; Feinberg 2007). A better understanding of action of alcohol on DNA methylation is pivotal for unraveling the pathogenesis of alcohol-related cancers.

Alcohol and DNA Methylation

Alcohol-induced organ damage reflects the genetic and epigenetic makeup of the individuals and the cumulative responses to alcohol exposure over time. Many alcohol-induced pathophysiological changes are long-lasting and persist even after discontinuation of alcohol intake. Although acetaldehyde, the first metabolite of ethanol, can form DNA adducts and causes sequence alteration of DNA, most of the short- or long-lasting effects of alcohol may be mediated through changes that do not involve DNA sequence alteration. Epigenetic mechanisms, which are generally sensitive to extrinsic input, have been well-documented in many other complex human diseases. Studies in the past few years have shown that epigenetic regulation of gene expression is an important mechanism for action of alcohol in the cell and alcohol-induced disorders (Shukla et al. 2008). Many environmental risk factors, such as age, diet, lifestyle, smoking, and stress which may also contribute to alcohol-related cancers, have been documented to cause epigenetic alterations. Thus, epigenetic modification may represent a critical mechanism for alcohol-induced cancers.

Alcohol exposure may also affect stem cells and tissue regeneration/repair through epigenetic mechanisms. Stem cell differentiation and tissue repair/regeneration are characterized by rapid, but well-synchronized patterns of, gene expression involving epigenetic processes in which the status of DNA methylation shifts dramatically, involving both loss of methylation and de novo methylation. DNA methylation has been suggested to be an important mechanism for cancer stem cell hypothesis (Feinberg et al. 2006; Iacobuzio-Donahue 2009; also see Chap. 11). For example, at the early neurulation of mouse embryo development, ethanol administration alters DNA methylation patterns (Liu et al. 2009). Many changes of DNA methylation during development and stem cell differentiation involve genes known to function in cell cycle, growth, apoptosis, and oxidative stress, all of which play a critical role in alcohol-induced organ damage and cancer. The effects of alcohol on epigenetic processes during tissue repair/regeneration and stem cell differentiation may cause undesirable changes in gene expression that, in turn, may alter the function of cells, contributing to the initiation and progression of cancers. Evidently, purely sequence-based genetic or genomic approaches to study gene regulation are not sufficient to explain the pathogenesis of alcohol-related cancers. The study of effects of alcohol on DNA methylation can provide valuable insights into the mechanisms of alcohol-induced cancers.

Effects of Alcohol on the Availability and Transfer of Methyl Groups

Chronic alcohol consumption is associated with abnormal methionine metabolism, increased plasma homocysteine level, decreased level of SAMe, and folate deficiency (Bleich and Hillemacher 2009; Seitz and Stickel 2007). As shown in Figs. 5.2 and 5.3, SAMe is the major methyl donor for DNA methylation. DNA is methylated by transferring the methyl group from SAMe to cytosine residues in the CpG dinucleotides. SAMe is primarily generated in the liver from L-methionine and ATP by methionine adenosyltransferase (MAT) isoforms, which are encoded by two genes, *MAT1A* and *MAT2A*. *MAT1A* encodes the isoenzymes MATI and MATIII, whereas *MAT2A* encodes the isoenzyme MATII. MATI and MATIII are mostly responsible for maintaining high intracellular SAMe levels in adult liver while MATII is predominantly active in fetal and regenerating liver tissues. *MAT1A* is the major gene responsible for producing SAMe used to methylate DNA. The transfer of the methyl group from SAMe

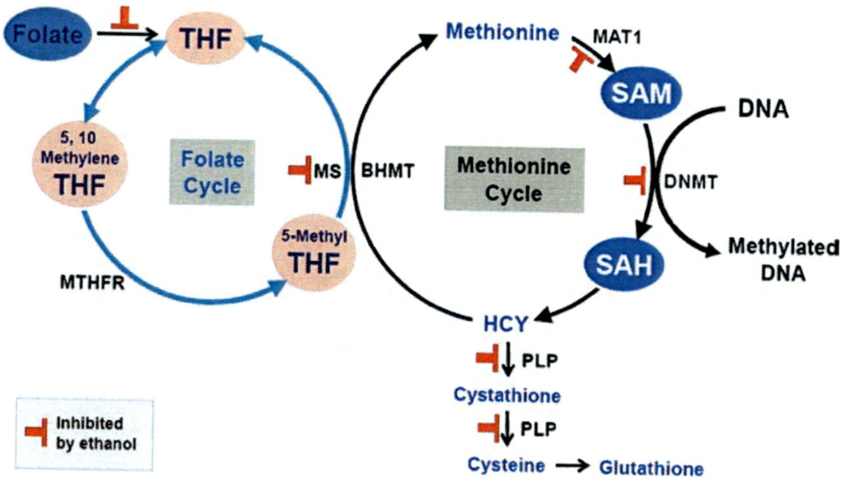

Fig. 5.3 Effects of ethanol on the transfer of methyl groups. Ethanol or its metabolite acetaldehyde affects several reactions and enzymes involved in the transfer of methyl groups. Ethanol inhibits folate absorption. Ethanol interacts with pyridoxal-5′ phosphate (PLP) and interrupts methyl group generation. Genetic variations of methylene tetrahydrofolate reductase (MTHFR) are associated with deficiencies in tetrahydrofolate (THF) production. Ethanol inhibits methionine synthase (MS) and increases homocysteine level. Ethanol inhibits methionine adenosyltransferase I (MAT1) and thus the synthesis of *S*-adenosylmethionine (SAM). Ethanol interferes with homocysteine disposal by inactivating cystathionine-β-synthase. Ethanol disrupts methyl group transfer onto the cytosine residues of DNA

generates *S*-adenosylhomocysteine (SAH), which subsequently becomes homocysteine. Homocysteine is either catabolized to cysteine, which is eliminated in urine, or remethylated to methionine to be further converted to SAMe.

The effects of ethanol on the availability and transfer of methyl groups may play a critical role in the development of alcohol-related cancers. Ethanol impairs the transfer of methyl group to the cytosine residues of DNA by reducing the levels and activity of DNMTs, resulting in DNA hypomethylation (Fig. 5.3). Ethanol metabolite acetaldehyde can also inhibit DNMT activity. Studies have shown that livers of *MAT1A* knockout mice had SAMe deficiency and increased expression of genes involved in proliferation, and consequently developed hepatomegaly, fatty liver, and eventually hepatocellular carcinoma (HCC). They also regenerated abnormally after partial hepatectomy and were more sensitive to developing steatosis in response to a methionine- and choline-deficient diet (Mato et al. 2008). It has been reported that during hepatocarcinogenesis or hepatectomy, *MAT1A* itself is severely downregulated due to the hypermethylation of its promoter (reviewed by Seitz and Stickel 2007). Overexpression of *MAT1A* in rat hepatoma cells resulted in growth arrest (Cai et al. 1998), whereas the addition of SAMe to the culture led to apoptosis (Yang et al. 2004). These observations suggest that ethanol may contribute to liver cancer development via its inhibition of MATI and MATIII activity as well as reducing SAMe levels (Fig. 5.3; reviewed by Seitz and Stickel 2007).

In addition to its effects on MAT and SAMe synthesis, ethanol also affects a number of other processes related to methyl group transfer. The conversion of homocysteine to methionine by methionine synthase is inhibited by ethanol, resulting in homocysteine accumulation. Ethanol also inactivates the enzyme cystathionine-β-synthase, which removes homocysteine through its transsulfuration to cystathionine, further disrupting the homocysteine disposal (Fig. 5.3). Furthermore, because cystathionine is used to generate the antioxidant glutathione (GSH), the decreased level of cystathionine by ethanol can reduce GSH generation leading to increased oxidative stress, which may, in turn, contribute to cancer pathogenesis (Fig. 5.3). GSH, a tripeptide synthesized predominantly in the liver from glycine, cysteine, and glutamate, is a major reservoir of cysteine and acts as a reducing agent and a major antioxidant. GSH is present in high abundance in cells and many extracellular fluids. Inside the cell, approximately 85–90% of GSH is freely distributed in cytosol, and the rest is confined in cellular organelles, such as mitochondria, endoplasmic reticulum (ER), and nuclear matrix. GSH is the most abundant nonprotein thiol in the cell and plays a pivotal role in cellular protection and many physiological reactions, including the synthesis of proteins and DNA, transport of amino acids, enzymatic activities, and control of the inflammatory cytokine-signaling pathways. Excessive ethanol intake can decrease GSH level by inhibiting hepatic GSH synthesis and the enzymatic activities involved in GSH-related peroxide detoxification, such as GSH peroxidase and glutathione *S*-transferase (GST), thus increasing the susceptibility of the liver to oxidative injury (Lieber 2000). Hepatic GSH depletion appears to precede the histological changes caused by alcohol-induced hepatotoxicity (Lieber 2000). In addition, studies have found associations between polymorphisms of GST gene and the susceptibility to various cancers, such as head and neck squamous cell carcinoma (HNSCC), HCC, renal and urinary bladder cell carcinoma, and cancers of breast, stomach, lung, and prostate (Di Pietro et al. 2010). Alcohol-induced GSH deficiency may play a significant role in the development of these cancers due to decreased cellular protection.

Another major site of actions of ethanol on methyl group transfer is folate metabolism cycle. Folates, a family of water-soluble B-class vitamins based on folic acid (pteorylglutamic acid), are required for the synthesis of nucleotide precursors (purines and pyrimidines) and the methylation of many essential biological substances, such as phospholipids, proteins, DNA, and neurotransmitters. Humans and other mammalians cannot synthesize folates de novo, and must obtain them from food via intestinal absorption. Folate deficiency, which affects 10% of Americans and is the most prevalent vitamin deficiency in the world, can be caused by reduced folate intake, malabsorption, altered metabolism, genetic defects, or other conditions. Earlier studies have demonstrated that chronic alcohol abuse is a major cause of folate deficiency, resulting from inadequate dietary intake, intestinal malabsorption, altered hepatobiliary metabolism, enhanced colonic metabolism, and increased renal excretion (reviewed by Hamid et al. 2009). Folates, mainly as N^5-methyl-tetrahydrofolate (THF), are transported through specialized transporters to the liver, the main storage site of folates in the body. After folates are secreted into the bile and transported to the small intestine, they can be reabsorbed. The pancreas, which is the second richest store of folates, and the kidneys may also play a significant role in folate homeostasis. The homeostasis of intracellular folates is important for the methyl group transfer reactions, as shown in Fig. 5.3. Folate (as N^5-methyl-THF) provides a methyl group to homocysteine to convert it to methionine. Folate, in the form of 5,10-methylene-tetrahydrofolate (5,10-CH_2-THF), also provides a methyl group to uracil and converts it to thymidine, which is used for DNA synthesis and repair. The enzyme methylene-tetrahydrofolate reductase (MTHFR) irreversibly converts 5,10-CH_2-THF to 5-methyl-THF, which then donates a methyl group to homocysteine to generate methionine. A common genetic variation (C677T) in *MTHFR* gene has been associated with increased risk to various cancers, including endometrial, breast, ovarian, esophageal, and gastric cancers. However, the variation has also been found to be associated with decreased risk for leukemia and colorectal cancer. The risk of cancer associated with *MTHFR* polymorphisms can be compensated by folate intake. The greater availability of 5,10-CH_2-THF, which can convert uracil to thymidine, reduces the genomic instability caused by compromised DNA synthesis and repair associated with the *MTHFR* polymorphism. The same *MTHFR* polymorphism and chronic alcohol abuse have been found to be linked to colorectal cancers (reviewed by Hamid et al. 2009).

Folate deficiency caused by chronic alcohol use can be attributed to the inhibition of folate uptake in the intestine and kidneys by disrupting the folate transport systems and to the inhibition of intestinal and renal expression of folate transporters (Fig. 5.3; reviewed by Seitz and Stickel 2007; Hamid et al. 2009). While first demonstrated 30 years ago by Halsted and colleagues that chronic use of alcohol caused malabsorption of folates, a recent study demonstrated that absorption of folic acid by the jejunum and cecum of ethanol-fed rats was decreased, and folate absorption and hepatic folate content in alcoholic monkeys were also significantly decreased (Hamid et al. 2009). Increased renal excretion is another contributing factor for decreased availability of dietary folate due to chronic alcohol use (Hamid et al. 2009).

Chronic alcohol use and folate deficiency appear to have a synergistic effect on the development of cancers. Ethanol can indirectly affect many oncogenic pathways through its effects on the transfer of methyl groups. In an epidemiological study of human colorectal cancers, the promoters of a number of tumor-suppressor and DNA repair genes were found to be hypermethylated which correlated with low folate intake and high alcohol intake (Jones and Laird 1999; Van Engeland et al. 2003). In addition, excess alcohol ingestion and low dietary folate intake have been implicated as interacting risk factors for several cancers of the oral cavity, pharynx, larynx, esophagus, liver, colon, rectum, and breast. Their link to cancers of the pancreas and lung has also been suspected. In addition to tumor-suppressor genes, dietary depletion of lipotropes, such as choline, methionine, betaine, SAMe, and folate, has been shown to cause hypomethylation in the promoters of oncogenes (e.g., *c-H-ras, c-K-ras, c-fos*) and DNA breaks, and lead to increased cancer incidence in rats (Cravo et al. 1996; Zapisek et al. 1992). It has also been shown in humans that high alcohol intake, combined with low-methionine and low-folate diets, increases the risk of colorectal cancer (Bingham 2006; Boffetta et al. 2006). Although the detailed mechanism is still unclear, folate deficiency has been found to increase DNA breaks in tumor-suppressor p53 gene and cause changes in some signaling pathways known to be important for tumorigenesis. These pathways include the wnt–APC pathway and pathways involved in cell adhesion, migration, and invasion (Crott et al. 2008). These effects of alcohol and folate deficiency may contribute to the initiation and progression of alcohol-related cancers.

Although it is clear that chronic alcohol ingestion alters availability and transfer of methyl group, its impact on DNA methylation appears to be complex. On one hand, patients with chronic alcohol dependence have elevated methylation in genomic DNA and in the promoter of α-synuclein and homocysteine-induced endoplasmic reticulum protein (HERP) (Bonsch et al. 2004, 2005, 2006; Bleich et al. 2006; Bleich and Hillemacher 2009). DNA methylation of the promoters of class I ADH genes is also elevated in an ethanol-treated human hepatoma cell line (Dannenberg et al. 2006). The expression of DNMT-3b is decreased in alcoholic patients and negatively correlated with blood alcohol concentration (Bonsch et al. 2006). This downregulation of DNMT-3b could be due to the feedback control of the increased genomic DNA methylation (Bonsch et al. 2006). On the other hand, ethanol seems to also cause demethylation in the promoters of some genes. In mouse cortical neurons, for example, chronic ethanol administration causes demethylation of CpG islands in the promoter of NMDA receptor NR2B gene (Ravindran and Ticku 2005; Biermann et al. 2009). Ethanol consumption increases DNA demethylation of normally hypermethylated imprinted regions in male gametes (Ouko et al. 2009). DNA demethylation associated with low-dietary folate intake can be also aggravated by high alcohol intake (Halsted et al. 2002). Although ethanol interferes with methyl group transfer and causes DNA hypomethylation, it remains unclear how ethanol causes DNA hypermethylation. The effect of ethanol on DNA methylation may depend on genomic context, cell type, target organ, and other variables.

Histone Modification

Chromatin structure is dynamically regulated to accommodate distinct phases of development, to selectively facilitate the expression of some genes while maintaining others in a quiescent state, to allow for DNA repair and replication, and to condense replicated chromosomes to assure their faithful segregation during cell division. The nucleosome, comprised of 146 base pairs of DNA wound around an octameric complex of histone proteins H2A, H2B, H3, and H4, represents the fundamental unit of chromatin (Fig. 5.4a). Interactions between nucleosomes dictate the degree to which chromatin is condensed as well as its accessibility to the machinery for replication, transcription, repair, and other processes. Genes within highly condensed "heterochromatin" regions are generally silenced, whereas uncondensed "euchromatin" is permissive for gene expression. The various states of chromatin are largely attributable to the posttranslational modification of histones. As depicted in Fig. 5.4b, these modifications primarily occur on the N-terminal histone "tail"

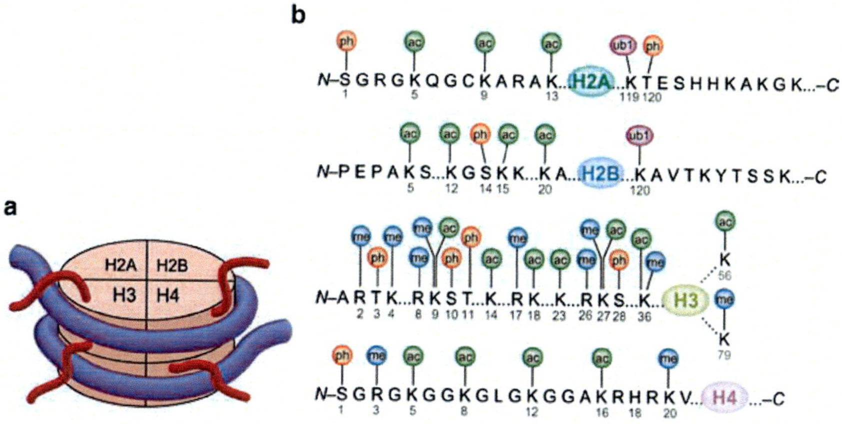

Fig. 5.4 Posttranslational modifications of histones. (**a**) Schematic depiction of a nucleosome, showing DNA (*blue*) wound around octameric histone core (*pink*) and protruding N- and C-terminal histone tails (*magenta*). (**b**) Summary of known sites of histone acetylation (ac), methylation (me), phosphorylation (ph), and ubiquitination (ub1). As shown, most sites reside with the N-terminal tails. Only a subset of these sites would be modified at a given time. Less frequently, modifications occur within the globular domains of histones (*ovals*) and C-terminal tails. [From Bhaumik et al. (2007); reprinted by permission from Macmillan Publishers Ltd: Nature Structural & Molecular Biology 14:1008–16, ©2007]

peptides, which protrude from the nucleosome structure, and include various extents of lysine methylation (mono-, di-, or tri-), lysine acetylation and lysine ubiquitination, arginine methylation (mono- or di-), and serine or threonine phosphorylation, among others (reviewed in Bhaumik et al. 2007).

Histone acetylation is associated with loosely packed chromatin and actively transcribed genes. This is thought to reflect the fact that acetylation (unlike methylation) neutralizes the positive charge on histone lysine residues and, thus, alleviates constraining interactions between histones and the negatively charged DNA. As depicted in Fig. 5.5, histone acetylation is determined by the opposing activities of histone acetyltransferases (HATs) and deacetylases (HDACs). Consistent with the association of histone acetylation and transcription, transcriptional coactivators (e.g., CBP/P300 and GCN5/PCAF) have been shown to possess HAT activity while transcriptional corepressor complexes typically contain subunits with HDAC activity. The latter include Zn^{2+}-dependent deacetylases and the NAD^{+}-dependent SIRT family deacetylases (Bhaumik et al. 2007; Kristensen et al. 2009; Zhong et al. 2010). Histone methylation, on the other hand, results from the action of histone methyltranferases (HMTs) and is reversed by histone demethylases (Fig. 5.5). Compared with enzymes involved in histone acetylation which are relatively few in number and promiscuous in terms of which lysines they can modify, HMTs and histone demethylases are typically specific for a single-histone residue and, consequently, are more numerous (Bhaumik et al. 2007; Kouzarides 2007).

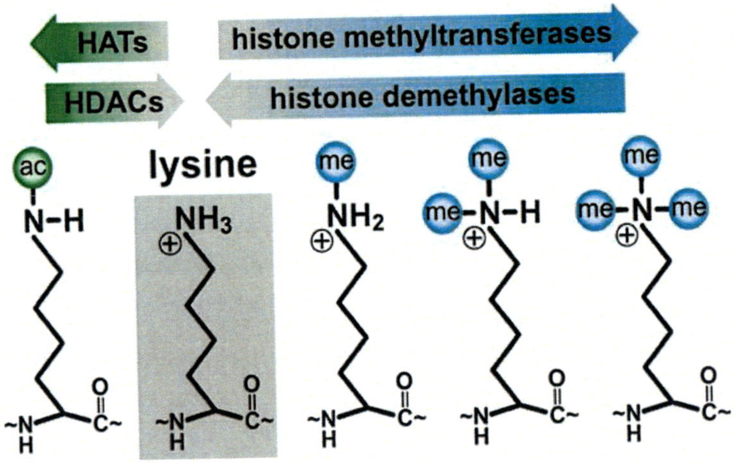

Fig. 5.5 Modification of histone lysine residues. Acetylation is mediated by histone acetyltransferases (HATs) and reversed by histone deacetylases (HDACs) while histone methyltransferases and demethylases determine if lysine is mono-, di-, or trimethylated. Although not shown, arginine residues can also be mono- or dimethylated

Given the large number of histone residues available for modification and the variety of modifications, the number of possible combinations capable of specifying various chromatin states has given rise to the notion of a "histone code" (Strahl and Allis 2000). Indeed, specific patterns of histone modification have been associated with distinct functional states of chromatin. For instance, methylation of H3K9 (i.e., lysine 9 of histone H3), H3K27, and H4K20 is generally associated with heterochromatin formation and transcriptional repression while methylation of H3K4 and H3K36 is associated with transcriptionally active chromatin regions. The modification of yet other histone residues is thought to play roles in establishing chromatin environments conducive to DNA replication (e.g., acetylation of H4 lysines), DNA repair (e.g., phosphorylation of H2AS129 and H4S1), and chromatin condensation during cell division (e.g., phosphorylation of H3S10 and H3T3). In general, histone modifications are thought to mediate these biological effects by a variety of mechanisms, including (1) influencing physical interaction of nucleosomes and, thus, the compactness of chromatin; (2) serving as docking sites for nonhistone proteins with various activities (e.g., HDACs); and (3) recruiting ATP-dependent chromatin-remodeling machines capable of promoting sliding, exchange, and eviction of histone octamers, alterations of the DNA path on the nucleosome surface, and other higher order changes to chromatin structure (Kouzarides 2007; Cvekl and Mitton 2010).

Histone Modifications and Cancer

Altered histone modification has been associated with a number of cancers. In many case, these are repressive histone modifications, which can lead to the silencing of tumor-suppressor genes and thereby promote cancer. For instance, elevated H3K27 methylation and associated repression of the gene encoding DACT3, a suppressor of oncogenic Wnt/β-catenin signaling, have been observed in colon cancers (Jiang et al. 2008; Ying and Tao 2009). Furthermore, EZH2, the methyltransferase responsible for H3K27 methylation, is frequently overexpressed in prostate cancers and the degree of overexpression has been correlated with the metastatic potential of these cancers (Varambally et al. 2002). The global loss of two repressive marks on histone 4, H4K16 acetylation and H4K20 methylation, has also been documented in a variety of cancers (Fraga et al. 2005b).

Various mutations of genes encoding histone-modifying enzymes have also been found to contribute to the development of cancer. Deregulation of histone acetylation results from mutation of HAT genes in a number of cancers. For example, mutations in the *p300* gene are linked to gastrointestinal tumors and aberrant CBP fusion proteins resulting from chromosomal translocations cause leukemia and uterine myomas. Similarly, fusion proteins of MLL, an HMT that is essential for H3K4 methylation, also arise from chromosomal translocations and are frequently associated with acute myeloid and lymphoid leukemias (Bhaumik et al. 2007).

The association of altered histone modification with cancer has spurred the development of cancer therapeutics aimed at correcting these aberrancies. In particular, the frequent occurrence of histone hypoacetylation and HDAC overexpression in various cancers has prompted the development and evaluation of HDAC inhibitors for cancer treatment. To date, one of these, vorinostat, has been approved for the treatment of cutaneous T-cell lymphoma while several others are in clinical development. In general, these promising therapeutics target the active sites of Zn^{2+}-dependent HDACs (as opposed to the NAD^{+}-dependent SIRT family of HDACs). Consistent with their ability to increase histone acetylation, HDAC inhibitors deter cancer cells, in part, by upregulating genes that encode cell cycle regulators, including the cyclin-dependent kinase inhibitor p21/WAF1, as well as proapoptotic proteins. Besides their histone-dependent effects on gene expression, HDAC inhibitors also promote hyperacetylation and, thereby, regulate the activity of various nonhistone proteins, including tumor-suppressor p53, which likely contributes to their effectiveness for treating cancer (reviewed in Kristensen et al. 2009; Lane and Chabner 2009).

Alteration of Histone Modification by Alcohol

Emerging evidence points to the potential of alcohol to exert its health effects by altering the state of chromatin. Acute alcohol administration to rats was shown to increase H3K9 acetylation in select tissues, including liver, lung, spleen, and testes, but not in others (e.g., kidney, brain, heart, stomach, colorectum), indicating that epigenetic effects of alcohol will likely vary by tissue (Kim and Shukla 2006). Consistent with these in vivo findings, Choudhury and Shukla (2008) found that alcohol also promotes the acetylation of H3K9 in primary hepatocyte cultures without affecting the acetylation status of other H3 lysines, including K14, K18, K23, or K27. Accompanying this increase in H3K9 acetylation, Pal-Bhadra et al. (2007) showed that there was an overall reduction of H3K9 methylation and a concomitant increase in H3K4 methylation in alcohol-treated hepatocyte cultures. At the individual gene level, genes whose promoters exhibited this predominant pattern were found to be transcriptionally active while those exhibiting the inverse pattern (i.e., increased H3K9 methylation and decreased H3K4 methylation) were silenced. In addition, acute alcohol exposure has been shown to promote the phosphorylation of H3S10 and H3S28 in liver, apparently mediated by mitogen-activated protein kinase p38 (Lee and Shukla 2007; Aroor et al. 2010). Together, these findings highlight the potential for alcohol to alter patterns of histone modification and the expression of associated genes, raising the possibility that oncogenes and/or tumor suppressors might be among the affected genes and represent a mechanism by which ethanol contributes to cancer.

Alcohol appears to affect histone modification by various mechanisms. Choudhury and Shukla (2008) showed that the ethanol-induced acetylation of H3K9 in hepatocytes depends on alcohol metabolism and could be explained by the direct stimulation of HAT activity by the ethanol metabolite acetate. It is also possible that alcohol promotes histone acetylation by impairing HDAC function. In this regard, chronic alcohol exposure has been shown to reduce the expression of the NAD^+-dependent HDAC SIRT1 by roughly 40% in rat liver (Lieber et al. 2008). In addition, the activity of SIRT1 and other SIRT family members may be further limited by the availability of NAD^+, which may be reduced by the oxidation of alcohol (Rawat 1968). Impairment of SIRT1 activity may have important implications for cancer as it has been recently shown to play an important role in the regulation of circadian genes, a number of which are involved in cell cycle control (Nakahata et al. 2008). Similarly, alcohol-mediated reduction of NAD^+ could impair SIRT6, which is an important regulator of genes encoding glycolytic enzymes (Zhong et al. 2010). The resulting upregulation of glycolysis could, in turn, promote tumorigenesis as many cancer cells rely on high rates of glycolysis, instead of aerobic respiration, to meet their metabolic needs, a phenomenon known as the Warburg effect (Kim and Dang 2006). Alcohol might also interfere with histone methylation. Hepatic SAMe levels were found to be reduced by 50% in patients with alcoholic liver disease (Lee et al. 2004). As SAMe is the requisite methyl donor for histone methylation and the liver is the principal site of SAMe production, this may affect histone methylation in the liver and perhaps other tissues as well.

MicroRNAs

Multiple classes of small nonprotein-coding RNAs (ncRNAs) have been identified in recent years and shown to be important regulators of gene expression. Among these, microRNAs (miRNAs) have attracted great interest due in part to the breadth of their regulatory influence as well as their potential to serve as biomarkers and/or therapeutic agents. These 21- to 23-nucleotide-long single-stranded RNAs are conserved among phylogenetically distant animals and have been shown to play integral roles in a broad spectrum of fundamental biological processes, including

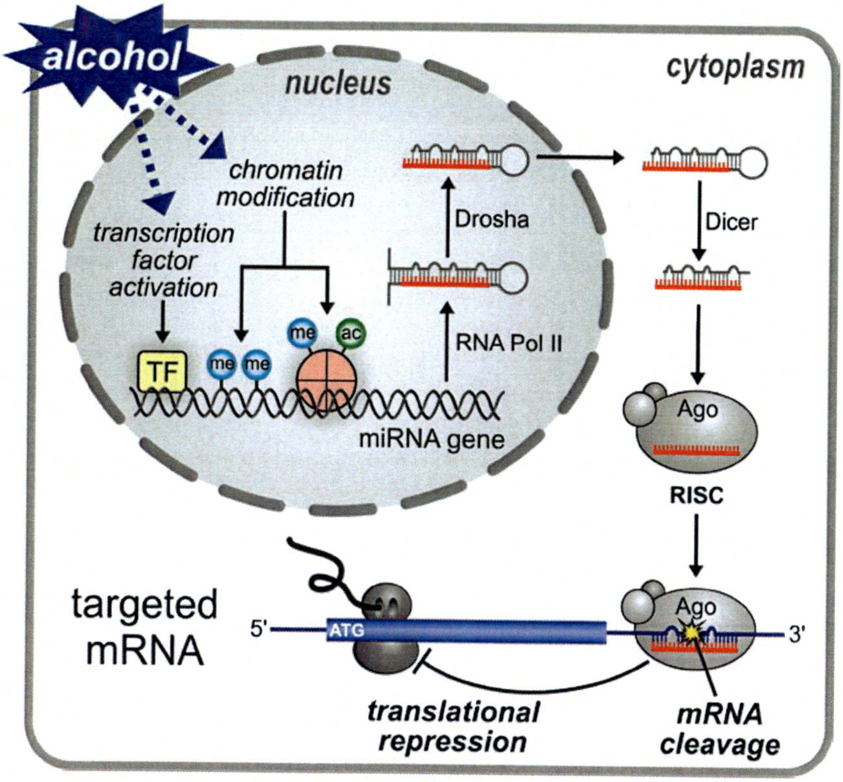

Fig. 5.6 miRNA biogenesis, mechanism of action, and possible alcohol effects. *Red* indicates miRNA at various stages of processing. Effects of alcohol on transcription factor (TF) activation or the modification of DNA and histones (*pink*) may result in altered miRNA expression. Abbreviations: *ac* acetylation, *Ago* Argonaut protein, *Pol* polymerase, *me* methylation, *RISC* RNA-induced silencing complex. (Adapted from Miranda et al. 2010)

cell cycle regulation, stem cell regeneration and differentiation, organogenesis, and oncogenic transformation.

Consistent with these diverse roles, the regulatory potential of miRNAs is substantial. More than 1,000 miRNAs are thought to exist in humans alone (http://microrna.sanger.ac.uk; Griffiths-Jones et al. 2008). miRNAs often act as "master" regulators, capable of targeting and silencing the expression of large collections of genes. These targeted genes are defined by short sequences typically found in their 3′ untranslated regions (UTRs) that are complementary to a given miRNA. Conversely, transcripts often harbor target sequences for multiple distinct miRNAs, thus creating the opportunity for complex miRNA-based regulatory networks to exist.

miRNAs are encoded either singly or in clusters by previously unrecognized endogenous genes or in some instances can be processed from introns excised from messenger RNAs as a result of splicing. As depicted in Fig. 5.6, primary miRNA transcripts possess internal complementarity and, thus, adopt stem-loop hairpin structures. These precursors are then successively cleaved by two ribonucleases, Drosha and Dicer, to yield an RNA duplex, one strand of which is the mature miRNA. In the cytoplasm, the miRNA associates with the Argonaute protein and additional accessory proteins, forming the so-called RNA-induced silencing complex (RISC). Serving as an adaptor, the miRNA guides this effector complex to mRNAs possessing a complementary 3′ UTR target sequence. Depending on the extent of complementarity, RISC then promotes posttranscriptional silencing typically by either repressing translation or effecting the Argonaute-catalyzed cleavage of the mRNA (Ambros 2003). Emerging evidence suggests that mammalian miRNAs might also mediate transcriptional gene silencing (TGS) as has been described in plants (Kim et al. 2008; Gonzalez et al. 2008). In this mechanism, an RNA-induced transcriptional silencing (RITS) complex, comprised of miRNA, Argonaute, and histone-modifying enzymes, **is targeted to nascent transcripts in the nucleus, where it modifies histones associated** with the corresponding gene in a manner that represses its expression.

MicroRNAs and Cancer

Numerous miRNAs have been shown to be involved in the regulation of virtually all known cancer-related signal transduction pathways, and altered expression of these miRNAs has been associated with a broad spectrum of cancers (Sotiropoulou et al. 2009). While the targets of many of these miRNAs remain to be determined, some have been shown to regulate the expression of well-known oncogenes and tumor suppressors. Therefore, dysregulation of these miRNAs can promote transformation and tumorigenicity. Such miRNAs themselves can be viewed as oncogenes and tumor suppressors. Examples include members of the let-7 family of miRNAs and miR-21. let-7 family members target several oncogenes, including RAS and MYC, and loss of these protective miRNAs is common in lung and breast cancer and other malignancies. On the other hand, miR-21 targets tumor suppressors PTEN and PDCD4, which govern cell proliferation and promote apoptosis, respectively. Overexpression of miR-21 and consequent reductions of these tumor suppressors are found in a wide variety of cancers (Visone and Croce 2009).

miRNAs have been found to be generally downregulated in a variety of human tumors (Lu et al. 2005), suggesting that miRNAs, in a collective sense, are antiproliferative. This notion is supported by recent evidence that rapid expansion of lymphocytes during immune responses is facilitated by the widespread truncation of mRNAs in their 3′ UTRs, resulting in the elimination of miRNA target sites (Sandberg et al. 2008). In cancer, defects in miRNA biogenesis could account for this global miRNA downregulation as knockdown of any of the three regulators of miRNA processing, Drosha, DGCR8, and Dicer1, promotes cellular transformation and tumorigenesis (Kumar et al. 2007). Indeed, *Dicer1* has been shown to be a tumor-suppressor gene and its monoallylic deletion is a common feature of naturally occurring human cancers (Kumar et al. 2009; Lambertz et al. 2010). Similarly, escape from miRNA regulatory control results in the elevated expression of the

Table 5.1 miRNAs dysregulated in cancers for which alcohol is a significant risk factor [Visone and Croce (2009) and references therein]

Cancer type	Upregulated miRNAs	Downregulated miRNAs
Hepatocellular carcinoma	10b, 18, 20, 21, 221, 222, 224	122, 145, 150, 199a, 199b, 200b, 214, 223
Esophageal cancer	25, 151, 424	29c, 99, 100, 140, 202, 203, 205
Colon cancer	20a, 21, 92, 106a, 203, 223	
Breast cancer	21, 155	10b, 125b, 145

HMGA2 oncogene in various tumors. In this case, chromosomal translocation eliminates the target sequence for miRNA let-7 from the 3′ UTR of the HMGA2 transcript, resulting in overexpression of HMGA2 (Mayr et al. 2007).

miRNA expression profiles for an array of cancers have been determined in recent years using microarrays. These profiles are providing important insights into the roles of miRNAs in cancer as well as their diagnostic and prognostic utility. A number of miRNAs are frequently dysregulated in many types of cancer (e.g., miR-21) while others are more specifically associated with certain cancers. In the case of some miRNAs, the degree to which their expression is altered is correlated with clinical or pathologic indicators of malignancy while others may be dysregulated in both malignant and premalignant cells, offering opportunities for early detection and insights into early pathogenesis (Calin and Croce 2006). miRNAs that are frequently up- or downregulated in cancers for which alcohol is a known risk factor are shown in Table 5.1.

HCC is of particular relevance to alcohol and has been the subject of several miRNA profiling studies. Murakami et al. (2006) identified three miRNAs that were overexpressed in HCC (miR-224, miR-18, and pre-miR-18) and five others that were underexpressed (miR-199a, miR-199a*, miR-200a, miR-125a, and miR-195) and furthermore demonstrated the effectiveness of a signature based on these miRNA in distinguishing HCC and non-HCC cases. In addition, they identified three miRNAs (miR-92, miR-20, and miR-18) whose expression was inversely correlated with the degree of HCC differentiation. In another study, Ladeiro et al. (2008) corroborated some of these findings and, furthermore, defined miRNA alterations that could be used to differentiate HCC (increased miR-21, miR-10b, and miR-222) and benign hepatocellular adenomas (decreased miR-200c and miR-203). Importantly, this study also revealed specific miRNA markers of alcohol-related HCC (decreased miR-126*) and HCC associated with hepatitis B viral exposure (increased miR-96).

Effect of Ethanol on miRNA Expression and Function

Given the breadth of processes that miRNAs are known to regulate, it seems likely that they will play important roles in alcohol-related pathologies, including cancer. Aside from the report by Ladeiro et al. (2008) discussed above, the role of miRNAs in alcohol-associated cancer remains largely unstudied. However, several recent investigations have identified miRNAs that are dysregulated in various models of

Table 5.2 miRNAs dysregulated as a result of alcohol exposure

Tissue	Upregulated miRNAs[a]	Downregulated miRNAs[a]	References
Alcoholic fatty liver (mouse)	320, 486, 705, 1224	27b, 182, 183, 199a-3p, 200a, 214, 322	Dolganiuc et al. (2009)
Fetal brain (mouse)	9, 10a, 10b, 30a-3p, 145, 152	29c, 30e-5p, 154, 200a, 296, 339, 362, 496	Wang et al. (2009)
Cultured fetal cerebral cortical neuroepithelial cells (mouse)	**None identified**	9, 21, 153, 335	Sathyan et al. (2007)
Supraoptic nucleus and striatal neurons (rat)	9	n/a	Pietrzykowski et al. (2008)
Caco-2 cells[b] and colon biopsies from ALD[c] patients (human)	212	n/a	Tang et al. (2008)

[a] *Underlined* miRNAs are similarly dysregulated in various cancers (Garzon et al. 2009; Ma and Weinberg 2008; Visone and Croce 2009)

[b] Human epithelial colorectal adenocarcinoma cell line

[c] Alcoholic liver disease

other alcohol-induced disorders (Table 5.2; reviewed in Miranda et al. 2010). These include two large-scale miRNA screens in animal models of alcoholic fatty liver (Dolganiuc et al. 2009) and fetal alcohol-exposed brains (Wang et al. 2009). In both studies, roughly 2–3% of the miRNAs evaluated were found to be significantly altered by ethanol; however, the collections of dysregulated miRNAs identified were largely nonoverlapping. Additional studies have implicated specific miRNAs in the mechanisms underlying alcohol tolerance (Pietrzykowski et al. 2008) and other pathological effects of alcohol, including gut leakiness (Tang et al. 2008) and aberrant proliferation and differentiation of neural stem cells (Sathyan et al. 2007). These early studies indicate that alcohol alters the abundances of a relatively small fraction of all miRNAs and that the specific miRNAs that are dysregulated depend on the tissue examined and undoubtedly a host of other factors. While several of the miRNAs identified in these alcohol studies (underlined in Table 5.2) have been found to be similarly dysregulated in various cancers, establishing a role for these and other miRNAs in alcohol-induced cancer will require examination of appropriate models of cancer or further analyses of well-documented clinical specimens.

How ethanol exposure might trigger alterations in miRNA levels, including those that influence cancer initiation and progression, remains to be determined. As depicted in Fig. 5.6, evidence presented in this chapter suggests that alcohol might influence miRNA expression as a result of its ability to alter patterns of DNA methylation and histone modification. In support of this possibility, several studies have identified tumor-suppressive miRNA genes that are silenced in certain cancers by CpG island hypermethylation and histone hypoacetylation (Huang et al. 2009; Toyota et al. 2008). Alternatively, dysregulation of miRNA levels by alcohol might reflect altered activation of transcription factors involved in miRNA gene expression (Fig. 5.6). In this regard, alcohol is known to alter the function of diverse signaling pathways with well-established roles in the regulation of gene expression, including those involving JAK kinases and STAT transcription factors (Weng et al. 2008), insulin and insulin-like growth factor receptors (Cohen et al. 2007; He et al. 2007), and multiple mitogen- and stress-activated protein kinases, including ERK1/2, p38, and JNK1/2 (Aroor et al. 2010).

Given (1) the potential of alcohol to dysregulate gene expression through the alteration of signal transduction mechanisms and DNA and histone modification systems, (2) the recent studies directly demonstrating the capacity of alcohol to change expression patterns of collections of miRNAs in a variety of tissues, and (3) the widespread involvement of miRNAs in known cancer pathways, it seems likely that alcohol-mediated perturbations of miRNAs will contribute to the genesis of alcohol-related cancers.

Future Directions

That the pathogenesis of alcohol-related cancers may involve alteration of epigenetic modification represents an exciting area for future alcohol research. Both genetic and epigenetic mechanisms are crucially important for susceptibility, initiation, progression, and pathogenesis of alcohol-induced organ damage. A better understanding of effects of alcohol on epigenetic regulation will complement information from genetic, genomic, and functional genomic studies. The information can also be integrated with other experimental and clinical measurements to identify complex system-level responses to alcohol. Together, they will improve our understanding of alcohol-related cancers and provide new prognostic, diagnostic, and therapeutic avenues. Epigenetic modifications are potentially reversible and more amenable to therapeutic interventions. For example, inhibition of DNMTs has been shown to reactivate the silenced tumor-suppressor genes (e.g., p16 and MLH1) and suppress tumor growth with little effects on normal cells in cultured cells or xenograft models (Ganesan et al. 2009). Two nucleoside analogue drugs that can inhibit DNMTs (5-azacytidine and 5-aza-2′-deoxycytidine) have been approved by FDA to treat certain hematological malignancies (Ganesan et al. 2009). The sites of epigenetic regulation could be ideal targets for the development of novel pharmacologic interventions if proven to be critically involved in the pathogenesis of alcohol-related cancers.

References

Ambros V (2003) MicroRNA pathways in flies and worms: growth, death, fat, stress, and timing. Cell 113:673–6.

Aroor AR, James TT, Jackson DE, Shukla SD (2010) Differential changes in MAP kinases, histone modifications, and liver injury in rats acutely treated with ethanol. Alcohol Clin Exp Res 34:1543–51.

Bartolomei MS (2009) Genomic imprinting: employing and avoiding epigenetic processes. Genes Dev 23:2124–33.

Bhaumik SR, Smith E, Shilatifard A (2007) Covalent modifications of histones during development and disease pathogenesis. Nat Struct Mol Biol 14:1008–16.

Biermann T, Reulbach U, Lenz B, Frieling H, Muschler M, Hillemacher T, Kornhuber J, Bleich S (2009) N-methyl-D-aspartate 2b receptor subtype (NR2B) promoter methylation in patients during alcohol withdrawal. J Neural Transm 116:615–22.

Bingham S (2006) The fibre-folate debate in colo-rectal cancer. Proc Nutr Soc 65:19–23.

Bjornsson HT, Brown LJ, Fallin MD, Rongione MA, Bibikova M, Wickham E, Fan JB, Feinberg AP (2007) Epigenetic specificity of loss of imprinting of the IGF2 gene in Wilms tumors. J Natl Cancer Inst 99:1270–3.

Bleich S, Hillemacher T (2009) Homocysteine, alcoholism and its molecular networks. Pharmacopsychiatry 42:S102–9.

Bleich S, Lenz B, Ziegenbein M, Beutler S, Frieling H, Kornhuber J, Bonsch D (2006) Epigenetic DNA hypermethylation of the HERP gene promoter induces down-regulation of its mRNA expression in patients with alcohol dependence. Alcohol Clin Exp Res 30:587–91.

Boffetta P, Hashibe M, Vecchia CL, Zatonski W, Rehm J (2006) The burden of cancer attributable to alcohol drinking. Int J Cancer 119:884–7.

Bonsch D, Lenz B, Fiszer R, Frieling H, Kornhuber J, Bleich S (2006) Lowered DNA methyltransferase (DNMT-3b) mRNA expression is associated with genomic DNA hypermethylation in patients with chronic alcoholism. J Neural Transm 113:1299–304.

Bonsch D, Lenz B, Kornhuber J, Bleich S (2005) DNA hypermethylation of the alpha synuclein promoter in patients with alcoholism. Neuroreport 16:167–70.

Bonsch D, Lenz B, Reulbach U, Kornhuber J, Bleich S (2004) Homocysteine associated genomic DNA hypermethylation in patients with chronic alcoholism. J Neural Transm 111:1611–6.

Cai J, Mao Z, Hwang JJ, Lu SC (1998) Differential expression of methionine adenosyltransferase genes influences the rate of growth of human hepatocellular carcinoma cells. Cancer Res 58:1444–50.

Calin GA, Croce CM (2006) MicroRNA-cancer connection: the beginning of a new tale. Cancer Res 66:7390–4.

Choudhury M, Shukla SD (2008) Surrogate alcohols and their metabolites modify histone H3 acetylation: involvement of histone acetyl transferase and histone deacetylase. Alcohol Clin Exp Res 32:829–39.

Cohen AC, Tong M, Wands JR, de la Monte SM (2007) Insulin and insulin-like growth factor resistance with neurodegeneration in an adult chronic ethanol exposure model. Alcohol Clin Exp Res 31:1558–73.

Cravo M, Pinto R, Fidalgo P, Chaves P, Gloria L, Nobre-Leitao C, Costa Mira F (1996) Global DNA hypomethylation occurs in the early stages of intestinal type gastric carcinoma. Gut 39:434–8.

Crott JW, Liu Z, Keyes MK, Choi SW, Jang H, Moyer MP, Mason JB (2008) Moderate folate depletion modulates the expression of selected genes involved in cell cycle, intracellular signaling and folate uptake in human colonic epithelial cell lines. J Nutr Biochem 19:328–35.

Cui H, Cruz-Correa M, Giardiello FM, Hutcheon DF, Kafonek DR, Brandenburg S, Wu Y, He X, Powe NR, Feinberg AP (2003) Loss of IGF2 imprinting: a potential marker of colorectal cancer risk. Science 299:1753–5.

Cvekl A, Mitton KP (2010) Epigenetic regulatory mechanisms in vertebrate eye development and disease. Heredity 105:135–51.

Dannenberg LO, Chen HJ, Tian H, Edenberg HJ (2006) Differential regulation of the alcohol dehydrogenase 1B (ADH1B) and ADH1C genes by DNA methylation and histone deacetylation. Alcohol Clin Exp Res 30:928–37.

Di Pietro G, Magno LA, Rios-Santos F (2010) Glutathione S-transferases: an overview in cancer research. Expert Opin Drug Metab Toxicol 6:153–70.

Dolganiuc A, Petrasek J, Kodys K, Catalano D, Mandrekar P, Velayudham A, Szabo G (2009) MicroRNA expression profile in Lieber-DeCarli diet-induced alcoholic and methionine choline deficient diet-induced nonalcoholic steatohepatitis models in mice. Alcohol Clin Exp Res 33:1704–10.

Edwards CA, Ferguson-Smith AC (2007) Mechanisms regulating imprinted genes in clusters. Curr Opin Cell Biol 19:281–9.

Feinberg AP (2007) An epigenetic approach to cancer etiology. Cancer J 13:70–4.

Feinberg AP, Ohlsson R, Henikoff S (2006) The epigenetic progenitor origin of human cancer. Nat Rev Genet 7:21–33.

Fraga MF, Ballestar E, Paz MF, Ropero S, Setien F, Ballestar ML, Heine-Suñer D, Cigudosa JC, Urioste M, Benitez J, Boix-Chornet M, Sanchez-Aguilera A, Ling C, Carlsson E, Poulsen P, Vaag A, Stephan Z, Spector TD, Wu YZ, Plass C, Esteller M (2005a) Epigenetic differences arise during the lifetime of monozygotic twins. Proc Natl Acad Sci USA 102:10604–9.

Fraga MF, Ballestar E, Villar-Garea A, Boix-Chornet M, Espada J, Schotta G, Bonaldi T, Haydon C, Ropero S, Petrie K, Iyer NG, Pérez-Rosado A, Calvo E, Lopez JA, Cano A, Calasanz MJ, Colomer D, Piris MA, Ahn N, Imhof A, Caldas C, Jenuwein T, Esteller M (2005b) Loss of acetylation at Lys16 and trimethylation at Lys20 of histone H4 is a common hallmark of human cancer. Nat Genet 37:391–400.

Ganesan A, Nolan L, Crabb SJ, Packham G (2009) Epigenetic therapy: histone acetylation, DNA methylation and anti-cancer drug discovery. Curr Cancer Drug Targets 9:963–81.

Garzon R, Calin GA, Croce CM (2009) MicroRNAs in Cancer. Annu Rev Med 60:167–79.

Gonzalez S, Pisano DG, Serrano M (2008) Mechanistic principles of chromatin remodeling guided by siRNAs and miRNAs. Cell Cycle 7:2601–8.

Griffiths-Jones S, Saini HK, van Dongen S, Enright AJ (2008) miRBase: tools for microRNA genomics. Nucleic Acids Res 36:D154-8.

Halsted CH, Villanueva JA, Devlin AM, Niemelä O, Parkkila S, Garrow TA, Wallock LM, Shigenaga MK, Melnyk S, James SJ (2002) Folate deficiency disturbs hepatic methionine metabolism and promotes liver injury in the ethanol-fed micropig. Proc Natl Acad Sci USA 99:10072–7.

Hamid A, Wani NA, Kaur J (2009) New perspectives on folate transport in relation to alcoholism-induced folate malabsorption – association with epigenome stability and cancer development. FEBS J 276:2175–91.

He J, de la Monte S, Wands JR (2007) Acute ethanol exposure inhibits insulin signaling in the liver. Hepatology 46:1791–800.

Huang YW, Liu JC, Deatherage DE, Luo J, Mutch DG, Goodfellow PJ, Miller DS, Huang TH (2009) Epigenetic repression of microRNA-129-2 leads to overexpression of SOX4 oncogene in endometrial cancer. Cancer Res 69:9038–46.

Iacobuzio-Donahue CA (2009) Epigenetic Changes in Cancer. Annu Rev Pathol Mech Dis 4:229–49.

Jiang X, Tan J, Li J, Kivimäe S, Yang X, Zhuang L, Lee PL, Chan MT, Stanton LW, Liu ET, Cheyette BN, Yu Q (2008) DACT3 is an epigenetic regulator of Wnt/β-catenin signaling in colorectal cancer and is a therapeutic target of histone modifications. Cancer Cell 13:529–41.

Jones PA, Laird PW (1999) Cancer epigenetics comes of age. Nat Genet 21:163–7.

Kim DH, Saetrom P, Snøve O Jr, Rossi JJ (2008) MicroRNA-directed transcriptional gene silencing in mammalian cells. Proc Natl Acad Sci USA 105:16230–5.

Kim JS, Shukla SD (2006) Acute in vivo effect of ethanol (binge drinking) on histone H3 modifications in rat tissues. Alcohol Alcohol 41:126–32.

Kim JW, Dang CV (2006) Cancer's molecular sweet tooth and the Warburg effect. Cancer Res 66:8927–30.

Kouzarides T (2007) Chromatin modifications and their function. Cell 128:693–705.

Kristensen LS, Nielsen HM, Hansen LL (2009) Epigenetics and cancer treatment. Eur J Pharmacol 625:131–42.

Kumar MS, Lu J, Mercer KL, Golub TR, Jacks T (2007) Impaired microRNA processing enhances cellular transformation and tumorigenesis. Nat Genet 39:673–7.

Kumar MS, Pester RE, Chen CY, Lane K, Chin C, Lu J, Kirsch DG, Golub TR, Jacks T (2009) Dicer1 functions as a haploinsufficient tumor suppressor. Genes Dev 23:2700–4.

Ladeiro Y, Couchy G, Balabaud C, Bioulac-Sage P, Pelletier L, Rebouissou S, Zucman-Rossi J (2008) MicroRNA profiling in hepatocellular tumors is associated with clinical features and oncogene/tumor suppressor gene mutations. Hepatology 47:1955–63.

Lambertz I, Nittner D, Mestdagh P, Denecker G, Vandesompele J, Dyer MA, Marine JC (2010) Monoallelic but not biallelic loss of Dicer1 promotes tumorigenesis in vivo. Cell Death Differ 17:633–41.
Lane AA, Chabner BA (2009) Histone deacetylase inhibitors in cancer therapy. J Clin Oncol 27:5459–68.
Lee TD, Sadda MR, Mendler MH, Bottiglieri T, Kanel G, Mato JM, Lu SC (2004) Abnormal hepatic methionine and glutathione metabolism in patients with alcoholic hepatitis. Alcohol Clin Exp Res 28:173–81.
Lieber CS, Leo MA, Wang X, Decarli LM (2008) Effect of chronic alcohol consumption on Hepatic SIRT1 and PGC-1α in rats. Biochem Biophys Res Commun 370:44–8.
Lee YJ, Shukla SD (2007) Histone H3 phosphorylation at serine 10 and serine 28 is mediated by p38 MAPK in rat hepatocytes exposed to ethanol and acetaldehyde. Eur J Pharmacol 573:29–38.
Lieber CS (2000) Alcohol: its metabolism and interaction with nutrients. Annu Rev Nutr 20:395–430.
Liu Y, Balaraman Y, Wang G, Nephew KP, Zhou FC (2009) Alcohol exposure alters DNA methylation profiles in mouse embryos at early neurulation. Epigenetics 4:500–11.
Lu J, Getz G, Miska EA, Alvarez-Saavedra E, Lamb J, Peck D, Sweet-Cordero A, Ebert BL, Mak RH, Ferrando AA, Downing JR, Jacks T, Horvitz HR, Golub TR (2005) MicroRNA expression profiles classify human cancers. Nature 435:834–8.
Ma L, Weinberg RA (2008) Micromanagers of malignancy: role of microRNAs in regulating metastasis. Trends Genet 24:448–56.
Mato JM, Martínez-Chantar ML, Lu SC (2008) Methionine metabolism and liver disease. Annu Rev Nutr 28:273–93.
Mayr C, Hemann MT, Bartel DP (2007) Disrupting the pairing between let-7 and Hmga2 enhances oncogenic transformation. Science 315:1576–9.
Miranda RC, Pietrzykowski AZ, Tang Y, Sathyan P, Mayfield D, Keshavarzian A, Sampson W, Hereld D (2010) MicroRNAs: master regulators of ethanol abuse and toxicity? Alcohol Clin Exp Res 34:575–87.
Murakami Y, Yasuda T, Saigo K, Urashima T, Toyoda H, Okanoue T, Shimotohno K (2006) Comprehensive analysis of microRNA expression patterns in hepatocellular carcinoma and non-tumorous tissues. Oncogene 25:2537–45.
Nakahata Y, Kaluzova M, Grimaldi B, Sahar S, Hirayama J, Chen D, Guarente LP, Sassone-Corsi P (2008) The NAD^+-dependent deacetylase SIRT1 modulates CLOCK-mediated chromatin remodeling and circadian control. Cell 134:329–40.
Ouko LA, Shantikumar K, Knezovich J, Haycock P, Schnugh DJ, Ramsay M (2009) Effect of alcohol consumption on CpG methylation in the differentially methylated regions of H19 and IG-DMR in male gametes: implications for fetal alcohol spectrum disorders. Alcohol Clin Exp Res 33:1615–27.
Pal-Bhadra M, Bhadra U, Jackson DE, Mamatha L, Park PH, Shukla SD (2007) Distinct methylation patterns in histone H3 at Lys-4 and Lys-9 correlate with up- & down-regulation of genes by ethanol in hepatocytes. Life Sci 81:979–87.
Pietrzykowski AZ, Friesen RM, Martin GE, Puig SI, Nowak CL, Wynne PM, Siegelmann HT, Treistman SN (2008) Posttranscriptional regulation of BK channel splice variant stability by miR-9 underlies neuroadaptation to alcohol. Neuron 59:274–87.
Ravindran CRM, Ticku MK (2005) Methylation of NMDA receptor NR2B gene as a function of age in the mouse brain. Neuroscience Letters 380: 223–8.
Rawat AK (1968) Effects of ethanol infusion on the redox state and metabolite levels in rat liver in vivo. Eur J Biochem 6:585–92.
Sakatani T, Kaneda A, Iacobuzio-Donahue CA, Carter MG, de Boom Witzel S, Okano H, Ko MS, Ohlsson R, Longo DL, Feinberg AP (2005) Loss of imprinting of Igf2 alters intestinal maturation and tumorigenesis in mice. Science 307:1976–8.
Sandberg R, Neilson JR, Sarma A, Sharp PA, Burge CB (2008) Proliferating cells express mRNAs with shortened 3′ untranslated regions and fewer microRNA target sites. Science 320:1643–7.

Sathyan P, Golden HB, Miranda RC (2007) Competing interactions between micro-RNAs determine neural progenitor survival and proliferation after ethanol exposure: evidence from an ex vivo model of the fetal cerebral cortical neuroepithelium. J Neurosci 27:8546–57.

Seitz HK, Stickel F (2007) Molecular mechanisms of alcohol-mediated carcinogenesis. Nat Rev Cancer 7:599–612.

Sharma S, Kelly TK, Jones PA (2010) Epigenetics in cancer. Carcinogenesis 31:27–36.

Shin T, Kraemer D, Pryor J, Liu L, Rugila J, Howe L, Buck S, Murphy K, Lyons L, Westhusin M (2002) A cat cloned by nuclear transplantation. Nature 415:859.

Shukla SD, Velazquez J, French SW, Lu SC, Ticku MK, Zakhari S (2008) Emerging role of epigenetics in the actions of alcohol. Alcohol Clin Exp Res 32:1525–34.

Sotiropoulou G, Pampalakis G, Lianidou E, Mourelatos Z (2009) Emerging roles of microRNAs as molecular switches in the integrated circuit of the cancer cell. RNA 15:1443–61.

Strahl BD, Allis CD (2000) The language of covalent histone modifications. Nature 403:41–5.

Tang Y, Banan A, Forsyth CB, Fields JZ, Lau CK, Zhang LJ, Keshavarzian A (2008) Effect of alcohol on miR-212 expression in intestinal epithelial cells and its potential role in alcoholic liver disease. Alcohol Clin Exp Res 32:355–64.

Toyota M, Suzuki H, Sasaki Y, Maruyama R, Imai K, Shinomura Y, Tokino T (2008) Epigenetic silencing of microRNA-34b/c and B-cell translocation gene 4 is associated with CpG island methylation in colorectal cancer. Cancer Res 68:4123–32.

Van Engeland M, Weijenberg MP, Roemen GM, Brink M, de Bruine AP, Goldbohm RA, van den Brandt PA, Baylin SB, de Goeij AF, Herman JG (2003) Effects of dietary folate and alcohol intake on promoter methylation in sporadic colorectal cancer: the Netherlands cohort study on diet and cancer. Cancer Res 63:3133–7.

Varambally S, Dhanasekaran SM, Zhou M, Barrette TR, Kumar-Sinha C, Sanda MG, Ghosh D, Pienta KJ, Sewalt RG, Otte AP, Rubin MA, Chinnaiyan AM (2002) The polycomb group protein EZH2 is involved in progression of prostate cancer. Nature 419:624–9.

Visone R, Croce CM (2009) MiRNAs and cancer. Am J Pathol 174:1131–8.

Wang LL, Zhang Z, Li Q, Yang R, Pei X, Xu Y, Wang J, Zhou SF, Li Y (2009) Ethanol exposure induces differential microRNA and target gene expression and teratogenic effects which can be suppressed by folic acid supplementation. Hum Reprod 24:562–79.

Weksberg R, Shuman C, Caluseriu O, Smith AC, Fei YL, Nishikawa J, Stockley TL, Best L, Chitayat D, Olney A, Ives E, Schneider A, Bestor TH, Li M, Sadowski P, Squire J (2002) Discordant KCNQ1OT1 imprinting in sets of monozygotic twins discordant for Beckwith-Wiedemann syndrome. Hum Mol Genet 11:1317–25.

Weng YI, Aroor AR, Shukla SD (2008) Ethanol inhibition of Angiotensin II-stimulated Tyr(705) and Ser(727) STAT3 phosphorylation in cultured rat hepatocytes: Relevance to activation of p42/44 mitogen-activated protein kinase. Alcohol 42:397–406.

Yang H, Sadda MR, Li M, Zeng Y, Chen L, Bae W, Ou X, Runnegar MT, Mato JM, Lu SC (2004) S-Adenosylmethionine and its metabolite methylthioadenosine induce apoptosis in HepG2 cells: role of protein phosphatase 1 and Bcl-x(S). Hepatology 40:221–31.

Ying Y, Tao Q (2009) Epigenetic disruption of the WNT/beta-catenin signaling pathway in human cancers. Epigenetics 4:307–12.

Zapisek WF, Cronin GM, Lyn-Cook BD, Poirier LA (1992) The onset of oncogene hypomethylation in the livers of rats fed methyl-deficient, amino acid-defined diets. Carcinogenesis 13:1869–72.

Zhang T-Y, Meaney MJ (2010) Epigenetics and the Environmental Regulation of the Genome and Its Function. Annu Rev Psychol 61:439–66.

Zhong L, D'Urso A, Toiber D, Sebastian C, Henry RE, Vadysirisack DD, Guimaraes A, Marinelli B, Wikstrom JD, Nir T, Clish CB, Vaitheesvaran B, Iliopoulos O, Kurland I, Dor Y, Weissleder R, Shirihai OS, Ellisen LW, Espinosa JM, Mostoslavsky R (2010) The histone deacetylase Sirt6 regulates glucose homeostasis via Hif1α. Cell 140:280–93.

Chapter 6
Alcohol, Cancer Genes, and Signaling Pathways

William C. Dunty Jr.

Abbreviations

ADH	Alcohol dehydrogenase
ALD	Alcoholic liver disease
ALDH	Aldehyde dehydrogenase
bFGF	Basic fibroblast growth factor
CYP2E1	Cytochrome P450E1
Cdk	Cyclin-dependent kinase
CRC	Colorectal cancer
ECM	Extracellular matrix
EGF	Epidermal growth factor
EMT	Epithelial-to-mesenchymal transition
ErbB2	v-erb-b2 Erythroblastic leukemia viral oncogene homolog 2
ERK	Extracellular signal-regulated kinase
ESCC	Esophageal squamous cell carcinoma
HCC	Hepatocellular carcinoma
HNSCC	Head and neck squamous cell carcinoma
FAS	Fetal alcohol syndrome
HBV	Hepatitis B virus
HCV	Hepatitis C virus
Hh	Hedgehog
HPE	Holoprosencephaly
JNK	c-jun N-terminal kinase
MAPK	Mitogen-activated protein kinase
MDM2	Murine double minute

W.C. Dunty Jr. (✉)
Division of Metabolism and Health Effects, National Institute on Alcohol Abuse and Alcoholism, National Institutes of Health, Bethesda, MD, USA
e-mail: duntyw@mail.nih.gov

S. Zakhari et al. (eds.), *Alcohol and Cancer*, DOI 10.1007/978-1-4614-0040-0_6,
© Springer Science+Business Media LLC, 2011

MMPs	Matrix metalloproteinases
NADH	Reduced nicotinamide adenine dinucleotide
NF-κB	Nuclear factor kappa-light-chain-enhancer of activated B cells
NIK	Nuclear factor-inducing kinase
OPN	Osteopontin
PKC	Protein kinase C
PLCγ	Phospholipase C gamma
Ptc	Patched
PTEN	Phosphatase and tensin homolog
p53	Tumor protein 53
Rb	Retinoblastoma protein
SAPK	Stress-activated protein kinase
Shh	Sonic hedgehog
Smo	Smoothen
TGFβ	Transforming growth factor beta
TNFα	Tumor necrosis factor alpha
uPA	Urokinase-type plasminogen activator
VEGF	Vascular endothelial growth factor
4-HNE	4-Hydroxynonenal

Introduction

According to the International Agency for Research on Cancer (IARC), alcohol and its metabolite acetaldehyde, are considered to be Group 1 carcinogens, defined as an agent (or mixture) with sufficient evidence of carcinogenicity in humans (Baan et al. 2007; Secretan et al. 2009). Both animal and in vitro studies have shown that acetaldehyde is genotoxic, capable of forming stable DNA adducts that cause DNA damage that may lead to cancer (reviewed by Brooks and Theruvathu 2005; Seitz and Stickel 2007). Although acetaldehyde is known to damage DNA, only a handful of studies have attempted to classify, on a molecular basis, tumor suppressor genes and oncogenes affected by alcohol consumption. This undertaking is often complicated by an inability to accurately quantify alcohol consumption in the context of identifying these molecular changes or by the presence of confounding variables such as tobacco use and viral infection in combination with alcohol use.

Although cancer genes underlie oncogenesis (see Chap. 2), it is the dysregulation of associated signaling pathways that arise from their functional disruption that confers a cancer phenotype upon cells. This premise holds true for most cancer causing agents such as alcohol, where they influence, among other carcinogenic mechanisms, signal transduction events within the cell (Fig. 6.1).

This chapter focuses on (1) the molecular classification of alcohol-related cancers and how they may relate to acquired traits that all cancer cells possess and (2) alcohol-related alterations in specific signaling pathways of the cell, which may contribute to malignancy. Relevant findings in other areas of alcohol research are also discussed and extrapolated, as they may enlighten our understanding of alcohol-associated carcinogenesis.

Alcohol and Mitogenic Signals

MAPK Pathway

Growth signaling pathways are dysregulated in virtually every type of human cancer. The Ras/Raf/MEK/MAPK signaling cascade is perhaps the best-known mediator of mitogenic responses to extracellular growth factors (Fig. 6.1). Its relevance to carcinogenesis is evident by the observation that dysregulation of MAPK signaling occurs in approximately one third of all human cancers (Dhillon et al. 2007).

The MAPK signaling cascade also plays a central role in the deleterious health effects associated with chronic alcohol abuse (Fig. 6.1; reviewed by Aroor and Shukla 2004). The pathway comprises at least three parallel cascades, including the p42/44 MAPK (also known as the extracellular signal-regulated kinases 1 and 2; ERK1/2), the p38 MAP kinase, and c-jun N-terminal kinase or stress-activated protein kinases (JNK/SAPK) (reviewed by Pimienta and Pascual 2007). In the context of alcohol-related tissue injury, MAPK signaling has been implicated in the areas of alcoholic liver injury, neuronal toxicity, cardiovascular disease, and immunity (reviewed by Aroor and Shukla 2004). Modulation of this pathway by alcohol is distinctive and dependent on several variables including cell and tissue type, duration of alcohol exposure, presence or absence of growth factors, and use of normal versus transformed cells (reviewed by Aroor and Shukla 2004). In the context of cancer, alcohol administered at physiologically relevant concentrations stimulates cell growth of the MCF-7 human breast cancer line in a MAPK-dependent manner (Izevbigie et al. 2002). Given the importance of the MAPK pathways in both malignancies (reviewed by Dhillon et al. 2007; Wagner and Nebreda 2009) and alcohol-induced tissue injuries, their potential involvement in alcohol-induced tumorigenesis requires further investigation.

RAS

A key component to MAPK signaling pathway is the oncogene *Ras* (Fig. 6.1), a member of a large superfamily of small GTPases, which function as molecular switches in signaling pathways involved in proliferation and survival (reviewed by Mitin et al. 2005). The three human *RAS* genes encode highly related proteins, designated H-Ras, N-Ras, and K-Ras. Activating mutations among these family members have been reported in a wide variety of human cancers (reviewed by Karnoub and Weinberg 2008).

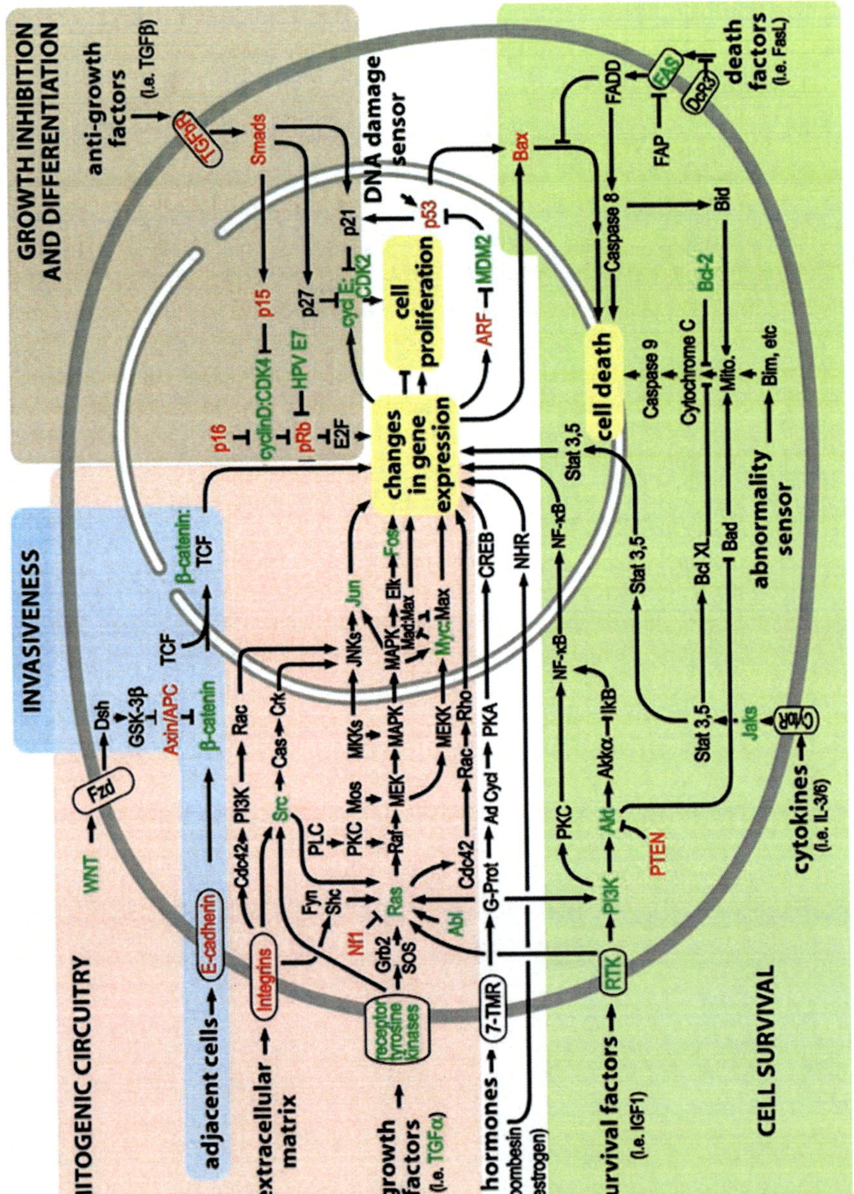
GROWTH INHIBITION AND DIFFERENTIATION
anti-growth factors
(i.e. TGFβ)
INVASIVENESS
MITOGENIC CIRCUITRY
adjacent cells
extracellular matrix
growth factors
(i.e. TGFα)
hormones
(i.e. bombesin estrogen)
survival factors
(i.e. IGF1)
CELL SURVIVAL
cytokines
(i.e. IL-3/6)
death factors
(i.e. FasL)
DNA damage sensor
abnormality sensor
changes in gene expression
cell proliferation
cell death
E-cadherin
Integrins
receptor tyrosine kinases
7-TMR
RTK
WNT
Fzd
Dsh
GSK-3β
Axin/APC
β-catenin
β-catenin: TCF
TCF
p16
cyclinD:CDK4
p15
pRb
HPV E7
E2F
p27
cycl E: CDK2
p21
p53
MDM2
ARF
Smads
TGFβR
Bax
FADD
FAS
DcR3
FAP
Bid
Caspase 8
Caspase 9
Cytochrome C
Bcl-2
Bcl XL
Bad
Mito.
Bim, etc
Stat 3,5
Jaks
CytoR
NF-κB
IkB
PKC
Akt
PI3K
PTEN
Ras
Raf
MEK
MAPK
MKKs
JNKs
Jun
Fos
Elk
Mad:Max
Myc:Max
MEKK
Rac
Rho
Cdc42
PKA
Ad Cycl
G-Prot
CREB
NHR
Abl
Nf1
Grb2
SOS
Fyn
Shc
Src
Cas
Crk
PLC
Mos

Fig. 6.1 The signal transduction circuitry of the mammalian cell. This diagram depicts only a subset of proteins that play critical roles in modulating the flow of signals through the various circuits operating within human cells. As delineated here by the various shadings, distinct subcircuits are responsible for regulating various cellular and biological responses. In addition to the mitogenic signaling circuit (*pink*) centered around Ras and coupled to a variety of extracellular inputs, other subcircuits mediate antigrowth and differentiation signals (*light brown*) or transmit cues to live or die by apoptosis (*light green*). Note that the circuit governing cancer cell invasiveness (*light blue)* overlaps with that of mitogenesis (*pink*), as a common set of proteins mediate both cellular processes. As for the genetic reprogramming of this circuitry in cancer cells, some of the proteins encoded by oncogenes (*green text*) and tumor suppressor genes (*red text*) known to be functionally altered are also indicated. Adapted from The Biology of Cancer © 2007 by R.A. Weinberg Garland Science/Taylor and Francis LLC and from *Cell,*100, Hanahan D, and Weinberg RA, *The Hallmarks of Cancer*, p. 57–70, (2000), with permission from Elsevier

Activating mutations have been seen preferentially in *K-Ras* following alcohol exposure. In pancreatic cancer, the frequency of *K-Ras* mutation is strongly associated with the patient's history of alcohol consumption (Malats et al. 1997). The risk of a somatic base-pair substitution within codon 12 of *K-Ras*, which renders the protein constitutively active, is 16 times higher in alcohol drinkers (>30 g per day) than non-drinkers who do not smoke [odds ratio (OR) = 16.00; $p < 0.024$] (Malats et al. 1997). **Similar findings have also been reported for esophageal cancer with a sevenfold** increased risk (OR = 7.22; $p < 0.001$) associated with alcohol use (Lyronis et al. 2008).

Estrogen Signaling

A strong association exists between circulating estrogen levels and the risk of breast cancer. Direct evidence for this causal relationship comes from observations that women with higher endogenous estrogen levels or postmenopausal women undergoing hormone replacement therapy (HRT) have an increased risk for the disease (reviewed by Key et al. 2001; Travis and Key 2003). In terms of alcohol use, both epidemiological and experimental evidence implicate enhanced estrogen signaling in alcohol-associated cancers of the breast. Meta-analyses of epidemiologic data demonstrate a dose-dependent increase for the risk of breast cancer associated with chronic alcohol consumption in both premenopausal and postmenopausal women (Longnecker 1994; Hamajima et al. 2002; Key et al. 2006; Allen et al. 2009; see Chap. 3). Some reports have suggested that effects of alcohol consumption on breast cancer risk may be greater in postmenopausal women who use hormone replacement therapy compared with nonusers (reviewed by Singletary and Gapstur 2001), though recent meta-analyses challenge this notion (Hamajima et al. 2002; Allen et al. 2009). In addition, studies have demonstrated a relationship between alcohol and breast cancer risk that varies by breast cancer subtype, with risks perhaps more pronounced for hormone (estrogen and progesterone) receptor-positive tumors (Suzuki et al. 2008; Li et al. 2010).

Estrogens are steroid compounds that function as potent promoters of cell proliferation in both normal and neoplastic breast epithelium (reviewed by Travis and Key 2003). Oxidative metabolites of estrogen may also directly damage DNA and thus contribute to the initiation processes of breast cancer (reviewed by Muti et al. 2006; Yager and Davidson 2006). Cellular effects of estrogen are mediated via binding to both intracellular and membrane-localized estrogen receptors (ER) (reviewed by Yager and Davidson 2006). Signal transduction pathways downstream of ligand binding consist of the following (Fig. 6.2): (1) a classical or "genomic" mechanism involving binding of estrogen to nuclear ER alpha (α) or beta (β), which then dimerize and bind to estrogen-response elements of DNA to regulate gene expression and (2) a nonclassical or "nongenomic" mechanism involving membrane-bound forms of ERs and the rapid activation of various protein kinases, such as MAPK, and secondary messengers, such as cyclic AMP (cAMP) (reviewed by Singh and Kumar 2005; Yager and Davidson 2006). Evidence of cross talk exists with pathways

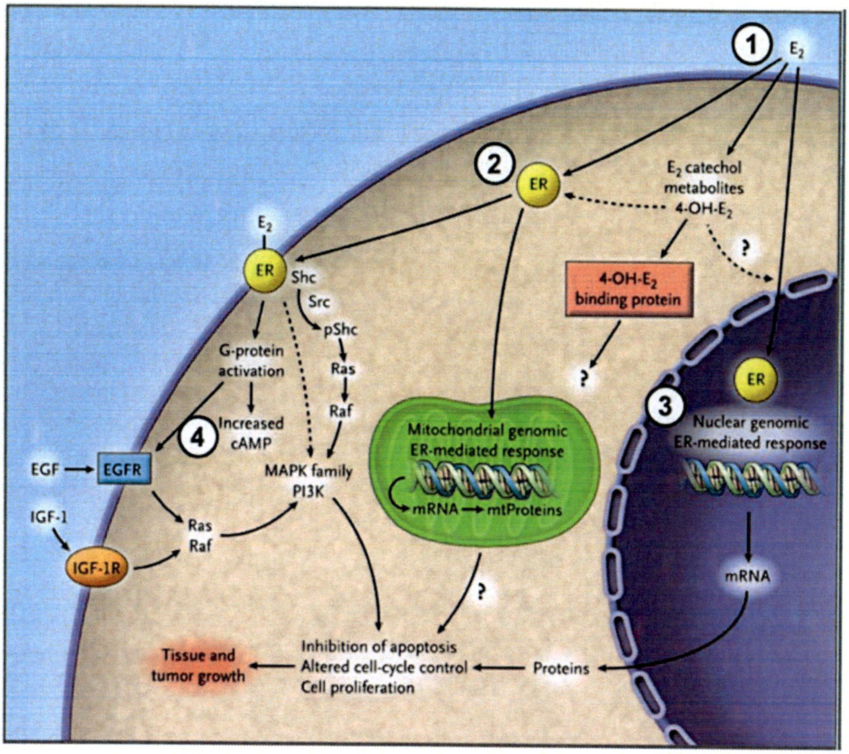

Fig. 6.2 Receptor-mediated estrogen-signaling pathways. A schematic representation of genomic and nongenomic mechanisms of estrogens signaling. Multiple levels at which alcohol has been reported to enhance estrogen signaling are denoted (*numbering*). See text for details. The abbreviation *cAMP* denotes cyclic AMP, *E2* estradiol, *4-OH-E2* 4-hydroxyestradiol, *ER* estrogen receptor, *EGF* epidermal growth factor, *EGFR* epidermal growth factor receptor, *IGF-1* insulin-like growth factor 1, *IGF-1R* insulin-like growth factor 1 receptor, *MAPK* mitogen-activated protein kinase, *mRNA* messenger RNA, *MPI3K* phosphoinositide 3 kinase, *mtProteins* mitochondrial proteins, and *pShc* phosphorylated Shc protein. Adapted from *N Engl J Med*, Estrogen Carcinogenesis in Breast Cancer, Yager JD, Davidson NE. Copyright © 2006 Massachusetts Medical Society. All rights reserved

downstream of other receptor tyrosine kinases (Fig. 6.2), complicating the means by which estrogen signaling controls proliferative and apoptotic processes within a cell.

On a mechanistic level, alcohol influences estrogen signaling at multiple points (Fig. 6.2; reviewed by Singletary and Gapstur 2001; Dumitrescu and Shields 2005). Alcohol consumption increases the level of circulating estrogens in both pre- and postmenopausal women (reviewed by Gill 2000; Singletary and Gapstur 2001), a proposed mechanism by which women may enhance their risk of breast cancer (Reichman et al. 1993; Ginsburg et al. 1996; Dorgan et al. 2001; Rinaldi et al. 2006). Levels of *aromatase*, a key enzyme responsible for the biosynthesis of estrogen, are altered by alcohol exposure in MCF-7 breast cancer cell (Etique et al. 2004a, b); consistent with the idea that ligand production may be enhanced by alcohol intake.

Moreover, alcohol may stimulate the proliferation of breast tumors by modulating levels of nuclear receptors for estrogen (Fan et al. 2000; Singletary et al. 2001; Etique et al. 2004a, b). Singletary and colleagues (2001) have shown that alcohol selectively **stimulates proliferation of ER+ but not ER– cultured human breast cancer cells** in vitro, an effect associated with elevated levels of ERα. Others have demonstrated a dose-dependent increase in the expression and transcriptional activity of ERα in MCF-7 breast cancer cells following alcohol treatment (Fan et al. 2000). Interestingly, alcohol downregulates the tumor suppressor protein BRCA1 while reversing the BRCA1-mediated inhibition of ERα activity (Fan et al. 2000), an additional putative mechanism by which alcohol intake may contribute to breast cancer development. Within the nucleus, alcohol treatment stimulates the transcription of estrogen responsive genes in MCF-7 cells, a ligand-independent, ERα mediated-event involving the cyclic AMP/protein kinase A (PKA) signaling pathway (Etique et al. 2007). Collectively, these data suggest that alcohol may stimulate estrogen signaling at multiple levels including both ligand-dependent and independent means (Fig. 6.2). Further investigation is warranted in understanding the cellular responses to enhanced estrogen signaling by alcohol, their contributions toward breast cancer development, and potential avenues of therapeutic interventions.

Alcohol and Insensitivity to Antigrowth Signals

Rb and Cell Cycle Control

To survive and replicate, cancer cells must avoid a variety of inhibitory mechanisms that protect normal tissues from excessive cell growth. In terms of cell cycle regulation, the hyperphosphorylation and inactivation of the Rb protein allows for E2F-mediated transcription of genes essential for DNA replication and progression into S phase.

Loss of Rb tumor suppressor activity has been linked to alcohol consumption. **Rb protein deficiency has been observed in ~20% of asymptomatic individuals at high risk for esophageal squamous cell carcinoma (ESCC) as defined by both alcohol consumption and cigarette smoking** (Contu et al. 2007). Loss of expression of *p16*^{INK4A} **is significantly correlated with a history of alcohol use** ($p=0.05$) in cases of head and neck squamous cell carcinoma (HNSCC; Ai et al. 2003). Absence of this Cdk inhibitor leads to inappropriate Rb phosphorylation and net loss of cell-cycle control (Fig. 6.1). In an independent study, Kraunz and colleagues (2006) revealed that duration of alcohol exposure, independent of intensity, predicts homozygous deletion of the *p16*^{INK4A} locus among long-term alcohol consumers (OR = 4.9).

Homozygous deletion or promoter methylation of the *p16*^{INK4A} locus have also been reported in almost 60% of hepatocellular carcinomas (HCC) associated with alcoholic liver cirrhosis (Table 6.1; Edamoto et al. 2003). Of importance, all 23 cases of HCCs associated with excessive alcohol consumption displayed at least one alteration in the Rb pathway (Table 6.1; e.g., *p16*^{INK4A} alteration, *p15*^{INK4B} promoter

Table 6.1 Alterations in the p53, RB1, and Wnt pathways in hepatocellular carcinomas

		RB1 pathway					p53 pathway				Wnt pathway
Etiology	No. of cases	*p16*[INK4A] alteration[a]	*p15*[INK4B] methylation	*RB1* alteration[b]	*Cyclin D1* **amplification**	At least one alteration	*p53* mutation	*p14*[ARF] alteration[a]	At least one alteration	Alterations in both RB1 and p53 pathways	β-catenin mutation
Hepatitis C	51	63%	20%[c]	25%	14%	82%	14%	6%	20%	20%	31%
Hepatitis B	26	54%	0%	38%	12%	69%	15%	27%	38%	35%	19%
Alcohol	*23*	*57%*	*26%*[d]	*44%*	*35%*	*100%*[e, f]	*13%*	*44%*[g]	*48%*[h]	*48%*[h]	*13%*
Total	100	59%	16%	33%	18%	83%	14%	20%	31%	30%	24%

[a]Homozygous deletion or promoter methylation
[b]Promoter methylation or loss of expression
[c]$p < 0.02$ HCV *versus* HBV
[d]$p < 0.01$ Alcohol *versus* HBV
[e]$p < 0.05$ Alcohol *versus* HCV
[f]$p < 0.005$ Alcohol *versus* HBV
[g]$p = 0.0002$ Alcohol *versus* HCV
[h]$p < 0.03$ Alcohol *versus* HCV. (Adapted from Edamoto et al. 2003)

methylation; *RB1* alteration, *cyclinD1* amplification). This effect was significantly more frequent than in HCCs associated with HBV or HCV infection ($p < 0.05$ and $p < 0.005$, respectively).

In addition to alterations in *Rb* and *p16*^{INK4A}, Edamoto and colleagues (2003) also reported that ~48% of all HCC examined carried at least one perturbation to the *p53* pathway (Table 6.1), a finding significantly more frequent than in HCCs associated with HCV status. Interestingly, alterations in both the *p53* and *Rb* pathways are very common, seen in almost half of all HCCs associated with alcohol consumption (Table 6.1). Concurrent loss of both tumor suppressor pathways is associated with malignant phenotypes in other cancers, such as astrocytomas (Ichimura et al. 2000) and oligodendrogliomas (Watanabe et al. 2001), and is linked to unfavorable prognosis in acute lymphoblastic leukemia and non-Hodgkins lymphoma (Gronbaek et al. 2000).

TGFβ Signaling

In cancer, the TGFβ-Smad signaling pathway is like the head of Janus. On one side, it is thought to exert antiproliferative effects as loss-of-function mutations to components of this pathway are common, particularly in human epithelial cancers. Tumor-suppressive activities of TGFβ have been attributed to its ability to induce apoptosis and regulate the cell cycle through transcriptional targets which inhibit cyclin–CDK complexes responsible for Rb phosphorylation (Fig. 6.3; reviewed by Jakowlew 2006; Massague 2008). On the other side, TGFβ also displays prooncogenic activity. This is particularly evident during the later stages of carcinogenesis as cancer cells have acquired mutations to downstream mediators of TGFβ's anti-growth effects (e.g., loss-of-function mutations to *p15*^{INK4B}, *p21*, or *Smad4*) and the role of TGFβ in tumor promotion becomes dominant (Fig. 6.3; reviewed by Jakowlew 2006; Massague 2008; Padua and Massague 2009). In fact, tumor cells often increase expression or production of TGFβ. Several studies have documented the protumorigenic role of TGFβ through its effects on the following: (1) local suppression of immune function, (2) promotion of angiogenesis, (3) production of autocrine mitogenic factors, and (4) induction of an epithelial-to-mesenchymal transition (EMT) (reviewed by Jakowlew 2006; Padua and Massague 2009; Tian and Schiemann 2009). The dichotomous nature of TGFβ signaling during carcinogenesis has been termed the "TGFβ paradox" (Tian and Schiemann 2009).

In alcoholic liver disease, TGFβ/Smad signaling represents a central mediator involved in multiple aspects of the injury response including inflammation, fibrogenesis, regeneration, and apoptosis (reviewed by Breitkopf et al. 2006; Meyer et al. 2010). Chronic alcohol consumption induces the production and release of TGFβ from Kupffer cells of the liver. A fibrogenic cytokine TGFβ causes subsequent activation and transdifferentation of hepatic stellate cells (HSC) into myofibroblasts, which deposit the extracellular matrix component collagen, a critical step in the development of liver fibrosis (reviewed by Wang et al. 2006; Meyer et al. 2010).

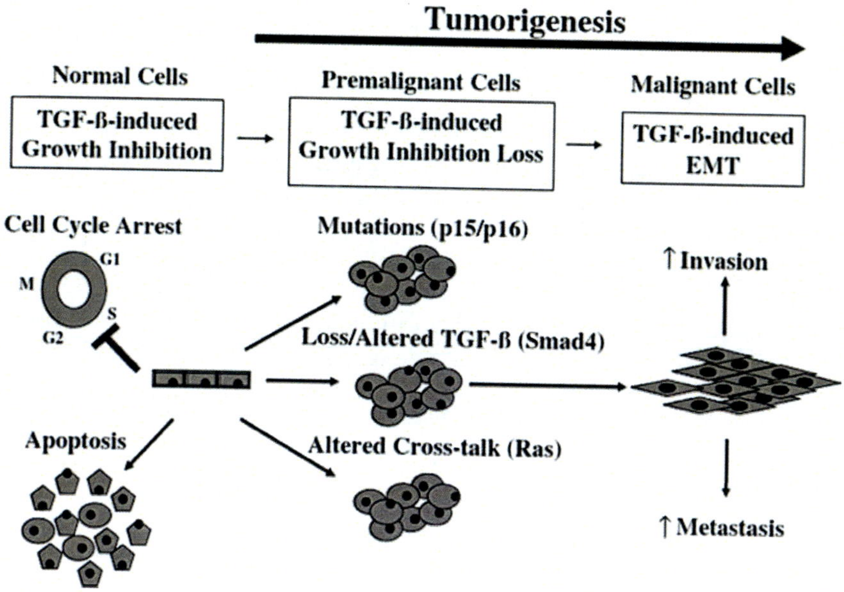

Fig. 6.3 TGFβ switches from being a tumor suppressor to a tumor promoter. In normal cells and those of early tumor stages, TGFβ inhibits tumor growth by inducing cell cycle arrest and apoptosis. As tumorigenesis advances and more mutations are acquired, the cells may become resistant to TGFβ-mediated growth inhibition. Eventually, these cells are incapable of eliciting inhibitory responses but remain able to respond to TGFβ with increased migration, invasion, and metastasis. With kind permission from Springer Science+Business Media: *Cancer Metastasis Rev*, Transforming growth factor-beta in cancer and metastasis, 25, 2006, 435–57, Jakowlew SB, Fig. 1

Alcohol also increases autocrine TGFβ expression in HSC. For hepatocytes which make up the bulk of the liver, TGFβ triggers apoptosis (Fig. 6.4), thereby providing physical space for HSC proliferation and ECM deposition. Ultimately, progressive fibrosis leads to scarring or cirrhosis of the liver, a condition that leads to HCC in a subset of individuals.

Hepatocytes that fail to succumb to cell death in response to TGFβ may undergo EMT, an important process involved at different stages of liver cancer progression (Fig. 6.4; reviewed by van Zijl et al. 2009a). The significance of EMT was initially recognized in the morphogenetic movements during embryogenesis, but more recently it has been recognized as an important mechanistic process for the progression and spread of epithelial cancers (reviewed by Thiery et al. 2009). TGFβ-mediated EMT of adult hepatocytes contributes to liver fibrogenesis (Zeisberg et al. 2007; Kaimori et al. 2007; Dooley et al. 2008), an early etiological event toward HCC development (Fig. 6.4). Van Zijl and colleagues (2009a) suggest that these nonmalignant hepatocytes may undergo phenotypic and functional changes to escape TGFβ-mediated apoptosis. Survival of hepatocyte-derived fibroblasts may result from EGF receptor and Src-mediated activation of PI3K/AKT pathways (Valdes et al. 2002; Murillo et al. 2005; Del Castillo et al. 2006) and dependent on

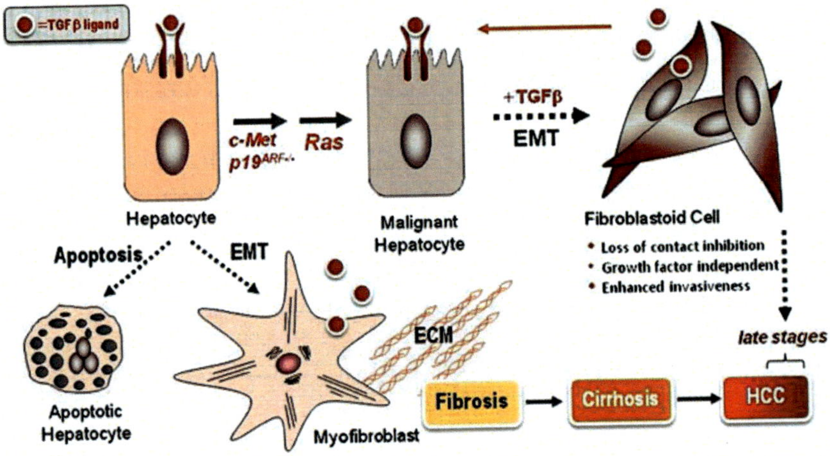

Fig. 6.4 The role of epithelial-to-mesenchymal transition (EMT) in hepatocellular carcinoma. Experimental evidence suggests that TGFβ-mediated EMT contributes to the progression of liver cancer at various time points. Hepatocytes that fail to succumb to cell death in response to TGFβ may undergo an EMT. These hepatocyte-derived myofibroblast-like cells contribute to liver fibrogenesis, an early etiological step toward hepatocellular carcinoma (HCC) development. After HCC has developed, malignant hepatocytes acquire invasive and metastatic abilities via TGFβ-mediated EMT. See text for details. *ECM* extracellular matrix

the transcriptional repressor *Snail1*(Franco et al. 2010; see Section "Discussion" below). Other groups have suggested that TGFβ-induced EMT endows hepatocytes with migratory and invasive properties during later stages of HCC progression (Fig. 6.4; reviewed by van Zijl et al. 2009a). Using immortalized c-Met hepatocytes, Gotzmann and colleagues (2002) demonstrated that TGFβ induces EMT in cooperation with oncogenic H-Ras, a transformation step leading to increased cellular invasiveness and malignancy. Subsequent studies of EMT in p19^{ARF} null hepatocytes implicated MAPK signaling in conferring tumor-promoting effects of TGFβ during later stages of liver tumorigenesis (Fischer et al. 2005). Establishment of autocrine and paracrine loops of TGFβ signaling underscore the importance of tumor–stroma cross talk between various cell types of the liver during HCC development (van Zijl et al. 2009b; Fig. 6.4). Overall, findings in both the alcohol as well as the cancer fields indicate that TGFβ-mediated EMT may be a key process in carcinoma aggressiveness and metastasis.

Alcohol and Apoptosis Evasion

Chronic alcohol consumption is associated with the induction of cell death in a variety of pathologies involving the developing brain and face (reviewed by Farber and Olney 2003; Sulik 2005; Ikonomidou 2009) and adult brain (Crews and Nixon 2009); in alcoholic myopathy (Fernandez-Sola et al. 2007); alcohol-induced liver disease (McVicker et al. 2007; Sastre et al. 2007) and pancreatitis (Gukovskaya et al. 2006). Alcohol-induced oxidative stress was shown to promote apoptosis leading to tissue damage that is in contrast to its role in carcinogenesis, where inhibiting cell death is a step toward malignancy. Despite this dichotomy, emerging evidence suggests that loss of apoptotic function does occur in alcohol-related cancers.

p53

The tumor suppressor protein *p53* not only inhibits cell proliferation following DNA damage but may lead to the transcriptional activation of apoptotic genes in case of irreparable DNA injury. p53 and its homologs p63 and p73 are members of a structurally related transcription factor family with unique biological functions during development and tumorigenesis (reviewed by Blandino and Dobbelstein 2004; Moll and Slade 2004). Inactivation of the p53 pathway is a crucial step in the acquisition of malignancy and occurs by a variety of means including the following: (1) mutations of the *p53* gene, (2) defects in regulators of p53 stability as seen in cases of *MDM2* amplification or loss of $p14^{ARF}$ function (e.g., Table 6.1), and (3) disruption of target genes that mediate the p53 response such as downstream components of the apoptotic machinery (reviewed by Vousden and Lu 2002).

As discussed in Chap. 4, ROS created during alcohol metabolism generate lipid peroxidation products such as 4-hydroxynonenal (4-HNE) among others (reviewed by Seitz and Stickel 2007). 4-HNE preferentially forms highly mutagenic DNA adducts at the third base of codon 249 for the human *p53* gene that is believed to be a unique mutational hotspot in HCC (Hu et al. 2002). Intriguingly, hepatocytes carrying the codon 249 mutation display stronger *p53* deficient phenotypes, such as increased resistance to apoptosis and a selective growth advantage, than hepatocytes with other *p53* alterations (Dumenco et al. 1995; Forrester et al. 1995).

Alcohol is a major etiological factor in the development of HCC, possibly contributing to the initiation, promotion, and progression of hepatocarcinogenesis (reviewed by Stickel et al. 2002; Morgan et al. 2004). Somatic mutations in *p53* have been clearly linked to HCC, with a frequency of mutation dependent on geographical location (reviewed by Hussain et al. 2007). Intriguingly, codon 249-specific mutations in *p53* (resulting in a G:C to T:A transversion) appear to be less common in other types of cancer and have been proposed as potential serum-derived biomarkers of liver cancer risk (Hussain et al. 2007).

Alcohol-associated mutations of *p53* may not be limited to liver cancer, although a direct association is hard to demonstrate as alcohol abuse is frequently associated with smoking (Blons and Laurent-Puig 2003). The prevalence of *p53* mutations in patients with invasive HNSCC is related to the level of exposure to cigarette smoke and to a lesser extent alcohol (Brennan et al. 1995). In this study, a higher incidence for *p53* mutations was observed in HNSCC tumors from patients who smoked cigarettes and used alcohol versus those who smoked but abstained from alcohol (58% vs. 33%, respectively; Brennan et al. 1995). Inadequate numbers of individuals who only drank and did not smoke precluded these investigators from evaluating the effect of alcohol consumption alone on *p53* in the absence of smoking. A separate study in a Taiwanese population found that alcohol drinkers exhibit a significantly higher incidence of *p53* mutations than nondrinkers, an effect that remains statistically significant after adjusting for tobacco use (Hsieh et al. 2001). For breast cancer, premenopausal women have an increased likelihood for *p53* mutations in association with alcohol consumption of 16 or more drinks per month (Freudenheim et al. 2004), although this relationship may not hold true for postmenopausal patients (Ali et al. 1999; Simao et al. 2002; Freudenheim et al. 2004).

PTEN

After *p53*, *PTEN* (phosphatase and tensin homolog deleted from chromosome 10) is one of the most commonly lost tumor suppressor genes in human malignancies (Salmena et al. 2008). PTEN is a nonredundant phosphoinositide phosphatase that is essential for inhibiting the highly oncogenic, prosurvival PI3K/AKT pathway (Fig. 6.1). Its phosphatase activity negatively regulates the intracellular levels of phosphatidylinositol-3,4,5 trisphosphate (PIP_3) and thus leads to the suppression of receptor tyrosine kinase or G protein-coupled receptor-mediated signaling in response to extracellular stimuli. Tumor-suppressive activities for PTEN impinge upon cellular processes essential to carcinogenesis including cell growth, survival, and proliferation (reviewed by Salmena et al. 2008; Chalhoub and Baker 2009). *PTEN* downregulation by siRNA enhances AKT prosurvival signaling and glucose uptake in response to insulin in 3T3-L1 adipocytes (Tang et al. 2005) and HepG2 hepatoma cells (Vinciguerra et al. 2008). Complete loss of PTEN function is generally associated with advanced cancers and metastases (Ali et al. 1999).

There is an emerging connection between PTEN and alcohol (reviewed by Vinciguerra and Foti 2008). Alcohol-induced liver injury has been associated with increased *PTEN* expression and function in hepatocytes from rats chronically fed alcohol (Yeon et al. 2003). Interestingly, exposure of HepG2 hepatoma cells to alcohol in culture also upregulates *PTEN* expression, subsequently sensitizing these cells to TNFα-induced cytotoxicity and cell death (Shulga et al. 2005). RNAi-mediated suppression of *PTEN* induction by alcohol rescues these cells by restoring TNFα-induced Akt and NF-κB activation, attenuating the p38 MAPK stress response, inhibiting caspase-3 activation, and preserving mitochondrial integrity and cell viability (Shulga et al. 2005). Acute alcohol exposure increases the association of PTEN with the PI3K regulatory (p85α) subunit, which results in attenuation of insulin-mediated survival signals through AKT (He et al. 2007). Thus, alcohol-mediated alterations of PTEN function are involved in the mechanism triggering alcohol-dependent hepatic insulin resistance and apoptosis (Fig. 6.5; Vinciguerra and Foti 2008).

Roles for PTEN in alcohol-related liver disease and malignancies are currently being investigated (Fig. 6.5). Several studies reported loss-of-function mutations, deletions, or diminished levels of PTEN protein in human HCC (reviewed by

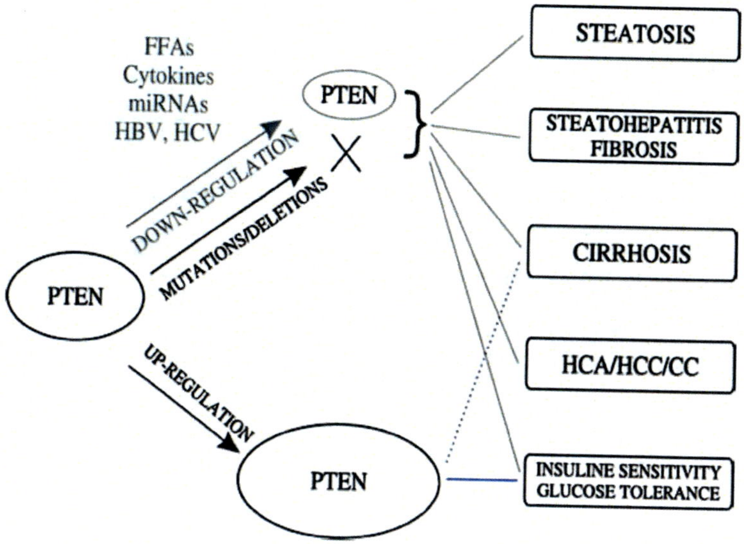

Fig. 6.5 Alcohol-induced PTEN alterations in the development and progression of a variety of liver disorders. The *dotted line* indicates a potential involvement of alcohol-induced PTEN upregulation in the development of liver cirrhosis. *FFA* free fatty acids, *miRNAs* microRNAs, *HBV/HCV* hepatitis B or C virus, *HCA* hepatocellular adenomas, *CC* cholangiocellular carcinomas, *HCC* hepatocellular carcinomas. Reprinted by permission from Mexico: Ediciones Medicina y Cultura: *Ann Hepatol*, PTEN at the crossroad of metabolic diseases and cancer in the liver, Vinciguerra M and Foti M (2008)

Vinciguerra and Foti 2008). Epigenetic silencing (Wang et al. 2007) and micro-RNA-mediated repression (Meng et al. 2007) of the PTEN locus may also contribute to hepatocarcinogenesis. Altered PTEN activity impinges on several hepatic and non-hepatic cellular processes crucial to cancer including apoptosis, cell cycle progression, EMT, cell–ECM interactions, cell–cell adhesion, chromosomal integrity, and DNA repair (reviewed by Vinciguerra and Foti 2008). Animal models have emphasized the importance of PTEN in liver carcinogenesis. Liver-specific knockout mice for *PTEN* (Horie et al. 2004; Stiles et al. 2004) display both hepatic steatosis (abnormal retention of lipids within the hepatocytes) and steatohepatitis (inflammation of the liver with concurrent fat accumulation), pathological conditions associated with alcoholic and nonalcoholic fatty liver diseases. Regardless of etiology, steatohepatitis may progress to cirrhosis of the liver and eventually lead to HCC. Indeed, all mice carrying hepatocyte-specific deletions of *PTEN* formed liver adenomas, with almost 70% of the animals eventually developing HCC (Horie et al. 2004). Together, data from both human and animal studies suggest that perturbations to PTEN's tumor suppressor activity represent a critical factor in hepatocarcinogenesis.

As PTEN is also known to function as a haploinsufficient tumor suppressor (reviewed by Salmena et al. 2008), it appears that enhanced, diminished and complete loss of PTEN activity are all important for the development and progression of several liver pathologies (Fig. 6.5; Vinciguerra and Foti 2008). Further research is needed to clarify the complexities of how alcohol-mediated regulation of PTEN contributes to the progression of ALD and cancer.

Alcohol and Tumor Angiogenesis

Few studies have examined the relationship between alcohol consumption and tumor angiogenesis. Cancer cells induce blood vessel growth by secreting various growth factors such as bFGF or VEGF. Recently, Tan and colleagues (2007) have shown that moderate alcohol consumption stimulates *VEGF* expression and subsequent tumor angiogenesis in a mouse tumor xenograft model. Alcohol consumption, equivalent to ~2 drinks per day in humans, by immunocompetent mice implanted with mouse melanoma cells causes a doubling of tumor volume, increased *VEGF* transcript and protein levels, and enhanced microvascular density (Tan et al. 2007). Consistent with these findings, epidemiological studies have linked alcohol consumption to increased risk of melanomas in humans (Freedman et al. 2003; Millen et al. 2004). Moreover, earlier studies utilizing a chick embryo chorioallantoic membrane model demonstrated that alcohol treatment at physiologically relevant levels (10–20 mM) increases intratumoral vascularity, *VEGF* expression, and intravasation of human fibrosarcoma cells (Gu et al. 2005). Similar findings were noted in a study investigating the cardiovascular-protective effects of moderate alcohol consumption in cultured vascular smooth muscles cells (Gu et al. 2001). Independent studies have also indicated that alcohol intake enhances angiogenesis in a rat model of choroidal neovascularization (Bora et al. 2006; Kaliappan et al. 2008). Recently, Morrow and colleagues (2008) have shown that alcohol enhances endothelial angiogenic activity in vitro through activation of a novel Notch/Angiopoietin-1 signaling pathway. Given the interplay between Notch and VEGF signaling during tumor angiogenesis (reviewed by Thurston and Kitajewski 2008), further investigation is needed to determine the potential involvement of this novel interaction in the etiology of alcohol-associated cancers. Altogether, these data suggest that alcohol-induced *VEGF* activity may represent an important mechanism of tumor progression associated with alcohol consumption.

Alcohol and Metastasis

Although uncontrolled cell proliferation allows cancer cells to amass, tissue invasion and metastasis are the traits that make many cancers lethal. To become metastatic, cancer cells must (1) deadhere from one another, usually accomplished via loss of adhesion molecules, (2) become migratory, (3) enter and survive transit in the circulatory system, (4) exit into new tissues, and (5) maintain growth and initiate angiogenesis at distant sites (reviewed by Chambers et al. 2002; Gupta and Massague 2006).

Recent evidence indicates that alcohol may stimulate cell-invasive and metastatic abilities by multiple mechanisms including disruption of epithelial adherens junctions, increases in cell motility, and degradation of the extracellular matrix (ECM).

Cell Adhesion and Motility

Cells in tissues are linked to one another and to the ECM by various types of cell junctions. *Adherens junctions* are areas of cell–cell adhesion comprised of transmembrane cadherin proteins and associated catenins proteins connected to the actin cytoskeleton. Cell–matrix interactions are mediated at *focal adhesions*, clusters of integrin receptors that bridge the actin cytoskeleton of the cell to the underlying ECM. Focal adhesions not only serves to provide the mechanical forces necessary for cell motility but functions as signaling centers influencing processes of cell proliferation, survival and motility. Disruptions to both types of cell junctions are implicated in cancer development.

Loss of E-cadherin. Few studies have examined alcohol's effects on cell–cell adhesion in the context of cancer. Meng and colleagues (2000) found that alcohol (40–80 mM) causes a dose-dependent loss of E-cadherin–catenins protein complexes, a phenomenon associated with enhanced migratory and invasive behaviors of MCF-7 breast cancer cells. Clinically, loss of E-cadherin-mediated adhesion is thought to contribute to the progression of many epithelial-derived malignancies including breast cancer (reviewed by Berx and Van Roy 2001; Cowin et al. 2005). Tumor-suppressive actions of E-cadherin may reside in the protein's ability to regulate Wnt pathway, modulate mitogenic signals, and influence epithelial cell polarity (reviewed by Jeanes et al. 2008). Interestingly, diminished expression of E-cadherin has been seen in patients with HCC (Shimoyama and Hirohashi 1991; Kozyraki et al. 1996; Endo et al. 2000), a phenomenon significantly associated with patient survival (Endo et al. 2000).

Induction of EMT. Loss of E-cadherin-mediated adhesion is an early event of the EMT, a biological program whereby epithelial cells deadhere from one another and become motile (Fig. 6.6; reviewed by Thiery 2002; Kang and Massague 2004; Thiery et al. 2009). EMT involves the simultaneous loss of epithelial markers and acquisition of mesenchymal markers, the net effect of which is a migratory phenotype (Fig. 6.6). Normally, the EMT program is used by cells of the early embryo during development and of the adult during processes such as wound healing. However, a growing body of evidence suggests that EMT is involved in the metastatic events of cancer (reviewed by Kang and Massague 2004; Thiery et al. 2009). Oncogenic pathways including Ras/MAPK, EGF, TGFβ, and Wnt/βcatenin signaling may induce EMT via activation of members of the Snail superfamily of transcriptional repressors (Fig. 6.6; reviewed by Kang and Massague 2004; Barrallo-Gimeno and Nieto 2005). Among their many targets, the *E-cadherin* locus is transcriptionally repressed by Snail proteins, an event leading to the loss of cell adhesion associated with EMT (reviewed by Thiery et al. 2009).

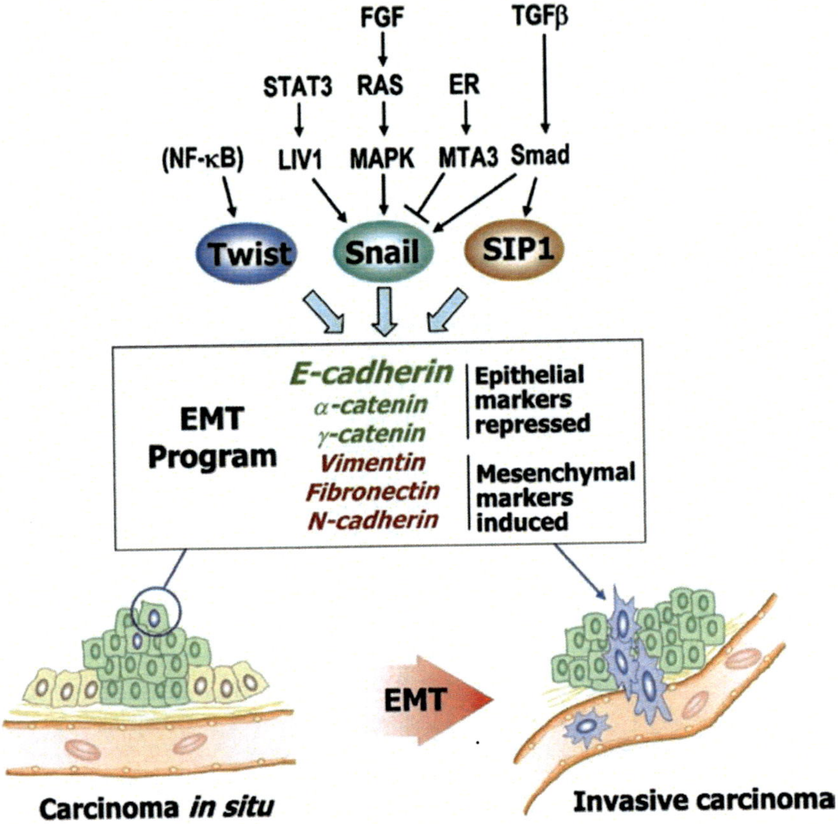

Fig. 6.6 Mediators of EMT. *Snail1* expression induces the loss of epithelial markers (e.g., E-cadherin) and the gain of mesenchymal markers (e.g., vimentin), which influence changes in cell shape and acquisition of motility and invasive properties. Reprinted from *Cell*, 118, Kang Y, Massague J, Epithelial-Mesenchymal Transitions: Twist in Development and Metastasis, 277–9, 2004, with permission from Elsevier

Recent findings suggest that alcohol may promote cancer by stimulating the EMT program in a *Snail1*-dependent manner. Alcohol-induced EMT events have been reported in keratinocytes (Chamulitrat et al. 2003) and breast epithelial cell lines (Robson et al. 2006), though mechanistic aspects were not experimentally addressed. Of particular importance, Forsyth and colleagues (2010) found that both colon and breast cancer cells exposed to alcohol upregulate signature EMT mesenchymal markers including vimentin and various matrix metalloproteinases (MMPs; Fig. 6.6). Alcohol's effects on EMT induction involved the expression, phosphorylation, and nuclear localization of *Snail1* (Forsyth et al. 2010). Moreover, alcohol-stimulated migration of cancer cells in vitro was dependent on EGFR and ERK1/2 signaling. Interestingly, *Snail1* RNA was found to be elevated in colonic mucosal biopsies from alcoholics (Forsyth et al. 2010). Forsyth and colleagues (2010) propose that alcohol-induced EMT mediated by Snail1 represents a novel mechanism for increased risk and progression of breast and colon cancers in alcoholics.

Although not experimentally addressed by these investigators, *Snail1* is a well-characterized target gene of the Wnt signaling pathway during both embryogenesis (Dale et al. 2006; Katoh 2006) and carcinogenesis (Yook et al. 2006; Dissanayake et al. 2007). The Wnt/βcatenin pathway influences numerous cellular processes during both embryo and cancer development through the transcriptional activation of target genes (reviewed by Reya and Clevers 2005). Emerging in vitro data indicate that Wnt-mediated effects on cell adhesion and migration contribute to cancer cell invasiveness (reviewed by Neth et al. 2007) and that these processes may be influenced by alcohol. Genetic and epigenetic alterations favoring constitutive activation of the Wnt pathway are seen in HCCs associated with alcohol-induced liver cirrhosis (Table 6.1; Edamoto et al. 2003) supporting a role for Wnt signaling in alcohol-related cancers. Epigenetic inactivation of *Sfrp1*, a secreted Wnt antagonist, has also been reported in HNSCC cases from both heavy and light alcohol drinkers, a phenomenon independent of tobacco use (Marsit et al. 2006). Further research should determine the importance of EMT and the role Wnt signaling may play in alcohol-related cancers.

L1CAM. Once believed to be a neuronal specific marker, the cell adhesion molecule L1CAM is now known to be upregulated in a variety of human malignancies including cancers of the breast, lung, brain, skin, kidney, ovary, and colon (reviewed by Raveh et al. 2009; Siesser and Maness 2009). L1CAM is among the transcriptional targets for Wnt/βcatenin signaling in colorectal cancer (CRC) cells (Gavert et al. 2005). Localization of L1CAM at the invasive front of human colorectal tumors along with the ADAM10, a metalloprotease that facilitates shedding of the L1CAM extracellular domain, is consistent with a role for L1CAM during advanced stages of tumorigenesis (Gavert et al. 2005; Raveh et al. 2009). Initial studies indicated that *L1CAM* and *ADAM10* co-expression confers enhanced motility (Gavert et al. 2005) and metastatic capacity of CRC cells to the liver (Gavert et al. 2007). Subsequent studies in glioma cells revealed an autocrine/paracrine stimulation of cell motility involving cleavage and release of the L1CAM extracellular domain (Yang et al. 2009). This proteolytic fragment then engages cell-surface integrins to stimulate motility in contrast to uncleaved cell surface forms of L1CAM, which would reduce the invasiveness due to adhesive interactions (Yang et al. 2009).

Phenotypic similarities between individuals with mutations in L1CAM responsible for the CRASH syndrome (corpus callosum hypoplasia, mental retardation, adducted thumbs, spastic paraplegia and hydrocephalus; reviewed by Fransen et al. 1995) and children with Fetal Alcohol Syndrome (FAS), imply that L1CAM may play a role in the etiology of both disorders. L1CAM was originally discovered as a critical regulator of neuronal migration, survival, and axon guidance (reviewed by Schmid and Maness 2008). Through a series of studies, Charness and colleagues have shown that (1) alcohol inhibits cell–cell adhesion mediated by human L1CAM and that such inhibition may contribute to the etiology of FAS (Ramanathan et al. 1996), (2) a number of primary-alcohols and small peptides that block alcohol-mediated inhibition of L1CAM also prevent alcohol-induced apoptosis and growth retardation during embryogenesis (Chen et al. 2001; Wilkemeyer et al. 2003; Zhou et al. 2004), and (3) alcohol-mediated disruption of L1CAM binding occurs within a specific pocket on the L1CAM molecule (Wilkemeyer et al. 2000; Arevalo et al. 2008). Similar finding of alcohol-mediated disruption of L1CAM function during CNS development have been reported by Bearer and her colleagues (reviewed by Bearer 2001).

Collectively, the data for L1CAM function in the nervous system and in cancer (reviewed by Schafer and Altevogt 2010) presents an intriguing question as to whether alcohol promotes tumorigenesis by altering L1CAM function as has been described in the case of FAS. Further experiments are needed to address the contribution of this mechanism to alcohol-related cancers, especially during the end stages of malignancies when a cell's metastatic ability is most fatal.

The Extracellular Matrix

The ECM provides structural support for cells. Components of the ECM such as various proteoglycans, glycoproteins, and fibrillar collagens serve as the molecular scaffold for cell adhesion and migration. During malignancy, the ECM not only provides physical barriers that tumor cells must circumvent but also may provide cues in the regulation of tumor dormancy versus metastatic growth (reviewed by Barkan et al. 2010) and in adhesion-mediated apoptosis (reviewed by Gilmore et al. 2009).

Matrix metalloproteinases. Alcohol effects on the ECM may promote metastasis. Several studies have suggested that matrix metalloproteinases (MMPs) are targets of alcohol (reviewed by Luo 2006). Secreted by cells, MMPs are zinc-dependent endopeptidases that degrade and remodel the ECM in association with various physiological and pathological processing including cancer metastasis (Fig. 6.7; reviewed by Deryugina and Quigley 2006). Initial work suggested that alcohol exposure increases the enzymatic activity of MMP-2 and/or MMP-9, but not their production in the lung and heart of rats (Lois et al. 1999; Partridge et al. 1999). Subsequent studies by Luo and colleagues (Aye et al. 2004) showed that physiologically relevant concentrations of alcohol (100–200 mg/dL) promote the conversion and release of biologically active forms of MMP-2 (59 and 62 kDa) from fibroblasts. Importantly, conditioned media from these alcohol-exposed fibroblasts significantly enhance the invasive potential of breast cancer cells and mammary epithelial cells overexpressing *ErbB2/HER2*, a member of the ErbB superfamily of receptor tyrosine kinases. This effect is dependent on MMP-2 activation mediated by protein kinase C (PKC) and JNK (Aye et al. 2004). A subsequent study by the same group revealed similar alcohol-induced activation of MMP-2 in breast cancer cells themselves, a phenomenon positively associated with ErbB2/HER2 status (Ke et al. 2006). In breast cancer, overexpression of the ErbB2 receptor is associated with increased disease recurrence and poor prognosis (reviewed by Jones and Buzdar 2009). Overexpression of *ErbB2* enhances the ability of alcohol to activate the JNK and p38 MAPK pathways during invasion of mammary-derived cells in vitro (Ma et al. 2003). Independent studies by Etique and colleagues (2006) revealed that alcohol

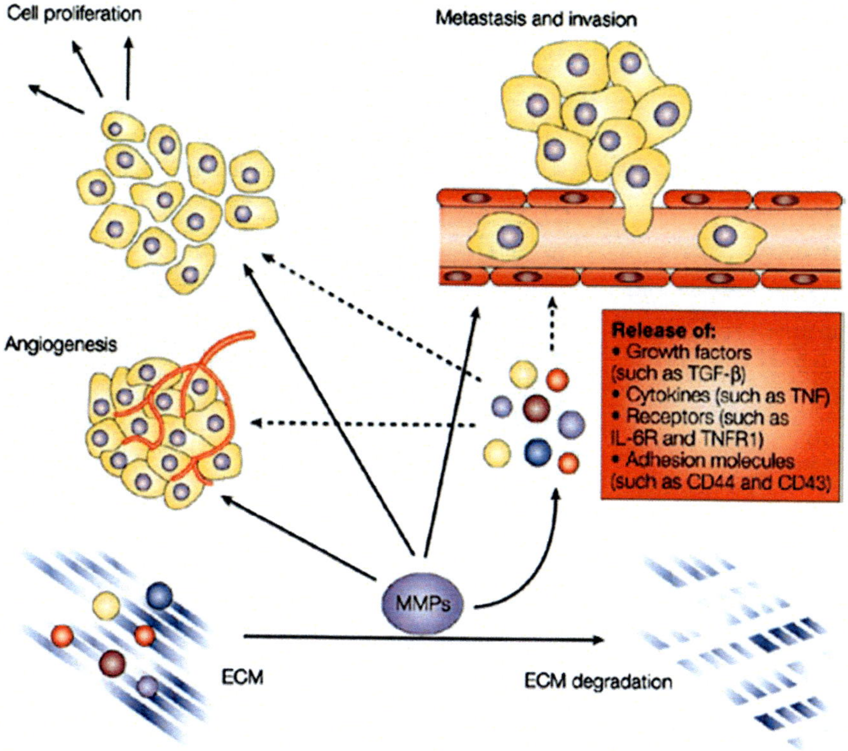

Fig. 6.7 MMPs promote tumorigenesis by several means. Matrix metalloproteinases (or MMPs) not only contribute to invasion and metastasis but also promote cancer cell proliferation by cleavage and release of various growth factors. MMPs increase the bioavailability of proangiogenic factors that promote tumor angiogenesis. Not pictured are MMPs' effects on apoptosis and immune suppression. Reprinted by permission from Macmillan Publishers Ltd: *Nat Rev Cancer*, Molecular mechanisms of glioma invasiveness: the role of proteases, Rao JS (2003)

stimulates the secretion of both MMP-2 and MMP-9 in the MCF-7 breast cancer cell line, although transcriptional activation of MMP-2 was observed, a discrepant finding with observations by the Luo group (Aye et al. 2004).

MMP-2 and MMP-9, or Gelatinase-A and -B respectively, are major contributors to the proteolytic degradation of ECM during tumor invasion (reviewed by Bjorklund and Koivunen 2005). Enhanced expression of MMP-2 and MMP-9 has been observed in cancers of the breast, lung, colon, skin, prostate, and ovary and has been positively associated with tumor progression (reviewed by Bjorklund and Koivunen 2005). Since MMPs not only regulate tissue invasion and intravasation but also are involved in several steps of cancer development including (1) promoting the growth of cancer cells, (2) regulating apoptosis, (3) promoting angiogenesis, (4) inhibiting the immune response to cancer cells, (5) contributing to the metastatic niche, and (6) regulating EMT (Fig. 6.7; reviewed by Egeblad and Werb 2002; Kessenbrock et al. 2010), more studies are warranted to understand the potential interaction of

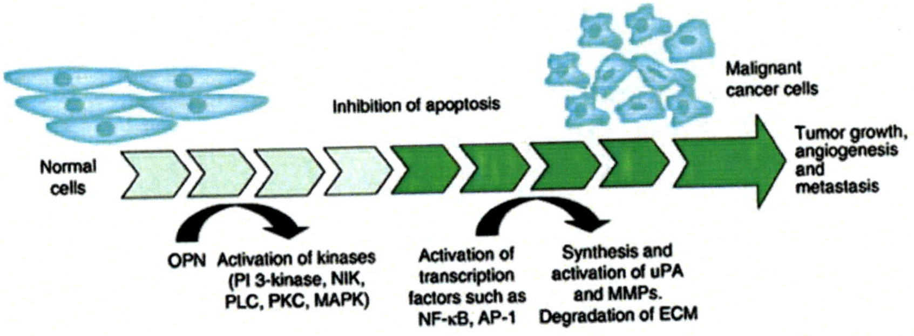

Fig. 6.8 Role of osteopontin (OPN) in tumor progression. Binding of OPN to either integrins or CD44 receptors induces the activation of various cellular kinases and nuclear translocation of transcription factors such as AP-1 and NF-κB. Ultimately, OPN contributes to carcinogenesis via its effects on cell survival and degradation of the ECM. Reprinted from *Trends Cell Biol*, 16, Rangaswami H, Bulbule A, Kundu GC, Osteopontin: role in cell signaling and cancer progression, 79–87, 2006, with permission from Elsevier

alcohol, MMPs, and cancer. This issue is of particular importance in breast cancer research where epidemiological data suggests that alcohol may enhance tumor growth and metastatic potential (Vaeth and Satariano 1998; Singletary and Gapstur 2001; Allen et al. 2009).

Osteopontin. Remodeling of the ECM is a complex and tightly regulated process. For example, MMPs are synthesized as inactive zymogens that require proteolytic removal of the prodomain for enzymatic activation. *Plasmin* is a serine protease released from the liver as the inactive zymogen *plasminogen*, which circulates in the blood. Apart from its function in dissolving fibrin blood clots, plasmin plays an important role in remodeling the ECM through cleavage and activation of MMPs.

An important upstream regulator of the plasmin–plasminogen system, osteopontin (OPN) is an arginine–glycine–aspartate (RGD) containing adhesive glycoprotein first identified in osteoblasts, but now known to be expressed in a variety of tissues (reviewed by Rangaswami et al. 2006). OPN activates many intracellular signaling pathways important for tumorigenesis, particularly those involving components of the plasmin–plasminogen system (Fig. 6.8; reviewed by Rangaswami et al. 2006). Binding of OPN to αvβ3 integrin receptors induces PI3K/Akt-dependent NF-κB activation and subsequent secretion of uPA in breast cancer cells (Das et al. 2005). Elevated expression of uPA or *urokinase-type plasminogen activator*, the serine protease responsible for converting plasminogen to plasmin, correlates with metastatic potential of several cancer types (Romer et al. 2004). Other studies suggest that OPN–integrin interactions also trigger uPA secretion and activation of MMP9 through both MAPK and nuclear factor inducing kinase (NIK)-mediated pathways (reviewed by Rangaswami et al. 2006). Furthermore, binding of OPN to CD44 cell surface receptors promotes cell survival and motility via activation of PLC-γ/PKC/Akt signaling pathways (Fig. 6.8). In summary, the role of OPN in ECM remodeling, controlling cell survival and motility positions it as a critical regulator of tumor growth and metastasis (Rangaswami et al. 2006).

In terms of alcohol, the plasmin–plasminogen system and OPN in particular are thought to contribute to the pathogenesis of alcoholic liver disease (reviewed by Seth et al. 2010). A series of molecular profiling studies by Seth and colleagues revealed significant upregulation of genes involved in OPN-mediated signaling, including OPN, OPN receptors (integrins, CD44), modulators (MMPs, thrombin), and downstream effectors (uPA, plasminogen) in liver samples of patients with alcoholic steatohepatitis and cirrhosis (Seth et al. 2003, 2006). OPN, a marker for metastatic progression in many cancers (reviewed by Rangaswami et al. 2006), may also serve as a biomarker of liver pathology for processes including inflammation (Banerjee et al. 2006b), fibrosis (Szalay et al. 2009), and hepatocarcinogenesis (Kim et al. 2006; Zhang et al. 2006). In rodent models of ALD, OPN plays an important role in disease progression, involved in both hepatic lipid accumulation (Lee et al. 2008) and neutrophil infiltration (Apte et al. 2005; Banerjee et al. 2006a, 2009) following chronic alcohol consumption. Further investigation is needed to define the role for increased hepatobiliary expression of *OPN* following alcohol consumption in alcohol-related cancer metastases.

Alcohol and Stem Cell Maintenance

Recent conceptual advances in cancer biology, such as the recognition that developmental signaling pathways including Wnt, Notch, Nodal, fibroblast growth factor (FGF), and Hedgehog (Hh) may be oncogenic when dysregulated, have arisen from the convergence of the fields of cancer and developmental biology (reviewed by Clevers 2006; Bailey et al. 2007; Jiang and Hui 2008; Strizzi et al. 2009). The concept of cancer stem cells exemplifies how these pathways may contribute to the self-renewal capabilities of stem cells in both the embryo and in tumors (reviewed by Reya and Clevers 2005; Pierfelice et al. 2008; Gotoh 2009; see Chap. 11). In addition to aberrant Wnt signaling serving as the initial transforming event in crypt stem cells of the intestines (reviewed by Reya and Clevers 2005; see Chap. 2, Fig. 3), other developmental pathways crucial to proper embyrogenesis also reemerge in cancer cells during tumorigenesis.

Hedgehog

The Hh family of secreted proteins controls a variety of processes essential for proper embryonic development and tissue homeostasis in the adult (reviewed by Jiang and Hui 2008). The hedgehog gene was first identified 30 years ago as a segment polarity gene that regulated cuticle patterning in *Drosophila* embryos (Nusslein-Volhard and Wieschaus 1980). Since then, numerous studies have focused on its role as a morphogen and on details of its signal transduction (Fig. 6.9). In mammals, three Hh proteins exist including Desert hedgehog, Indian hedgehog,

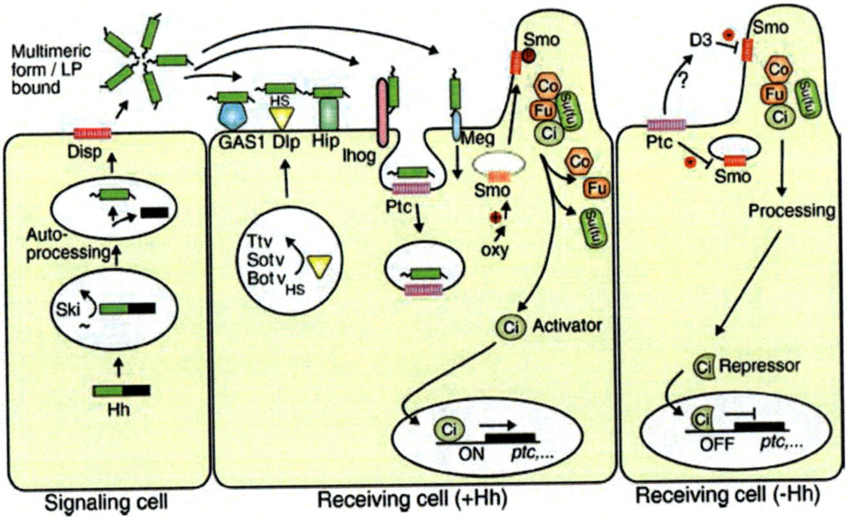

Fig. 6.9 Hedgehog signaling. Hh protein maturation (*left cell*) involves autoprocessing of full-length hedgehog (Hh) precursor protein to generate an N-terminal fragment that once modified with cholesterol at the carboxyl end (*red loop*) and palmitate at the amino end is secreted by Dispatched (Disp), forming multimers of fully active signaling molecules. In the absence of Hh ligand (*right cell*) the Patched (Ptc) receptor inhibits the activity of Smoothened (Smo) protein, a key regulator for nuclear transmission of the Hh signal. Interactions with the cytoplasmic proteins Fused (Fu)/Supressor of Fused (Sufu) convert various Ci/Gli to transcriptional repressors. In the Hh receiving cell (*middle cell*), several molecules may interact with Hh to modulate its signal including Growth-arrest specific 1 (Gas1) and Dally-like protein (Dlp). Binding of Hedgehog (Hh) ligand results in a derepression of Smo, allowing for its translocation to the mammalian cilium. Phosphorylation of Smo results in the functional dissociation of the Fu/Sufu complex. Transcriptionally active forms of Ci/Gli accumulate and enter the nucleus to promote target gene expression. Pathway constructed from combined *Drosophila* and mammalian data. Reprinted from *Genome Biol*, 9, Burglin TR, The hedgehog protein family, 2008, with permission from BioMed Central Ltd

and Sonic hedgehog (Shh). In the absence of a general Hh ligand, the Hh receptor Patched (Ptc) inhibits the protein Smoothen (Smo), a seven-pass G-protein-coupled receptor that serves as the key mediator of the signal transduction pathway. Details of how Ptc inhibits Smo are still not clear. In the presence of extracellular Hh, binding of ligand to the Ptc receptor relieves this inhibition, allowing Smo to translocate to the primary cillum of mammalian cells. This event eventually leads to the conversion of Ci/Gli transcription factors to active forms, thereby promoting target gene expression (Fig. 6.9). As an additional layer of pathway regulation, proteolytic cleavage of a precursor form and modification by cholesterol produces the mature 20-kDa N-terminal signaling ligand, which may then be secreted to elicit both autocrine or paracrine responses (Fig. 6.9).

Both disruptions in Hh signaling and exposure to alcohol in utero cause holoprosencephaly (HPE), a birth defect involving loss of midline structures of the brain and face (reviewed by Cohen and Shiota 2002; Roessler and Muenke 2003). In both mice and men, mutations in genes involving the Hh pathway (e.g., *Ptch, Shh, Gas1, Disp*) are commonly linked to HPE. Abnormalities consistent with HPE are also seen in children with Fetal Alcohol Syndrome (reviewed by Sulik 2005). In animal models, alcohol exposure downregulates *Shh* and other components of the signaling pathway, while addition of exogenous Shh or cholesterol itself rescues FAS-like phenotypes, suggesting that inhibition of Shh signaling is a major consequence of prenatal alcohol exposure (Ahlgren et al. 2002; Li et al. 2007; Loucks and Ahlgren 2009).

In contrast to its suppression by alcohol in the embryo, the Hh pathway is activated in a variety of human cancers (reviewed by Pasca di Magliano and Hebrok 2003; Jiang and Hui 2008; Yang et al. 2010). Loss-of-function mutations in *PTCH* and gain-of-function mutations in *SMO*, both which would result in constitutive activation of the Hh pathway, are seen in patients with basal cell carcinomas, medulloblastomas, and rhabdomyosarcomas (Xie et al. 1998; Wicking et al. 1999; Kappler et al. 2004), whereas in other cancers (e.g., prostate, lung, gastrointestinal tract, breast, and brain) Hh pathway components are not genetically altered and their growth remains ligand dependent (reviewed by Jiang and Hui 2008). Hh signaling activation seen in human malignancies may promote cell growth and/or survival (reviewed by Varjosalo and Taipale 2008), regulate a variety of adult stem cells (reviewed by Jiang and Hui 2008), and maintain cancer stem cells (reviewed by Yang et al. 2010). Of interest to alcohol-related cancers, specific downregulation of Gli-2 by antisense oligonucleotide technology inhibits the proliferation of various HCC cell lines and may provide a useful therapeutic option for the treatment of HCC (Kim et al. 2007). Importantly, Hh pathway activation has been observed in both mouse and human alcoholic liver disease (Jung et al. 2008).

Concluding Remarks

Both alcohol and cancer researchers have contributed to our understanding of how cancer genes and signaling pathways are involved in the etiology of alcohol-attributable cancers. Alcohol clearly regulates oncogenic signaling pathways, though the effects may depend on the cell and tissue type and the duration and level of exposure. Understanding how alcohol modulates cell proliferation, survival, motility, and angiogenesis may aid in the development of therapeutic strategies for the prevention and treatment of alcohol-associated cancers. Given the increased cancer risks associated with alcohol consumption, more work is needed to further elucidate the cellular and molecular mechanisms of alcohol-mediated carcinogenesis.

References

Ahlgren SC, Thakur V, Bronner-Fraser M (2002) Sonic hedgehog rescues cranial neural crest from cell death induced by ethanol exposure. Proc Natl Acad Sci U S A 99:10476–81.

Ai L, Stephenson KK, Ling W, Zuo C, Mukunyadzi P, Suen JY, Hanna E, Fan CY (2003) The p16 (CDKN2a/INK4a) tumor-suppressor gene in head and neck squamous cell carcinoma: a promoter methylation and protein expression study in 100 cases. Mod Pathol 16:944–50.

Ali IU, Schriml LM, Dean M (1999) Mutational spectra of PTEN/MMAC1 gene: a tumor suppressor with lipid phosphatase activity. J Natl Cancer Inst 91:1922–32.
Allen NE, Beral V, Casabonne D, Kan SW, Reeves GK, Brown A, Green J (2009) Moderate alcohol intake and cancer incidence in women. J Natl Cancer Inst 101:296–305.
Apte UM, Banerjee A, McRee R, Wellberg E, Ramaiah SK (2005) Role of osteopontin in hepatic neutrophil infiltration during alcoholic steatohepatitis. Toxicol Appl Pharmacol 207:25–38.
Arevalo E, Shanmugasundararaj S, Wilkemeyer MF, Dou X, Chen S, Charness ME, Miller KW (2008) An alcohol binding site on the neural cell adhesion molecule L1. Proc Natl Acad Sci U S A 105:371–5.
Aroor AR, Shukla SD (2004) MAP kinase signaling in diverse effects of ethanol. Life Sci 74:2339–64.
Aye MM, Ma C, Lin H, Bower KA, Wiggins RC, Luo J (2004) Ethanol-induced in vitro invasion of breast cancer cells: the contribution of MMP-2 by fibroblasts. Int J Cancer 112:738–46.
Baan R, Straif K, Grosse Y, Secretan B, El Ghissassi F, Bouvard V, Altieri A, Cogliano V (2007) Carcinogenicity of alcoholic beverages. Lancet Oncol 8:292–3.
Bailey JM, Singh PK, Hollingsworth MA (2007) Cancer metastasis facilitated by developmental pathways: Sonic hedgehog, Notch, and bone morphogenic proteins. J Cell Biochem 102:829–39.
Banerjee A, Apte UM, Smith R, Ramaiah SK (2006a) Higher neutrophil infiltration mediated by osteopontin is a likely contributing factor to the increased susceptibility of females to alcoholic liver disease. J Pathol 208:473–85.
Banerjee A, Burghardt RC, Johnson GA, White FJ, Ramaiah SK (2006b) The temporal expression of osteopontin (SPP-1) in the rodent model of alcoholic steatohepatitis: a potential biomarker. Toxicol Pathol 34:373–84.
Banerjee A, Rose R, Johnson GA, Burghardt RC, Ramaiah SK (2009) The influence of estrogen on hepatobiliary osteopontin (SPP1) expression in a female rodent model of alcoholic steatohepatitis. Toxicol Pathol 37:492–501.
Barkan D, Green JE, Chambers AF (2010) Extracellular matrix: A gatekeeper in the transition from dormancy to metastatic growth. Eur J Cancer.
Barrallo-Gimeno A, Nieto MA (2005) The Snail genes as inducers of cell movement and survival: implications in development and cancer. Development 132:3151–61.
Bearer CF (2001) L1 cell adhesion molecule signal cascades: targets for ethanol developmental neurotoxicity. Neurotoxicology 22:625–33.
Berx G, Van Roy F (2001) The E-cadherin/catenin complex: an important gatekeeper in breast cancer tumorigenesis and malignant progression. Breast Cancer Res 3:289–93.
Bjorklund M, Koivunen E (2005) Gelatinase-mediated migration and invasion of cancer cells. Biochim Biophys Acta 1755:37–69.
Blandino G, Dobbelstein M (2004) p73 and p63: why do we still need them? Cell Cycle 3:886–94.
Blons H, Laurent-Puig P (2003) TP53 and head and neck neoplasms. Hum Mutat 21:252–7.
Bora PS, Kaliappan S, Xu Q, Kumar S, Wang Y, Kaplan HJ, Bora NS (2006) Alcohol linked to enhanced angiogenesis in rat model of choroidal neovascularization. FEBS J 273:1403–14.
Breitkopf K, Godoy P, Ciuclan L, Singer MV, Dooley S (2006) TGF-beta/Smad signaling in the injured liver. Z Gastroenterol 44:57–66.
Brennan JA, Boyle JO, Koch WM, Goodman SN, Hruban RH, Eby YJ, Couch MJ, Forastiere AA, Sidransky D (1995) Association between cigarette smoking and mutation of the p53 gene in squamous-cell carcinoma of the head and neck. N Engl J Med 332:712–7.
Brooks PJ, Theruvathu JA (2005) DNA adducts from acetaldehyde: implications for alcohol-related carcinogenesis. Alcohol 35:187–93.
Burglin TR (2008) The hedgehog protein family. Genome Biology 9:241.
Chalhoub N, Baker SJ (2009) PTEN and the PI3-kinase pathway in cancer. Annu Rev Pathol 4:127–50.
Chambers AF, Groom AC, MacDonald IC (2002) Dissemination and growth of cancer cells in metastatic sites. Nat Rev Cancer 2:563–72.

Chamulitrat W, Schmidt R, Chunglok W, Kohl A, Tomakidi P (2003) Epithelium and fibroblast-like phenotypes derived from HPV16 E6/E7-immortalized human gingival keratinocytes following chronic ethanol treatment. Eur J Cell Biol 82:313–22.

Chen SY, Wilkemeyer MF, Sulik KK, Charness ME (2001) Octanol antagonism of ethanol teratogenesis. FASEB J 15:1649–51.

Clevers H (2006) Wnt/beta-catenin signaling in development and disease. Cell 127:469–80.

Cohen MM, Jr., Shiota K (2002) Teratogenesis of holoprosencephaly. Am J Med Genet 109:1–15.

Contu SS, Contu PC, Damin DC, Fagundes RB, Bevilacqua F, Rosa AS, Prolla JC, Moreira LF (2007) pRB expression in esophageal mucosa of individuals at high risk for squamous cell carcinoma of the esophagus. World J Gastroenterol 13:1728–31.

Cowin P, Rowlands TM, Hatsell SJ (2005) Cadherins and catenins in breast cancer. Curr Opin Cell Biol 17:499–508.

Crews FT, Nixon K (2009) Mechanisms of neurodegeneration and regeneration in alcoholism. Alcohol Alcohol 44:115–27.

Dale JK, Malapert P, Chal J, Vilhais-Neto G, Maroto M, Johnson T, Jayasinghe S, Trainor P, Herrmann B, Pourquie O (2006) Oscillations of the snail genes in the presomitic mesoderm coordinate segmental patterning and morphogenesis in vertebrate somitogenesis. Dev Cell 10:355–66.

Das R, Philip S, Mahabeleshwar GH, Bulbule A, Kundu GC (2005) Osteopontin: it's role in regulation of cell motility and nuclear factor kappa B-mediated urokinase type plasminogen activator expression. IUBMB Life 57:441–7.

Del Castillo G, Murillo MM, Alvarez-Barrientos A, Bertran E, Fernandez M, Sanchez A, Fabregat I (2006) Autocrine production of TGF-beta confers resistance to apoptosis after an epithelial-mesenchymal transition process in hepatocytes: Role of EGF receptor ligands. Exp Cell Res 312:2860–71.

Deryugina EI, Quigley JP (2006) Matrix metalloproteinases and tumor metastasis. Cancer Metastasis Rev 25:9–34.

Dhillon AS, Hagan S, Rath O, Kolch W (2007) MAP kinase signalling pathways in cancer. Oncogene 26:3279–90.

Dissanayake SK, Wade M, Johnson CE, O'Connell MP, Leotlela PD, French AD, Shah KV, Hewitt KJ, Rosenthal DT, Indig FE et al. (2007) The Wnt5A/protein kinase C pathway mediates motility in melanoma cells via the inhibition of metastasis suppressors and initiation of an epithelial to mesenchymal transition. J Biol Chem 282:17259–71.

Dooley S, Hamzavi J, Ciuclan L, Godoy P, Ilkavets I, Ehnert S, Ueberham E, Gebhardt R, Kanzler S, Geier A et al. (2008) Hepatocyte-specific Smad7 expression attenuates TGF-beta-mediated fibrogenesis and protects against liver damage. Gastroenterology 135:642–59.

Dorgan JF, Baer DJ, Albert PS, Judd JT, Brown ED, Corle DK, Campbell WS, Hartman TJ, Tejpar AA, Clevidence BA et al. (2001) Serum hormones and the alcohol-breast cancer association in postmenopausal women. J Natl Cancer Inst 93:710–5.

Dumenco L, Oguey D, Wu J, Messier N, Fausto N (1995) Introduction of a murine p53 mutation corresponding to human codon 249 into a murine hepatocyte cell line results in growth advantage, but not in transformation. Hepatology 22:1279–88.

Dumitrescu RG, Shields PG (2005) The etiology of alcohol-induced breast cancer. Alcohol 35:213–25.

Edamoto Y, Hara A, Biernat W, Terracciano L, Cathomas G, Riehle HM, Matsuda M, Fujii H, Scoazec JY, Ohgaki H (2003) Alterations of RB1, p53 and Wnt pathways in hepatocellular carcinomas associated with hepatitis C, hepatitis B and alcoholic liver cirrhosis. Int J Cancer 106:334–41.

Egeblad M, Werb Z (2002) New functions for the matrix metalloproteinases in cancer progression. Nat Rev Cancer 2:161–74.

Endo K, Ueda T, Ueyama J, Ohta T, Terada T (2000) Immunoreactive E-cadherin, alpha-catenin, beta-catenin, and gamma-catenin proteins in hepatocellular carcinoma: relationships with tumor grade, clinicopathologic parameters, and patients' survival. Hum Pathol 31:558–65.

Etique N, Chardard D, Chesnel A, Flament S, Grillier-Vuissoz I (2004b) Analysis of the effects of different alcohols on MCF-7 human breast cancer cells. Ann N Y Acad Sci 1030:78–85.

Etique N, Chardard D, Chesnel A, Merlin JL, Flament S, Grillier-Vuissoz I (2004a) Ethanol stimulates proliferation, ERalpha and aromatase expression in MCF-7 human breast cancer cells. Int J Mol Med 13:149–55.

Etique N, Grillier-Vuissoz I, Flament S (2006) Ethanol stimulates the secretion of matrix metalloproteinases 2 and 9 in MCF-7 human breast cancer cells. Oncol Rep 15:603–8.

Etique N, Flament S, Lecomte J, Grillier-Vuissoz I (2007) Ethanol-induced ligand-independent activation of ERalpha mediated by cyclic AMP/PKA signaling pathway: an in vitro study on MCF-7 breast cancer cells. Int J Oncol 31:1509–18.

Fan S, Meng Q, Gao B, Grossman J, Yadegari M, Goldberg ID, Rosen EM (2000) Alcohol stimulates estrogen receptor signaling in human breast cancer cell lines. Cancer Res 60:5635–9.

Farber NB, Olney JW (2003) Drugs of abuse that cause developing neurons to commit suicide. Brain Res Dev Brain Res 147:37–45.

Fernandez-Sola J, Preedy VR, Lang CH, Gonzalez-Reimers E, Arno M, Lin JC, Wiseman H, Zhou S, Emery PW, Nakahara T et al. (2007) Molecular and cellular events in alcohol-induced muscle disease. Alcohol Clin Exp Res 31:1953–62.

Fischer AN, Herrera B, Mikula M, Proell V, Fuchs E, Gotzmann J, Schulte-Hermann R, Beug H, Mikulits W (2005) Integration of Ras subeffector signaling in TGF-beta mediated late stage hepatocarcinogenesis. Carcinogenesis 26:931–42.

Forrester K, Lupold SE, Ott VL, Chay CH, Band V, Wang XW, Harris CC (1995) Effects of p53 mutants on wild-type p53-mediated transactivation are cell type dependent. Oncogene 10:2103–11.

Forsyth CB, Tang Y, Shaikh M, Zhang L, Keshavarzian A (2010) Alcohol stimulates activation of snail, epidermal growth factor receptor signaling, and biomarkers of epithelial-mesenchymal transition in colon and breast cancer cells. Alcohol Clin Exp Res 34:19–31.

Franco DL, Mainez J, Vega S, Sancho P, Murillo MM, de Frutos CA, Del Castillo G, Lopez-Blau C, Fabregat I, Nieto MA (2010) Snail1 suppresses TGF-beta-induced apoptosis and is sufficient to trigger EMT in hepatocytes. J Cell Sci 123:3467–77.

Fransen E, Lemmon V, Van Camp G, Vits L, Coucke P, Willems PJ (1995) CRASH syndrome: clinical spectrum of corpus callosum hypoplasia, retardation, adducted thumbs, spastic paraparesis and hydrocephalus due to mutations in one single gene, L1. Eur J Hum Genet 3:273–84.

Freedman DM, Sigurdson A, Doody MM, Rao RS, Linet MS (2003) Risk of melanoma in relation to smoking, alcohol intake, and other factors in a large occupational cohort. Cancer Causes Control 14:847–57.

Freudenheim JL, Bonner M, Krishnan S, Ambrosone CB, Graham S, McCann SE, Moysich KB, Bowman E, Nemoto T, Shields PG (2004) Diet and alcohol consumption in relation to p53 mutations in breast tumors. Carcinogenesis 25:931–9.

Gavert N, Conacci-Sorrell M, Gast D, Schneider A, Altevogt P, Brabletz T, Ben-Ze'ev A (2005) L1, a novel target of beta-catenin signaling, transforms cells and is expressed at the invasive front of colon cancers. J Cell Biol 168:633–42.

Gavert N, Sheffer M, Raveh S, Spaderna S, Shtutman M, Brabletz T, Barany F, Paty P, Notterman D, Domany E et al. (2007) Expression of L1-CAM and ADAM10 in human colon cancer cells induces metastasis. Cancer Res 67:7703–12.

Gill J (2000) The effects of moderate alcohol consumption on female hormone levels and reproductive function. Alcohol Alcohol 35:417–23.

Gilmore AP, Owens TW, Foster FM, Lindsay J (2009) How adhesion signals reach a mitochondrial conclusion – ECM regulation of apoptosis. Curr Opin Cell Biol 21:654–61.

Ginsburg ES, Mello NK, Mendelson JH, Barbieri RL, Teoh SK, Rothman M, Gao X, Sholar JW (1996) Effects of alcohol ingestion on estrogens in postmenopausal women. JAMA 276:1747–51.

Gotoh N (2009) Control of stemness by fibroblast growth factor signaling in stem cells and cancer stem cells. Curr Stem Cell Res Ther 4:9–15.

Gotzmann J, Huber H, Thallinger C, Wolschek M, Jansen B, Schulte-Hermann R, Beug H, Mikulits W (2002) Hepatocytes convert to a fibroblastoid phenotype through the cooperation of TGF-beta1 and Ha-Ras: steps towards invasiveness. J Cell Sci 115:1189–202.
Gronbaek K, de Nully Brown P, Moller MB, Nedergaard T, Ralfkiaer E, Moller P, Zeuthen J, Guldberg P (2000) Concurrent disruption of p16INK4a and the ARF-p53 pathway predicts poor prognosis in aggressive non-Hodgkin's lymphoma. Leukemia 14:1727–35.
Gu JW, Bailey AP, Sartin A, Makey I, Brady AL (2005) Ethanol stimulates tumor progression and expression of vascular endothelial growth factor in chick embryos. Cancer 103:422–31.
Gu JW, Elam J, Sartin A, Li W, Roach R, Adair TH (2001) Moderate levels of ethanol induce expression of vascular endothelial growth factor and stimulate angiogenesis. Am J Physiol Regul Integr Comp Physiol 281:R365–72.
Gukovskaya AS, Mareninova OA, Odinokova IV, Sung KF, Lugea A, Fischer L, Wang YL, Gukovsky I, Pandol SJ (2006) Cell death in pancreatitis: effects of alcohol. J Gastroenterol Hepatol 21 Suppl 3:S10–3.
Gupta GP, Massague J (2006) Cancer metastasis: building a framework. Cell 127:679–95.
Hamajima N, Hirose K, Tajima K, Rohan T, Calle EE, Heath CW, Jr., Coates RJ, Liff JM, Talamini R, Chantarakul N et al. (2002) Alcohol, tobacco and breast cancer – collaborative reanalysis of individual data from 53 epidemiological studies, including 58,515 women with breast cancer and 95,067 women without the disease. Br J Cancer 87:1234–45.
He J, de la Monte S, Wands JR (2007) Acute ethanol exposure inhibits insulin signaling in the liver. Hepatology 46:1791–800.
Horie Y, Suzuki A, Kataoka E, Sasaki T, Hamada K, Sasaki J, Mizuno K, Hasegawa G, Kishimoto H, Iizuka M et al. (2004) Hepatocyte-specific Pten deficiency results in steatohepatitis and hepatocellular carcinomas. J Clin Invest 113:1774–83.
Hsieh LL, Wang PF, Chen IH, Liao CT, Wang HM, Chen MC, Chang JT, Cheng AJ (2001) Characteristics of mutations in the p53 gene in oral squamous cell carcinoma associated with betel quid chewing and cigarette smoking in Taiwanese. Carcinogenesis 22:1497–503.
Hu W, Feng Z, Eveleigh J, Iyer G, Pan J, Amin S, Chung FL, Tang MS (2002) The major lipid peroxidation product, trans-4-hydroxy-2-nonenal, preferentially forms DNA adducts at codon 249 of human p53 gene, a unique mutational hotspot in hepatocellular carcinoma. Carcinogenesis 23:1781–9.
Hussain SP, Schwank J, Staib F, Wang XW, Harris CC (2007) TP53 mutations and hepatocellular carcinoma: insights into the etiology and pathogenesis of liver cancer. Oncogene 26:2166–76.
Ichimura K, Bolin MB, Goike HM, Schmidt EE, Moshref A, Collins VP (2000) Deregulation of the p14ARF/MDM2/p53 pathway is a prerequisite for human astrocytic gliomas with G1-S transition control gene abnormalities. Cancer Res 60:417–24.
Ikonomidou C (2009) Triggers of apoptosis in the immature brain. Brain Dev 31:488–92.
Izevbigie EB, Ekunwe SI, Jordan J, Howard CB (2002) Ethanol modulates the growth of human breast cancer cells in vitro. Exp Biol Med (Maywood) 227:260–5.
Jakowlew SB (2006) Transforming growth factor-beta in cancer and metastasis. Cancer Metastasis Rev 25:435–57.
Jeanes A, Gottardi CJ, Yap AS (2008) Cadherins and cancer: how does cadherin dysfunction promote tumor progression? Oncogene 27:6920–9.
Jiang J, Hui CC (2008) Hedgehog signaling in development and cancer. Dev Cell 15:801–12.
Jones KL, Buzdar AU (2009) Evolving novel anti-HER2 strategies. Lancet Oncol 10:1179–87.
Jung Y, Brown KD, Witek RP, Omenetti A, Yang L, Vandongen M, Milton RJ, Hines IN, Rippe RA, Spahr L, et al. (2008) Accumulation of hedgehog-responsive progenitors parallels alcoholic liver disease severity in mice and humans. Gastroenterology 134:1532–43.
Kaimori A, Potter J, Kaimori JY, Wang C, Mezey E, Koteish A (2007) Transforming growth factor-beta1 induces an epithelial-to-mesenchymal transition state in mouse hepatocytes in vitro. J Biol Chem 282:22089–101.
Kaliappan S, Jha P, Lyzogubov VV, Tytarenko RG, Bora NS, Bora PS (2008) Alcohol and nicotine consumption exacerbates choroidal neovascularization by modulating the regulation of complement system. FEBS Lett 582:3451–8.

Kang Y, Massague J (2004) Epithelial-mesenchymal transitions: twist in development and metastasis. Cell 118:277–9.

Kappler R, Bauer R, Calzada-Wack J, Rosemann M, Hemmerlein B, Hahn H (2004) Profiling the molecular difference between Patched- and p53-dependent rhabdomyosarcoma. Oncogene 23:8785–95.

Karnoub AE, Weinberg RA (2008) Ras oncogenes: split personalities. Nat Rev Mol Cell Biol 9:517–31.

Katoh M (2006) Cross-talk of WNT and FGF signaling pathways at GSK3beta to regulate beta-catenin and SNAIL signaling cascades. Cancer Biol Ther 5:1059–64.

Ke Z, Lin H, Fan Z, Cai TQ, Kaplan RA, Ma C, Bower KA, Shi X, Luo J (2006) MMP-2 mediates ethanol-induced invasion of mammary epithelial cells over-expressing ErbB2. Int J Cancer 119:8–16.

Kessenbrock K, Plaks V, Werb Z (2010) Matrix Metalloproteinases: Regulators of the Tumor Microenvironment. 141:52–67.

Key J, Hodgson S, Omar RZ, Jensen TK, Thompson SG, Boobis AR, Davies DS, Elliott P (2006) Meta-analysis of studies of alcohol and breast cancer with consideration of the methodological issues. Cancer Causes Control 17:759–70.

Key TJ, Verkasalo PK, Banks E (2001) Epidemiology of breast cancer. Lancet Oncol 2:133–40.

Kim J, Ki SS, Lee SD, Han CJ, Kim YC, Park SH, Cho SY, Hong YJ, Park HY, Lee M et al. (2006) Elevated plasma osteopontin levels in patients with hepatocellular carcinoma. Am J Gastroenterol 101:2051–9.

Kim Y, Yoon JW, Xiao X, Dean NM, Monia BP, Marcusson EG (2007) Selective down-regulation of glioma-associated oncogene 2 inhibits the proliferation of hepatocellular carcinoma cells. Cancer Res 67:3583–93.

Kozyraki R, Scoazec JY, Flejou JF, D'Errico A, Bedossa P, Terris B, Fiorentino M, Bringuier AF, Grigioni WF, Feldmann G (1996) Expression of cadherins and alpha-catenin in primary epithelial tumors of the liver. Gastroenterology 110:1137–49.

Kraunz KS, McClean MD, Nelson HH, Peters E, Calderon H, Kelsey KT (2006) Duration but not intensity of alcohol and tobacco exposure predicts p16INK4A homozygous deletion in head and neck squamous cell carcinoma. Cancer Res 66:4512–5.

Lee JH, Banerjee A, Ueno Y, Ramaiah SK (2008) Potential relationship between hepatobiliary osteopontin and peroxisome proliferator-activated receptor alpha expression following ethanol-associated hepatic injury in vivo and in vitro. Toxicol Sci 106:290–9.

Li CI, Chlebowski RT, Freiberg M, Johnson KC, Kuller L, Lane D, Lessin L, O'Sullivan MJ, Wactawski-Wende J, Yasmeen S et al. (2010) Alcohol consumption and risk of postmenopausal breast cancer by subtype: the women's health initiative observational study. J Natl Cancer Inst 102:1422–31.

Li YX, Yang HT, Zdanowicz M, Sicklick JK, Qi Y, Camp TJ, Diehl AM (2007) Fetal alcohol exposure impairs Hedgehog cholesterol modification and signaling. Lab Invest 87:231–40.

Lois M, Brown LA, Moss IM, Roman J, Guidot DM (1999) Ethanol ingestion increases activation of matrix metalloproteinases in rat lungs during acute endotoxemia. Am J Respir Crit Care Med 160:1354–60.

Longnecker MP (1994) Alcoholic beverage consumption in relation to risk of breast cancer: meta-analysis and review. Cancer Causes Control 5:73–82.

Loucks EJ, Ahlgren SC (2009) Deciphering the role of Shh signaling in axial defects produced by ethanol exposure. Birth Defects Res A Clin Mol Teratol 85:556–67.

Luo J (2006) Role of matrix metalloproteinase-2 in ethanol-induced invasion by breast cancer cells. J Gastroenterol Hepatol 21 Suppl 3:S65–8.

Lyronis ID, Baritaki S, Bizakis I, Krambovitis E, Spandidos DA (2008) K-ras mutation, HPV infection and smoking or alcohol abuse positively correlate with esophageal squamous carcinoma. Pathol Oncol Res 14:267–73.

Ma C, Lin H, Leonard SS, Shi X, Ye J, Luo J (2003) Overexpression of ErbB2 enhances ethanol-stimulated intracellular signaling and invasion of human mammary epithelial and breast cancer cells in vitro. Oncogene 22:5281–90.

Malats N, Porta M, Corominas JM, Pinol JL, Rifa J, Real FX (1997) Ki-ras mutations in exocrine pancreatic cancer: association with clinico-pathological characteristics and with tobacco and alcohol consumption. PANK-ras I Project Investigators. Int J Cancer 70:661–7.

Marsit CJ, McClean MD, Furniss CS, Kelsey KT (2006) Epigenetic inactivation of the SFRP genes is associated with drinking, smoking and HPV in head and neck squamous cell carcinoma. Int J Cancer 119:1761–6.

Massague J (2008) TGFbeta in Cancer. Cell 134:215–30.

McVicker BL, Tuma DJ, Casey CA (2007) Effect of ethanol on pro-apoptotic mechanisms in polarized hepatic cells. World J Gastroenterol 13:4960–6.

Meng F, Henson R, Wehbe-Janek H, Ghoshal K, Jacob ST, Patel T (2007) MicroRNA-21 regulates expression of the PTEN tumor suppressor gene in human hepatocellular cancer. Gastroenterology 133:647–58.

Meng Q, Gao B, Goldberg ID, Rosen EM, Fan S (2000) Stimulation of cell invasion and migration by alcohol in breast cancer cells. Biochem Biophys Res Commun 273:448–53.

Meyer C, Meindl-Beinker NM, Dooley S (2010) TGF-beta signaling in alcohol induced hepatic injury. Front Biosci 15:740–9.

Millen AE, Tucker MA, Hartge P, Halpern A, Elder DE, Guerry Dt, Holly EA, Sagebiel RW, Potischman N (2004) Diet and melanoma in a case-control study. Cancer Epidemiol Biomarkers Prev 13:1042–51.

Mitin N, Rossman KL, Der CJ (2005) Signaling interplay in Ras superfamily function. Curr Biol 15:R563-74.

Moll UM, Slade N (2004) p63 and p73: roles in development and tumor formation. Mol Cancer Res 2:371–86.

Morgan TR, Mandayam S, Jamal MM (2004) Alcohol and hepatocellular carcinoma. Gastroenterology 127:S87–96.

Morrow D, Cullen JP, Cahill PA, Redmond EM (2008) Ethanol stimulates endothelial cell angiogenic activity via a Notch- and angiopoietin-1-dependent pathway. Cardiovasc Res 79:313–21.

Murillo MM, del Castillo G, Sanchez A, Fernandez M, Fabregat I (2005) Involvement of EGF receptor and c-Src in the survival signals induced by TGF-beta1 in hepatocytes. Oncogene 24:4580–7.

Muti P, Rogan E, Cavalieri E (2006) Androgens and estrogens in the etiology and prevention of breast cancer. Nutr Cancer 56:247–52.

Neth P, Ries C, Karow M, Egea V, Ilmer M, Jochum M (2007) The Wnt signal transduction pathway in stem cells and cancer cells: influence on cellular invasion. Stem Cell Rev 3:18–29.

Nusslein-Volhard C, Wieschaus E (1980) Mutations affecting segment number and polarity in Drosophila. Nature 287:795–801.

Padua D, Massague J (2009) Roles of TGFbeta in metastasis. Cell Res 19:89–102.

Partridge CR, Sampson HW, Forough R (1999) Long-term alcohol consumption increases matrix metalloproteinase-2 activity in rat aorta. Life Sci 65:1395–402.

Pasca di Magliano M, Hebrok M (2003) Hedgehog signalling in cancer formation and maintenance. Nat Rev Cancer 3:903–11.

Pierfelice TJ, Schreck KC, Eberhart CG, Gaiano N (2008) Notch, neural stem cells, and brain tumors. Cold Spring Harb Symp Quant Biol 73:367–75.

Pimienta G, Pascual J (2007) Canonical and alternative MAPK signaling. Cell Cycle 6:2628–32.

Ramanathan R, Wilkemeyer MF, Mittal B, Perides G, Charness ME (1996) Alcohol inhibits cell-cell adhesion mediated by human L1. J Cell Biol 133:381–90.

Rangaswami H, Bulbule A, Kundu GC (2006) Osteopontin: role in cell signaling and cancer progression. Trends Cell Biol 16:79–87.

Rao JS (2003) Molecular mechanisms of glioma invasiveness: the role of proteases. Nat Rev Cancer 3:489–501.

Raveh S, Gavert N, Ben-Ze'ev A (2009) L1 cell adhesion molecule (L1CAM) in invasive tumors. Cancer Lett 282:137–45.

Reichman ME, Judd JT, Longcope C, Schatzkin A, Clevidence BA, Nair PP, Campbell WS, Taylor PR (1993) Effects of alcohol consumption on plasma and urinary hormone concentrations in premenopausal women. J Natl Cancer Inst 85:722–7.

Reya T, Clevers H (2005) Wnt signalling in stem cells and cancer. Nature 434:843–50.

Rinaldi S, Peeters PH, Bezemer ID, Dossus L, Biessy C, Sacerdote C, Berrino F, Panico S, Palli D, Tumino R et al. (2006) Relationship of alcohol intake and sex steroid concentrations in blood in pre- and post-menopausal women: the European Prospective Investigation into Cancer and Nutrition. Cancer Causes Control 17:1033–43.

Robson EJ, Khaled WT, Abell K, Watson CJ (2006) Epithelial-to-mesenchymal transition confers resistance to apoptosis in three murine mammary epithelial cell lines. Differentiation 74:254–64.

Roessler E, Muenke M (2003) How a Hedgehog might see holoprosencephaly. Hum Mol Genet 12 Spec No 1:R15–25.

Romer J, Nielsen BS, Ploug M (2004) The urokinase receptor as a potential target in cancer therapy. Curr Pharm Des 10:2359–76.

Salmena L, Carracedo A, Pandolfi PP (2008) Tenets of PTEN tumor suppression. Cell 133:403–14.

Sastre J, Serviddio G, Pereda J, Minana JB, Arduini A, Vendemiale G, Poli G, Pallardo FV, Vina J (2007) Mitochondrial function in liver disease. Front Biosci 12:1200–9.

Schafer MK, Altevogt P (2010) L1CAM malfunction in the nervous system and human carcinomas. Cell Mol Life Sci.

Schmid RS, Maness PF (2008) L1 and NCAM adhesion molecules as signaling coreceptors in neuronal migration and process outgrowth. Curr Opin Neurobiol 18:245–50.

Secretan B, Straif K, Baan R, Grosse Y, El Ghissassi F, Bouvard V, Benbrahim-Tallaa L, Guha N, Freeman C, Galichet L et al. (2009) A review of human carcinogens – Part E: tobacco, areca nut, alcohol, coal smoke, and salted fish. Lancet Oncol 10:1033–4.

Seitz HK, Stickel F (2007) Molecular mechanisms of alcohol-mediated carcinogenesis. Nat Rev Cancer 7:599–612.

Seth D, D'Souza El-Guindy NB, Apte M, Mari M, Dooley S, Neuman M, Haber PS, Kundu GC, Darwanto A, de Villiers WJ et al. (2010) Alcohol, signaling, and ECM turnover. Alcohol Clin Exp Res 34:4–18.

Seth D, Gorrell MD, Cordoba S, McCaughan GW, Haber PS (2006) Intrahepatic gene expression in human alcoholic hepatitis. J Hepatol 45:306–20.

Seth D, Leo MA, McGuinness PH, Lieber CS, Brennan Y, Williams R, Wang XM, McCaughan GW, Gorrell MD, Haber PS (2003) Gene expression profiling of alcoholic liver disease in the baboon (*Papio hamadryas*) and human liver. Am J Pathol 163:2303–17.

Shimoyama Y, Hirohashi S (1991) Cadherin intercellular adhesion molecule in hepatocellular carcinomas: loss of E-cadherin expression in an undifferentiated carcinoma. Cancer Lett 57:131–5.

Shulga N, Hoek JB, Pastorino JG (2005) Elevated PTEN levels account for the increased sensitivity of ethanol-exposed cells to tumor necrosis factor-induced cytotoxicity. J Biol Chem 280:9416–24.

Siesser PF, Maness PF (2009) L1 cell adhesion molecules as regulators of tumor cell invasiveness. Cell Adh Migr 3:275–7.

Simao TA, Ribeiro FS, Amorim LM, Albano RM, Andrada-Serpa MJ, Cardoso LE, Mendonca GA, de Moura-Gallo CV (2002) TP53 mutations in breast cancer tumors of patients from Rio de Janeiro, Brazil: association with risk factors and tumor characteristics. Int J Cancer 101:69–73.

Singh RR, Kumar R (2005) Steroid hormone receptor signaling in tumorigenesis. J Cell Biochem 96:490–505.

Singletary KW, Frey RS, Yan W (2001) Effect of ethanol on proliferation and estrogen receptor-alpha expression in human breast cancer cells. Cancer Lett 165:131–7.

Singletary KW, Gapstur SM (2001) Alcohol and breast cancer: review of epidemiologic and experimental evidence and potential mechanisms. JAMA 286:2143–51.

Stickel F, Schuppan D, Hahn EG, Seitz HK (2002) Cocarcinogenic effects of alcohol in hepatocarcinogenesis. Gut 51:132–9.

Stiles B, Wang Y, Stahl A, Bassilian S, Lee WP, Kim YJ, Sherwin R, Devaskar S, Lesche R, Magnuson MA et al. (2004) Liver-specific deletion of negative regulator Pten results in fatty liver and insulin hypersensitivity [corrected]. Proc Natl Acad Sci U S A 101:2082–7.
Strizzi L, Hardy KM, Seftor EA, Costa FF, Kirschmann DA, Seftor RE, Postovit LM, Hendrix MJ (2009) Development and cancer: at the crossroads of Nodal and Notch signaling. Cancer Res 69:7131–4.
Sulik KK (2005) Genesis of alcohol-induced craniofacial dysmorphism. Exp Biol Med (Maywood) 230:366–75.
Suzuki R, Orsini N, Mignone L, Saji S, Wolk A (2008) Alcohol intake and risk of breast cancer defined by estrogen and progesterone receptor status – a meta-analysis of epidemiological studies. Int J Cancer 122:1832–41.
Szalay G, Sauter M, Haberland M, Zuegel U, Steinmeyer A, Kandolf R, Klingel K (2009) Osteopontin: a fibrosis-related marker molecule in cardiac remodeling of enterovirus myocarditis in the susceptible host. Circ Res 104:851–9.
Tan W, Bailey AP, Shparago M, Busby B, Covington J, Johnson JW, Young E, Gu JW (2007) Chronic alcohol consumption stimulates VEGF expression, tumor angiogenesis and progression of melanoma in mice. Cancer Biol Ther 6:1211–7.
Tang X, Powelka AM, Soriano NA, Czech MP, Guilherme A (2005) PTEN, but not SHIP2, suppresses insulin signaling through the phosphatidylinositol 3-kinase/Akt pathway in 3T3-L1 adipocytes. J Biol Chem 280:22523–9.
Thiery JP (2002) Epithelial-mesenchymal transitions in tumour progression. Nat Rev Cancer 2:442–54.
Thiery JP, Acloque H, Huang RY, Nieto MA (2009) Epithelial-mesenchymal transitions in development and disease. Cell 139:871–90.
Thurston G, Kitajewski J (2008) VEGF and Delta-Notch: interacting signalling pathways in tumour angiogenesis. Br J Cancer 99:1204–9.
Tian M, Schiemann WP (2009) The TGF-beta paradox in human cancer: an update. Future Oncol 5:259–71.
Travis RC, Key TJ (2003) Oestrogen exposure and breast cancer risk. Breast Cancer Res 5:239–47.
Vaeth PA, Satariano WA (1998) Alcohol consumption and breast cancer stage at diagnosis. Alcohol Clin Exp Res 22:928–34.
Valdes F, Alvarez AM, Locascio A, Vega S, Herrera B, Fernandez M, Benito M, Nieto MA, Fabregat I (2002) The epithelial mesenchymal transition confers resistance to the apoptotic effects of transforming growth factor Beta in fetal rat hepatocytes. Mol Cancer Res 1:68–78.
van Zijl F, Mair M, Csiszar A, Schneller D, Zulehner G, Huber H, Eferl R, Beug H, Dolznig H, Mikulits W (2009b) Hepatic tumor-stroma crosstalk guides epithelial to mesenchymal transition at the tumor edge. Oncogene 28:4022–33.
van Zijl F, Zulehner G, Petz M, Schneller D, Kornauth C, Hau M, Machat G, Grubinger M, Huber H, Mikulits W (2009a) Epithelial-mesenchymal transition in hepatocellular carcinoma. Future Oncol 5:1169–79.
Varjosalo M, Taipale J (2008) Hedgehog: functions and mechanisms. Genes Dev 22:2454–72.
Vinciguerra M, Foti M (2008) PTEN at the crossroad of metabolic diseases and cancer in the liver. Ann Hepatol 7:192–9.
Vinciguerra M, Veyrat-Durebex C, Moukil MA, Rubbia-Brandt L, Rohner-Jeanrenaud F, Foti M (2008) PTEN down-regulation by unsaturated fatty acids triggers hepatic steatosis via an NF-kappaBp65/mTOR-dependent mechanism. Gastroenterology 134:268–80.
Vousden KH, Lu X (2002) Live or let die: the cell's response to p53. Nat Rev Cancer 2:594–604.
Wagner EF, Nebreda AR (2009) Signal integration by JNK and p38 MAPK pathways in cancer development. Nat Rev Cancer 9:537–49.
Wang JH, Batey RG, George J (2006) Role of ethanol in the regulation of hepatic stellate cell function. World J Gastroenterol 12:6926–32.
Wang L, Wang WL, Zhang Y, Guo SP, Zhang J, Li QL (2007) Epigenetic and genetic alterations of PTEN in hepatocellular carcinoma. Hepatol Res 37:389–96.

Watanabe T, Yokoo H, Yokoo M, Yonekawa Y, Kleihues P, Ohgaki H (2001) Concurrent inactivation of RB1 and TP53 pathways in anaplastic oligodendrogliomas. J Neuropathol Exp Neurol 60:1181–9.
Wicking C, Smyth I, Bale A (1999) The hedgehog signalling pathway in tumorigenesis and development. Oncogene 18:7844–51.
Wilkemeyer MF, Chen SY, Menkari CE, Brenneman DE, Sulik KK, Charness ME (2003) Differential effects of ethanol antagonism and neuroprotection in peptide fragment NAPVSIPQ prevention of ethanol-induced developmental toxicity. Proc Natl Acad Sci U S A 100:8543–8.
Wilkemeyer MF, Sebastian AB, Smith SA, Charness ME (2000) Antagonists of alcohol inhibition of cell adhesion. Proc Natl Acad Sci U S A 97:3690–5.
Xie J, Murone M, Luoh SM, Ryan A, Gu Q, Zhang C, Bonifas JM, Lam CW, Hynes M, Goddard A et al. (1998) Activating Smoothened mutations in sporadic basal-cell carcinoma. Nature 391:90–2.
Yager JD, Davidson NE (2006) Estrogen carcinogenesis in breast cancer. N Engl J Med 354:270–82.
Yang L, Xie G, Fan Q, Xie J (2010) Activation of the hedgehog-signaling pathway in human cancer and the clinical implications. Oncogene 29:469–81.
Yang M, Adla S, Temburni MK, Patel VP, Lagow EL, Brady OA, Tian J, Boulos MI, Galileo DS (2009) Stimulation of glioma cell motility by expression, proteolysis, and release of the L1 neural cell recognition molecule. Cancer Cell Int 9:27.
Yeon JE, Califano S, Xu J, Wands JR, De La Monte SM (2003) Potential role of PTEN phosphatase in ethanol-impaired survival signaling in the liver. Hepatology 38:703–14.
Yook JI, Li XY, Ota I, Hu C, Kim HS, Kim NH, Cha SY, Ryu JK, Choi YJ, Kim J et al. (2006) A Wnt-Axin2-GSK3beta cascade regulates Snail1 activity in breast cancer cells. Nat Cell Biol 8:1398–406.
Zhang H, Ye QH, Ren N, Zhao L, Wang YF, Wu X, Sun HC, Wang L, Zhang BH, Liu YK et al. (2006) The prognostic significance of preoperative plasma levels of osteopontin in patients with hepatocellular carcinoma. J Cancer Res Clin Oncol 132:709–17.
Zeisberg M, Yang C, Martino M, Duncan MB, Rieder F, Tanjore H, Kalluri R (2007) Fibroblasts derive from hepatocytes in liver fibrosis via epithelial to mesenchymal transition. J Biol Chem 282:23337–47.
Zhou FC, Sari Y, Powrozek TA, Spong CY (2004) A neuroprotective peptide antagonizes fetal alcohol exposure-compromised brain growth. J Mol Neurosci 24:189–99.

Chapter 7
Alcohol, Retinoic Acid, and Cancer

Svetlana Radaeva

Abbreviations

ADH	Alcohol dehydrogenase
ALD	Alcoholic liver disease
AP-1	Activating protein 1
APC	Adenomatous polyposis coli
APL	Promyelocytic leukemia
ATRA	All-*trans*-RA
COX-2	Cyclooxygenase-2
CRABP	Cellular retinoic acid-binding protein
CRBP	Cellular retinol-binding protein
ECS	Embryonic stem cells
FABP	Fatty acid binding protein
FFA	Free fatty acid
HAT	Histone acetylase
HDAC	Histone deacetylase
HSC	Hepatic stellate cells
LRAT	Lecithin retinol acyltransferase
PPAR	Peroxisome proliferator-activated receptor
RA	Retinoic acid
RALDH	Retinaldehyde dehydrogenase
RAR	Retinoic acid receptors
RARE	Retinoic acid response element
RBP4	Retinol binding protein 4
RE	Retinyl ester

S. Radaeva (✉)
Division of Metabolism and Health Effects, National Institute on Alcohol Abuse and Alcoholism, National Institutes of Health, Bethesda, MD, USA
e-mail: sradaeva@mail.nih.gov

S. Zakhari et al. (eds.), *Alcohol and Cancer*, DOI 10.1007/978-1-4614-0040-0_7,
© Springer Science+Business Media, LLC 2011

REH Retinylester hydrolase
ROH Retinol
RXR Retinoid X receptors
SC Stem cells

Introduction

The first observation potentially linking alcohol consumption and vitamin A deficiency was published over 70 years ago (Patek and Haig 1939). Since then, numerous studies have provided solid evidence that alcohol indeed interferes with vitamin A and its analogs, collectively termed retinoids, both in experimental models and in humans. In addition, many experimental and epidemiological studies demonstrated that such interferences might result in impaired tissue regeneration and cancer development. Furthermore, since vitamin A deficiency (or excess) increases the risk for a number of human cancers, and since alcohol impairs the body's retinoid homeostasis, interactions between vitamin A and alcohol may represent central mechanisms by which alcohol induces multiorgan pathology and carcinogenesis.

Retinoids and Carcinogenesis

Carcinogenesis can be considered as gradual accumulation of genetic and epigenetic aberrations resulting in the dysregulation of cellular homeostasis (Karamouzis and Papavassiliou 2005), which requires the correct balance between cellular proliferation and differentiation. The control of cell proliferation is linked to cell specialization (von Wangenheim and Peterson 2008). During differentiation, cycling embryonic cells acquire the ability to perform specialized functions. Terminal differentiation is the end stage of this process where cells irreversibly lose their proliferative capacity, a form of negative control of growth (Gudas 1992). The highly coordinated process of cell proliferation, differentiation and death is tightly controlled during embryogenesis and adulthood. The loss of this control, manifested as an acquisition of aberrant differentiation, invariably accompanied by increased proliferation and survival, is a hallmark of carcinogenesis (Harris 2004). Carcinogenesis proceeds as a series of stepwise neoplastic transformations from normal cells to premalignant lesions to localized carcinoma and, finally, to metastatic disease (Tallman and Wiernik 1992). One of the systems that possess the unique ability to modulate the growth and differentiation of normal, premalignant, and malignant epithelial and mesenchymal cells in vitro and in vivo is retinoid signaling, placing retinoids at the center of cancer regulation (Fig. 7.1). As early as 1925, Wolbach and Howe found that retinoids are needed for the proper maintenance of normal epithelial differentiation; vitamin A deficiency caused the replacement normal mucociliary epithelia in bronchi by a squamous metaplastic and eventually keratinizing

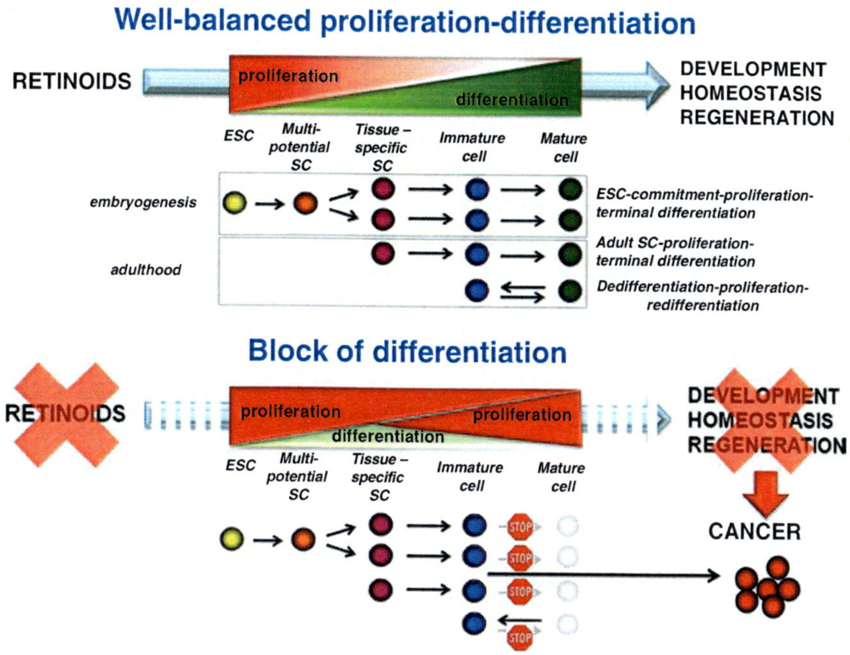

Fig. 7.1 Retinoids control the body's flexible cell renewal system via balanced regulation of proliferation and differentiation. The loss of this control results in a block of cell differentiation and unbalanced proliferation that eventually leads to the development of cancer. *ESC* embryonic stem cell, *SC* stem cell

epithelium, leading to malignant carcinoma. More direct morphologic evidence implicating vitamin A in carcinogenesis was provided in 1955, when Lasnitzki reported identical histological changes in prostate tissue after exposure to either the carcinogen 3-methylcholanthrene or vitamin-A-depleted culture medium (Lasnitzki 1955). Current data from experimental animals, epidemiology, cellular models, and clinical trials undoubtedly demonstrated that loss of retinoid activity or responsiveness is associated with carcinogenesis of the lung, head and neck, liver, pancreas, breast, gastric, colon, and many other organs (Niles 2004; Wald et al. 1980; Poulain et al. 2009; Yang et al. 2002; Okuno et al. 2004). Also, the association between cancer, retinoids, and alcohol is becoming more evident. Esophageal adenocarcinoma, hepatocellular carcinoma (HCC), lung, pancreas, and colon cancer are among malignancies that were strongly linked to alterations in differentiation/proliferation status due to changes in retinoid levels in the presence of alcohol (Seitz 2009; Seitz and Stickel 2006; Wang 2005; Shiraishi-Yokoyama et al. 2006; Jaster et al. 2003).

Most of the evidence indicates that retinoids act at the stage of tumor promotion rather than initiation (Lotan 1996) (see Chap. 1). The promotion stage involves the expansion of initiated cells to form a premalignant lesion that ultimately gives rise to a malignant tumor. According to a well-accepted hypothesis, the cellular origin of cancer, the initiated cells, could arise either from preexisting mature cells that underwent **dedifferentiation and retained the ability to proliferate, or from organ-specific adult stem cells that underwent maturation arrest, processes influenced by retinoids.** For example, retinoids induce end-stage redifferentiation and apoptosis in the pancreatic ductal adenocarcinoma DSL-6AIC1 cell line originated from dedifferentiated pancreatic acinar cells (Brembeck et al. 1998; El-Metwally and Pour 2007). Similarly, retinoids stimulate terminal differentiation in the poorly differentiated papillary thyroid carcinoma cell line, KTC-1, and suppress the growth and aberrant squamous phenotype of head and neck cell carcinoma both in vitro and in vivo (Kurebayashi et al. 2000; Higuchi et al. 2003; Satake et al. 2003). In addition, retinoids induce differentiation of cancer stem cells. The best example is the treatment of acute promyelocytic leukemia (APL) with retinoids, which removes the maturation block of transit-amplifying precursors of the myelocytic lineage, changing the clinical course of disease from highly lethal to highly curable (Freemantle et al. 2003). Interestingly, in alcoholic liver disease (ALD), retinoids may be simultaneously involved in the promotion of hepatic malignant lesions of different origins. Retinoids have been implicated in the development of both well-differentiated HCC originating from initiated mature hepatocytes in cirrhotic liver (dedifferentiation hypothesis) as well as in poorly differentiated HCC arising from liver stem cells, or oval cells (maturation arrest hypothesis) (Breitkopf et al. 2009; Naves et al. 2001; Sano et al. 2005). In addition to their ability to cause oncogenic transformation of epithelial cells, retinoids play a central role in tumor stroma production and thus control tumor progression and invasion by regulating the expression of matrix metalloproteinases, transforming growth factor-β, and cell-cycle regulatory proteins (Bogos et al. 2008).

In line with their broad capacity to cause differentiation, retinoids can inhibit the progression of premalignant lesions to malignant stages and reverse the carcinogenic process. Animal experiments have shown the preventive effects of retinoids on chemical- or radiation-induced carcinogenesis in various organs (Okuno et al. 2004; Mccormick et al. 1981; De Luca et al. 1996; Harisiadis et al. 1978). Retinoids have been reported to reduce second malignancies in the liver, aerodigestive tract, or breast (Hong and Sporn 1997; Sun and Lotan 2002; Freemantle et al. 2003). They have also proven effective in the treatment of certain malignancies such as APL, juvenile chronic myelogenous leukemia, mycosis fungoides, Kaposi's sarcoma, and high-risk neuroblastoma (reviewed by Cheer and Foster 2000; Reynolds and Lemons 2001). The chemopreventive and therapeutic activity of retinoids is attributed to the following: inhibition of proliferation, induction of differentiation, destruction of the cells, or imposition to senesce (Christov 2009).

Importantly, the beneficial effects of retinoids are not restricted to specific car-cinogens, but rather to the type of organs involved (Okuno et al. 2004). Thus, the exciting opportunity of the wealth of information available on the biochemical and molecular mechanisms underlying the retinoids' biological activities avails itself to alcohol–cancer research. However, alcohol-potentiating effects on retinoid toxicity create additional complexities that need to be understood. While retinoid toxicity is already a serious problem that limits retinoids' full potential use in oncology, alcohol is one of the most common aggravating factors of systemic and local vitamin A toxicity (Leo and Lieber 1999). For example, high doses of vitamin A (>100,000 IU/day) are hepatotoxic and can lead to liver cirrhosis when taken over a period of weeks or months; chronic alcohol consumption further exacerbates this intrinsic hepatotoxicity, leading to liver damage even at a low vitamin A dose of 500–10,000 IU/day, a range of doses commonly found in commercial supplements (Dan et al. 2005).

The observations that vitamin A dysregulation causes cancer and its restoration reverses neoplastic transformation have led to the hypothesis that physiological levels of retinoids guard the organism against the development of premalignant and malignant lesions (Sun and Lotan 2002). Therefore, the impairment of this guardian at systemic and local level by alcohol may underlie numerous alcohol-induced deleterious effects that are known to promote chronic organ diseases at multiple sites and increase the risk of cancer development. The mechanisms through which alcohol interferes with retinoids are extremely complex, tissue-specific, and still not fully understood. Understanding the effect of retinoids on the cellular and stromal components of individual organs in the presence of alcohol will yield useful clues for cancer prevention.

The Molecular Basis of Retinoid Action in Tumors

Vitamin A is a generic term for compounds possessing the biological activity of all-*trans*-retinol (Blomhoff and Blomhoff 2006). Structurally, vitamin A comprises a hydrophobic β-ionone ring and a conjugated isoprenoid lateral chain containing a polar group. The term "retinoids" includes both naturally occurring forms of vitamin A and many synthetic analogs of retinol (Debier and Larondelle 2005). Retinoids are essential for vision, reproduction, embryonic development, immune responses, growth and differentiation, and maintenance of the general health of the organism (Blomhoff and Blomhoff 2006). In animal tissues, different forms of vitamin A are found: retinol, retinal, retinyl esters (RE) and retinoic acid (RA). Among retinoids, RA is the most potent form and is responsible for mediating most of the nonvisual functions of this class of compounds (Kurlandsky et al. 1995). RA is a powerful regulator of gene expression, and its functions are tightly controlled at many levels by proteins involved in RA transport, metabolism, and signaling. These proteins are expressed in a unique, tissue-specific pattern and are induced by RA, which provides a feedback mechanism that regulates its cellular levels. Any exogenous or endogenous changes that unbalance the control over RA functions can lead to aberrant cellular growth and increase the risk of cancer development. Alcohol represents a serious threat to the integrity of RA system because of its numerous interferences with retinoids systemic and intracellular routes.

Retinoic Acid Production and Homeostasis

RA is a small lipophilic molecule (300 Da) derived from vitamin A and must be taken in diet in the form of retinyl esters (animal products) and carotenoids (plants), since animals cannot synthesize vitamin A. Regardless of the dietary source, retinoids

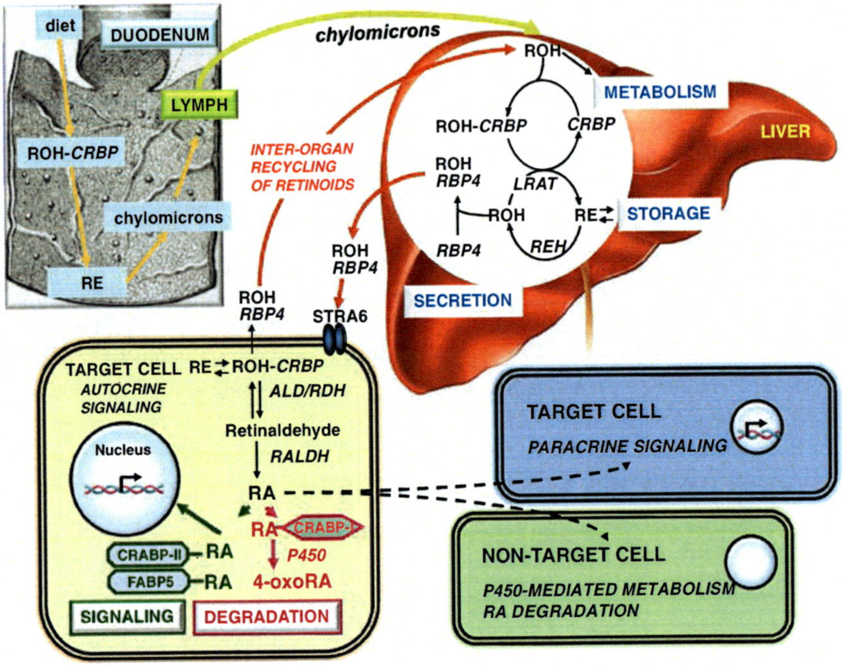

Fig. 7.2 Absorption, distribution, and metabolism of retinoids. STRA6 is the membrane receptor for the RBP4-ROH complex. *ADH* alcohol dehydrogenases, *CRABP* cellular retinoic acid-binding protein, *CRBP* cellular retinol-binding protein, *LRAT* lecithin retinol acyltransferase, *RA* retinoic acid, *RALDH* retinaldehyde dehydrogenases, *RBP4* retinol-binding protein 4, *REH* retinyl ester hydrolase, *ROH* retinol

undergo a series of metabolic conversions in the duodenum and are incorporated into chylomicrons as RE (Buletic et al. 2006) (Fig. 7.2). The chylomicrons are secreted into the lymphatic system and eventually are taken up by hepatocytes. During or shortly after uptake, the chylomicrons-derived RE are hydrolyzed and **the unesterified retinol is reesterified with long-chain fatty acids, predominantly** palmitic, stearic, and oleic acid, to form hepatic RE stores. In fact, up to 80% of the total RE in the body is stored in hepatic stellate cells (HSC) (Napoli 1996). Upon demand, RE is hydrolyzed to retinol, which is released into the bloodstream and circulates bound to serum retinol-binding protein 4 (RBP4). The concentration of **unesterified "free" retinol is tightly regulated. Kinetic studies have shown that each** molecule of retinol circulates several times between plasma and liver before undergoing irreversible disposal (Ross and Zolfaghari 2004). This recycling process provides an ideal means for the liver to constantly sample and adjust the concentration of retinol available for peripheral tissues. Animals fed diets containing a wide range **of vitamin A have nearly constant levels of circulating unesterified retinol, while RE levels are more reflective of dietary vitamin A intake. In humans, the concentra**tion of plasma retinol remained nearly constant (1.7–2 μmol/L) even as total liver retinol varied by >15-fold (Ross and Zolfaghari 2004). Retinol is taken up by target extrahepatic tissues (eye, skin, kidney, testis, lung, bone marrow, adipose tissue, brain) via interactions with the membrane receptor for RBP4, STRA6. In cells, retinoids are bound to proteins that solubilize and stabilize them in aqueous environments, thus contributing to retinoid homeostasis (metabolism, storage, and transport). Several binding proteins for retinol, retinaldehyde, and RA have been identified in vertebrates, including cellular retinol-binding proteins (CRBP), cellular RA-binding proteins (CRABP) and fatty acid binding proteins (FABP). In target cells, retinol can be either esterified by lecithin–retinol acyltransferase (LRAT) and stored as retinol esters, or converted to the biological active form all-*trans*-RA (ATRA) in a two-step reaction. The first step involves the reversible oxidation of retinol to retinaldehyde by several alcohol dehydrogenases (ADHs) and retinol dehydrogenases (RDHs) (Duester 2008). Genetic studies suggest that at least three ADHs (ADH1, ADH3, and ADH4) and two RDHs (RDH1 and RDH10) play a role in RA synthesis. The second step in RA synthesis is the irreversible oxidation of retinaldehyde to RA by several classes of cytosolic retinaldehyde dehydrogenases (RALDH1, RALDH2, RALDH3, and RALDH4), which display tissue-specific patterns of expression (Crabb et al. 2001; Napoli 1996; Lin et al. 2003; Kedishvili et al. 1997). Once synthesized, RA is sequestered in the cytoplasm by binding to CRABPI and CRABPII. While binding to CRABP II stimulates the entry of RA into the nucleus, where it activates RA-dependent transcription, binding to CRABP I reduces cellular responses to RA by promoting its degradation (Napoli et al. 1995). Degradation of RA is also an important balancing mechanism that protects cells from excessive RA stimulation (Taimi et al. 2004). It is catalyzed by at least three cytochrome P450 hydroxylases (CYP26A1, CYP26B1, and CYP26C1) that repeatedly hydroxylate RA and its metabolites into increasingly less active and readily excreted water-soluble products (Blomhoff and Blomhoff 2006). In addition to degradation, ATRA can also be isomerized into less active isoforms, 9-*cis*-RA and 13-*cis*-RA.

Once RA is formed, two general models, paracrine and autocrine, have been proposed to describe RA actions and metabolism (Fig. 7.2). In the paracrine model, RA is generated in one cell and then secreted into circulation and taken up either by target cells, where it causes pharmacological action, or by nontarget cells (that express cytochrome P450), where it is further oxidized and degraded. In the autocrine model, RA is synthesized, exerts pharmacological action, and is metabolized in the same cell (Thatcher and Isoherranen 2009). In plasma, RA circulates bound to albumin at a concentration of 1–10 nmol/L (Miano and Berk 2000). Experimental and clinical pharmacokinetic studies show peak plasma levels of RA occurring 2 h after oral administration and near-complete plasma clearance after 6 h.

Association of abnormal retinoic acid levels with carcinogenesis. Changes in RA availability due to dysregulation of retinoid metabolism and transport are associated with carcinogenesis. For example, greatly reduced levels of retinol and retinyl esters, and a corresponding aberrantly low expression of the enzyme LRAT, have been shown in a wide variety of cancers including HCC, kidney, prostate, breast, oral cavity, and skin malignancies (De Luca et al. 1984; Guo et al. 2001, 2002; Sheren-Manoff et al. 2006; Zhan et al. 2003; Hayden and Satre 2002). Methylation-silenced expression of RALDH2 (ALDH1a2) and lower RA levels are reported in prostate cancer (Kim et al. 2005). Reexpression of a wild-type gene in prostate cancer cell line DU145 resulted in decreased colony formation and inhibition of cell growth, consistent with a tumor suppressor function. Alterations in the level of CRABPs that control the actual concentration of RA in cells have also been implicated in cancer development. Overexpression of CRABP II in RA-resistant carcinoma SC115 cell line restored the cells responsiveness to RA-induced growth inhibition both in culture and in physiologically relevant models of breast cancer (Manor et al. 2003).

Retinoic Acid Interaction with Nuclear Receptors

RA acts as a signaling molecule and regulates gene expression by binding to two subclasses of nuclear receptors, retinoic acid receptors (RARα, β, and γ isotypes) and retinoid X receptors (RXRα, β and γ isotypes), encoded by distinct genes (Soprano et al. 2004). RXR and RAR form stable heterodimers required for high-affinity binding to DNA sequences, called retinoic acid response elements (RAREs) or retinoid X response elements, located within the promoter of target genes. Upon DNA binding, RXR–RAR heterodimers regulate the gene expression of RA target genes in a ligand-dependent manner. RXR is also able to form heterodimers with other nuclear receptors such as the thyroid receptor (TR), vitamin D receptor (VDR), peroxisome proliferator-activated receptor (PPAR), and several orphan receptors (Karamouzis and Papavassiliou 2005). This allows cross talk and cross-modulation of multiple signaling pathways by RA (Minucci and Pelicci 1999). The existence of six nuclear retinoid receptors whose combination leads to a complex repertoire of heterodimeric form also contributes to extremely diverse biological outcomes of retinoid action in different cell populations. Indeed, RA directs the growth and patterning of many vertebrate structures during embryogenesis, while it inhibits cellular growth during tumor progression in adulthood. An interesting clue to a possible basis for the pleiotropic action of RA has recently been provided by the observation that in cells expressing high CRABP II and low FABP5, RA activates the RAR, while in the presence of the reverse ratio, RA activates the PPARβ/δ (Schug et al. 2007) (Fig. 7.3). Remarkably, RA signaling through RAR or PPARβ/δ commits the cell to opposite fates: terminal differentiation, growth arrest, apoptosis and antitumor activity versus cell survival, proliferation, and tumor growth, respectively. These observations raise the possibility that RA resistance of some tumors may result from the targeting of RA to PPARβ/δ, rather than RAR, and that this behavior may stem from the deregulation of expression of the two RA-binding proteins, CRABP-II and FABP5 (Schug et al. 2008).

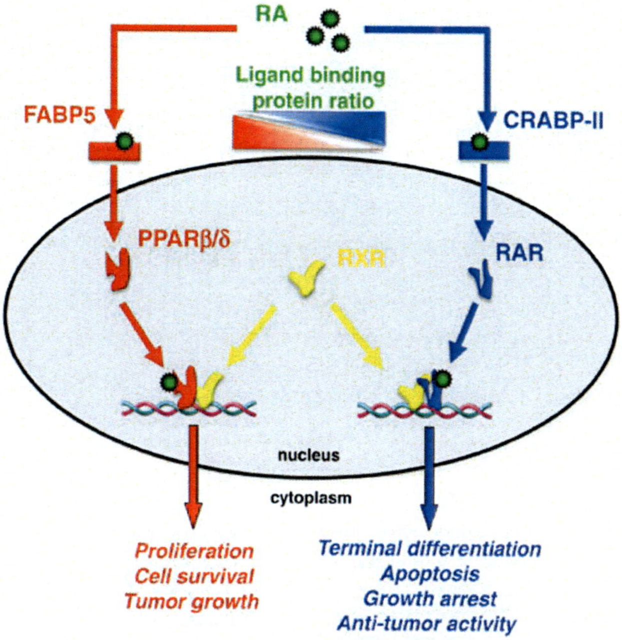

Fig. 7.3 Diverse combinations of retinoic acid nuclear receptors commit cells to opposite fates. In cells expressing high CRABP-II and low FABP5, RA activates the RAR, whereas in the presence of the reverse ratio (i.e., low CRABP-II and high FABP5), RA activates PPARβ/γ. This leads to opposite cellular outcomes: either apoptosis, growth arrest, and anticancer activity or survival, proliferation, and tumor growth, respectively. In both situations, RXR is the indispensable dimerization partner of the nuclear receptor involved. (Modified from Michalik and Wahli 2007; License Number: 2517760612919, License Agreement from Elsevier provided by CCC)

Nuclear Retinoic Acid Receptor Coregulators

The ability of retinoid receptors to modulate gene expression results from a complex and dynamic interaction with a coactivator/corepressor complex (Bastien et al. 2000). In the absence of the ligand, the RAR–RXR heterodimer is constitutively bound to DNA on RAREs and associated with the corepressor complex that induces transcriptional silencing of target genes (Fig. 7.4). Transrepression occurs through the recruitment of histone deacetylases (HDACs), which prevent the opening of chromatin, which is associated with the deacetylation of nucleosomes (Vigushin and Coombes 2004). On the contrary, RA binding induces conformational changes, releasing the corepressor and allowing recruitment of a coactivator complex with histone acetylase activity (HATs). This leads to histone acetylation and activation of transcription. The corepressors and coactivators are not exclusive to retinoid nuclear

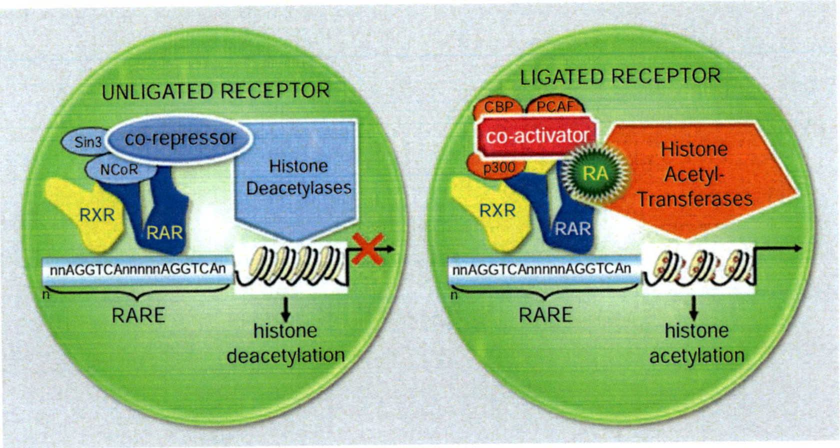

Fig. 7.4 The retinoic acid receptor regulates gene transcription by recruiting coactivators and corepressors. Unligated RAR is assembled with the corepressor complex (histone deacetylase, NCoR, Sin 3) inhibiting gene transcription. When the receptor interacts with RA, the affinity of RXR–RAR for the corepressor complex is lower than for the activator complex (p300, CBP, PCAF, histone acetyltransferase) leading to histone acetylation and gene transcription

receptors and are shared with other DNA-binding transcriptional factors, contributing to specificity in the biological responses of cells in which these regulatory elements are present.

Malfunction of Retinoic Acid Receptors in Cancer

Alterations in the level of expression or functional activity of retinoid nuclear receptors are associated with a variety of cancers despite normal vitamin A levels. The loss of RARβ expression has been associated with tumor progression and is frequently found in a variety of carcinomas such as esophageal, prostate, breast, and lung, as well as premalignant lesions, suggesting that such deregulation could represent an initiative mechanism through which tumor cells escape from normal cellular homeostasis (Lotan et al. 2000; Zhang et al. 2001; Picard et al. 1999; Albrechtsson et al. 2002; Martinet et al. 2000). While RARβ has been widely recognized as a tumor suppressor gene, a number of reports suggest that the loss of RARα and RARγ may also be important (Soprano et al. 2004). In addition, a malfunction of RXR has been observed in many tumors. Because RXR forms heterodimers with many different nuclear receptors, its alterations have a multitude of effects (Niles 2004). Upregulation of RXRγ has been observed in Barrett's esophagus and associated adenocarcinoma as well as in human thyroid carcinoma (Brabender et al. 2004;

Haugen et al. 2004), whereas decreased RXRα has been reported in non-small lung cancer (Brabender et al. 2002). Mechanistically, it was demonstrated that the conditional disruption of the RXR gene in mouse prostatic epithelium resulted in developmental and functional abnormalities as well as preneoplastic lesions, which consequently progressed to low- and high-grade prostatic intraepithelial neoplasms (Niles 2004).

The mechanism by which retinoid nuclear receptors become inactivated in cancer cells is often via epigenetic changes. Hypermethylation in the RARβ promoter has been found in 48 of 50 invasive breast cancers and in 8 of 14 ductal carcinomas in situ, but was not detected in normal breast tissue (Evron et al. 2001). In vitro treatment of breast cancer cells with demethylating agent 5-aza-2′-deoxycytidine leads to demethylation within the RARβ promoter and the reexpression of RARβ (Esteller et al. 2002; Mongan and Gudas 2007). The overwhelming correlation between the disruption of RAR signaling due to chromosomal translocations and leukemia very strongly links histone deacetylase-mediated transcription repression to the pathogenesis of leukemias (Chakraborty et al. 2001). Indeed, a reciprocal gene translocation between the RARα gene and one of several distinct gene loci, including the promyelocytic leukemia and promyelocytic zinc finger genes, rearrange gene encoding transcription factors that recruit corepressors (Collins 2008). The HDAC-inhibiting agent trichostatin-A can restore RA signaling and the terminal differentiation in the AML1-ETO leukemic cells (Wang et al. 1999).

Modes of Retinoic Acid Action

The precise mechanisms by which RA regulates biological processes is not yet fully understood, although it has become clear that RA is capable of working via multiple genomic mechanisms as well as interacting with other intracellular signaling systems, providing a basis for its extremely broad and pleiotropic actions. The effects of RA on cell growth and differentiation result primarily from its ability to regulate the expression of specific genes (Love and Gudas 1994). RA modulates the transcription of more than 500 genes through several distinct mechanisms, which include direct and indirect gene activation as well as inhibition of gene expression (Balmer and Blomhoff 2002) (Fig. 7.5).

Direct activation of RARE-containing genes. The classical cascade by which RA regulates the expression of direct target genes includes the activation of its nuclear receptors, which then bind to retinoic acid response elements (RARE) in the promoter regions of direct target genes and activate their transcription. Direct target genes encode other transcriptional factors, certain orphan receptors, and proteins involved in RA transport, metabolism, and signaling. The fact that some of the RA direct target genes are transcriptional factors adds further complexity, as these factors can subsequently regulate the expression of a certain subset of indirect target genes that are part of a cell-type-dependent differentiation program.

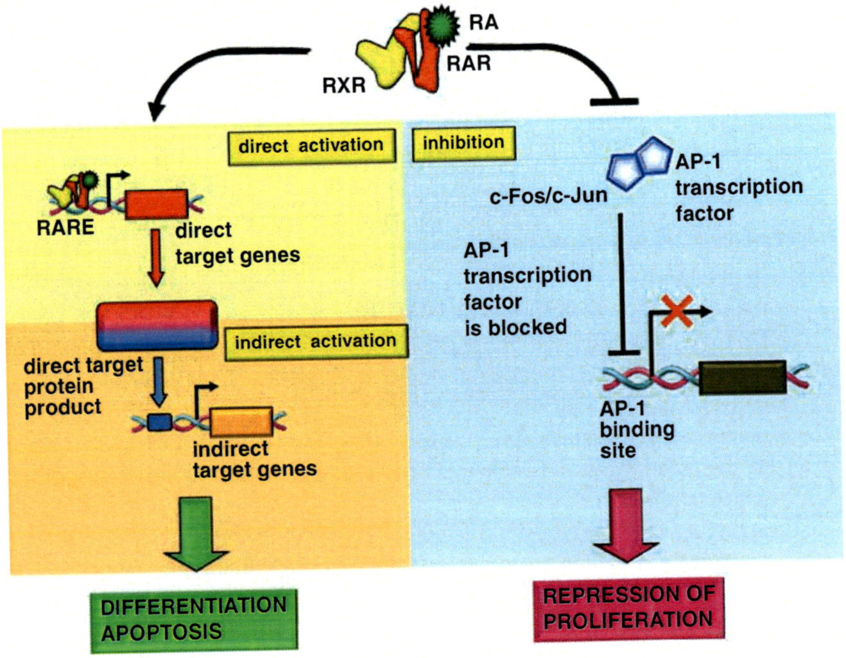

Fig. 7.5 Genomic mechanisms of RA action include (1) direct and (2) indirect gene activation as well as (3) inhibition of gene expression

Indirect gene activation through the intermediary signaling protein. The indirect target genes regulated by RA include growth factors and growth factor receptors such as the transforming growth factor β, fibroblast growth factors, epidermal growth factor, tumor necrosis factor, platelet-derived growth factor-α, interleukin-2, BMP, and hepatocyte growth factor that are expressed in a tissue-specific mode (Balmer and Blomhoff 2002). Growth factors are major growth-regulatory molecules that control the morphogenesis of many organs and the pathogenesis of a number of diseases, including cancer. The involvement of RA with such large numbers of diverse but complementary signaling pathways that control cell growth may explain why the impairment of RA signaling results in the sequence of events, which enable cells to escape normal controls of cellular proliferation (Mongan and Gudas 2007). There are no uniform responses of a particular pathway to retinoids. However, in general, it appears that retinoid-induced differentiation is accompanied by a dramatic decrease in the rate of proliferation due to direct induction of the cell cycle-regulatory genes, coordinating cell G1 arrest, and transition into differentiation (Boyle 2001). One of the central mechanisms by which RA modulates cell-cycle progression is by increasing the rate of proteolytic turnover of key regulatory proteins of the cell cycle, cyclin D1, and cyclin E (Dimberg et al. 2002; Langenfeld et al. 1997). RA also contributes to cell cycle arrest by enhancing the expression and posttranslational stability of key cyclins and cyclin-dependent kinases, including p21(waf1/cip1) and p27(kip1) (Liu et al. 1996; Zancai et al. 1998).

Inhibition of gene expression. Another genomic mechanism for the modulatory effects of RA is the transrepression of non-RARE genes. For example, retinoids exhibit antineoplastic activities through transrepression of activating protein 1 (AP-1), a heterodimeric transcriptional factor composed of protooncogenes c-Jun and c-Fos, the activity of which is often associated with cell proliferation and tumor progression (Blomhoff and Blomhoff 2006). Mechanisms proposed to explain the anti-AP1 activity of retinoids include the following: (1) both RAR/RXR and AP1 compete for limited amounts of common coactivators, such as CBP or p300 and (2) inhibition of the JNK signaling pathway (Buletic et al. 2006).

Nongenomic effects of retinoic acid. In addition to the retinoid nuclear receptor-mediated gene activation, RA can exert its effects in a "nonclassical" or "nongenomic" action. RA signaling synergizes and converges with major pathways known to regulate proliferation, differentiation, and apoptosis, such as protein kinase C, mitogen-activated protein kinase, phosphoinositide-3 kinase and Akt, cAMP, Bcl-2 family proteins, and others. For example, RA has been shown to modulate PKC activity by binding directly to the C2-domain of PKCα (Ochoa et al. 2003).

The Retinoic Acid System and Alcohol

RA regulates a complex interplay of genomic and nongenomic signaling mechanisms associated with such fundamental cellular functions as proliferation, differentiation, tumorigenesis and apoptosis, and the integrated actions of these processes have a pivotal role for tissue homeostasis and health. Alcohol interferes with RA at many levels and, therefore, has the potential to dysregulate this system, leading to aberrant growth pattern and eventually to carcinogenesis (Fig. 7.6).

Alcohol impairs retinoic acid synthesis and transport. A long-standing observation that alcoholics with cirrhosis may suffer from night blindness related to vitamin A deficiency (Patek and Haig 1939). Alcohol dramatically changes vitamin A and RA availability and thus can impact carcinogenesis. RA deficiency in alcoholics results from poor dietary intake and decreased absorption of retinoids, and the significant overlap in metabolic pathways of alcohol and retinol, the alcohol form of vitamin A. Alcohol and retinol can be oxidized by similar, and sometimes identical, enzymes. It has been reported that even social drinking (1.4 drinks) suppresses the catalytic efficiency of retinol oxidation by 73% in hepatic cytosol, resulting in the significant inhibition of RA synthesis (Parlesak et al. 2000). In addition to the competitive inhibition of RA biosynthesis, prolonged ethanol consumption decreases tissue RA concentrations by enhancing its catabolism through the induction of cytochrome P450 enzymes and increasing mobilization of retinoids from the liver to extrahepatic tissues (Leo and Lieber 1999; Liu et al. 2001; Wang 2005). As a result, alcohol profoundly depletes hepatic retinoids and alters their distribution in other tissues (Mobarhan et al. 1991). Rats fed alcohol for 4–6 weeks showed 60% decline in hepatic vitamin A levels (Lieber 2003), which became severe (72%) after 7–9 weeks

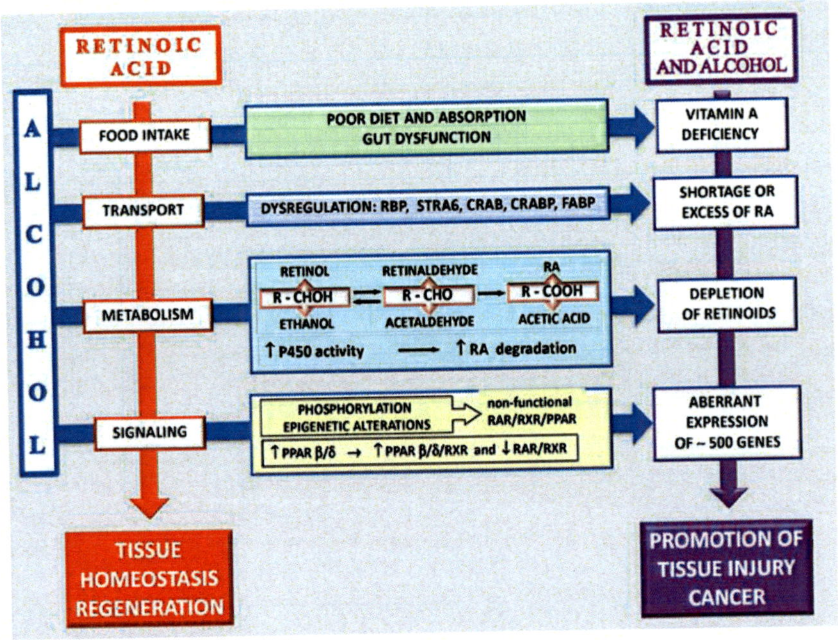

Fig. 7.6 Alcohol interferes with RA at many levels and can dysregulate this system, leading to multiorgan pathology and carcinogenesis. Alcohol consumption is commonly associated with a poor diet, gut dysfunction, and deficiency of vitamin A, the RA precursor. Ethanol and retinol share chemical similarities and can be oxidized by similar, and sometimes the same, enzymes. Thus, the presence of ethanol has the potential to inhibit the RA synthesis by substrate competition. Chronic ethanol consumption also induces P450 enzymes that in turn increase RA degradation. In addition, ethanol changes the expression of proteins involved in RA transport and signaling, leading to an unbalanced cell differentiation and proliferation and increasing the likelihood of cancer

of alcohol administration. At the same time, levels of vitamin A in the esophagus and colon were elevated. In alcoholics with oropharyngeal cancer, a normal retinoid concentration was found in oral mucosa adjacent to malignant tissue (Leo et al. 1995). In an epidemiologic study, the increased risk of cancer associated with cigarettes and alcohol was also enhanced with ingestion of foods containing retinol (Graham et al. 1990). It has been suggested that tissue-specific increases in Stra6 and CrbpI expression during alcohol administration may underlie a site-specific elevation of retinoids (Kane et al. 2010). Similarly, both marginal excess or shortage of RA due to alcohol during development caused numerous embryonic malformations such as cleft palate, neural tube defects, and limb and facial malformations (similar to those observed in FAS children), emphasizing the importance of physiological levels of retinoids for proper embryonic development (Yelin et al. 2007; Marrs et al. 2009; Kane et al. 2010). In addition to directly affecting RA metabolism and transport, alcohol may also affect plasma retinol concentration and its organ distribution indirectly through LPS-induced inflammation that reduces the level of RBP mRNA in the liver, resulting in the impairment of the transport of retinol from the liver to plasma (Rosales et al. 1996).

Retinoic acid signaling and alcohol. Alcohol affects the expression and activation of RA receptors, which in turn can impair the signaling events and induce harmful effects on cell survival and differentiation (Kumar et al. 2010). Recent developments indicate that ethanol induces epigenetic alterations, particularly acetylation, methylation of histones and hypo- and hypermethylation of DNA, and thus can contribute to the aberrancy of retinoid nuclear receptor function and increased risk of cancer development (Shukla and Aroor 2006; Shukla et al. 2008). Also, alcohol may promote mitogenic responses and survival pathways through the upregulation of PPARβ/δ and FABP5 (Pang et al. 2009; Westerbacka et al. 2007), which would favor the formation of PPARβ/δ/RXR rather than RAR/RXR.

A great gap still exists in our knowledge concerning the organ-specific effects of alcohol on RA availability, the function of each component of its signaling and RA interactions with the common intracellular pathways.

Retinoic Acid Promotes Nongenotoxic Alcohol-Related Carcinogenesis

Carcinogenesis promoted by nongenotoxic carcinogens such as alcohol is closely related to the continuous cycles of tissue injury and repair driven by interactions between many different cell types and, therefore, depend on cell-to-cell communication via signaling factors such as cytokines and growth factors (Roberts and Kimber 1999; Stickel et al. 2002). RA influences these processes, as it controls cell proliferation-or-differentiation decisions, exerts its effects on cells of different origin (e.g., epithelial, stromal, and inflammatory), and acts both as an autocrine and paracrine factor. Therefore, the dysregulation of RA signaling would have dramatic impact on tissue regenerative responses. Interestingly, changes in gene expression in initiated cells either due to mutations or non-DNA related stimulations can themselves impair RA signaling, which in turn would further amplify the aberrancy of initiated cells, leading to neoplastic transformation and cancer. For example, mutations in the tumor suppressor gene adenomatous polyposis coli (APC), which underlie the earliest stages of colorectal carcinogenesis, result in RA signaling deficiencies through two independent mechanisms that involve impaired RA biosynthesis and enhanced RA catabolism. Specifically, retinol dehydrogenases (RDHs) were found to be reduced in human colon adenomas and adenocarcinomas carrying mutated APC. The introduction of wild type APC into colon tumor cells increased cellular RA production by promoting degradation of the transcriptional corepressor C-terminal binding protein-1 (CtBP1), thereby allowing expression of intestinal RDHs, which are required for retinoic acid production and intestinal differentiation (Nadauld et al. 2005, 2006). In addition, increased expression of CYP26A1, the major retinoic acid-metabolizing cytochrome P450 enzyme in the intestine, occurs as a direct consequence of mutations in APC (Shelton et al. 2006). The loss of RA production in APC mutants leads to consequences such as the stabilization and accumulation of β-catenin, dysregulation of cyclooxygenase-2 (COX-2) expression, and the uncontrolled activation of cell proliferation programs (Eisinger et al. 2007).

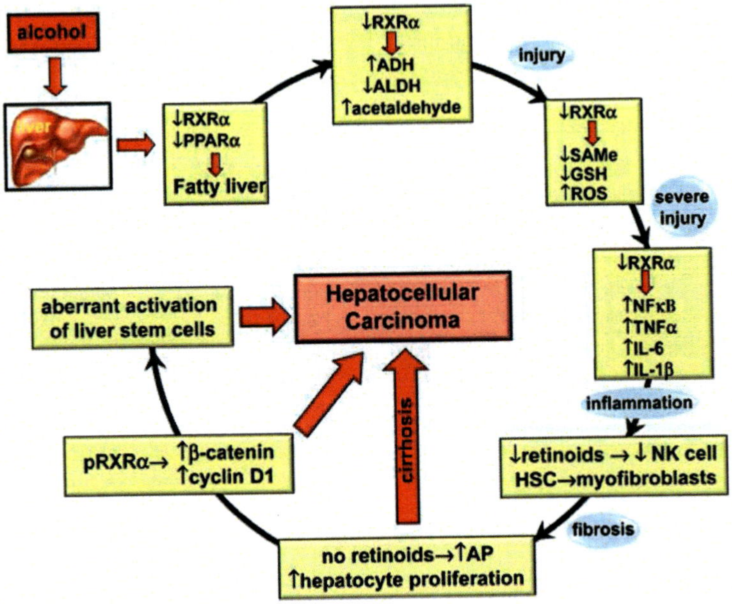

Fig. 7.7 RA promotes the evolution of early, curable stages of alcohol-induced tissue injury to irreversible end-stage disease and cancer

In the case of alcohol consumption, cellular hyperproliferation at early stages of colorectal carcinogenesis was thought to be related to acetaldehyde-induced cell injury, as acetaldehyde and crypt cell production rates showed a significant positive correlation (Simanowski et al. 2001). However, this important alteration in cell cycle behavior could also be due to RA deficiency, and acetaldehyde may contribute by preventing its generation (Seitz 2000; Simanowski et al. 2001). In fact, alcohol in the concentration range that results from the consumption of 1–2 drinks by an adult markedly impairs acute intracellular RA formation by inhibiting cytosolic retinol oxidation in colon (Parlesak et al. 2000). Thus, emerging data indicate that alcohol-induced impaired RA signaling should be considered a new promoting factor in alcohol-associated carcinogenesis that has the potential to induce defects in cell terminal differentiation, growth control, and programmed cell death, thereby increasing the likelihood of cancer.

Retinoic Acid Signaling, Alcohol, and Hepatocarcinogenesis

The liver can provide an interesting example of how the multilayered involvement of RA signaling in pathophysiological processes can promote the evolution of early, curable stages of alcohol-induced tissue injury to irreversible end-stage disease and cancer (Fig. 7.7).

Normal liver. In the adult liver, expression of different RA signaling components is dependent on cell type and organ physiology. Hepatocytes throughout the liver parenchyma express Crbp, Raldh2, RARs, and RXRs, whereas the key catabolic P450 enzyme is expressed almost exclusively by hepatocytes located in the centrilobular zone (Zhai et al. 2001; Wojcik et al. 1988; Shin et al. 2002). HSC cells constantly express Crbp, Raldh1, RARs, and RXRs and are capable of the induction of Raldh2 and production of RA in response to liver injury (Zhai et al. 2001; Radaeva et al. 2007). The higher density of HSC in the periportal zone of the liver lobule, in contrast to the location of P450 enzymes in hepatocytes near central vein, suggests the opposite distribution of catabolic and synthetic enzymes of the RA metabolic pathway and, therefore, the gradient in the RA concentration in the adult liver.

Early stages of ALD. The first signs of the involvement of the dysregulated RA pathway can be traced to fatty liver, an early stage of ALD, which is associated with deranged fatty acid metabolism, severe free fatty acid (FFA) overload and increased synthesis of triacylglycerol. Under normal conditions, RA cooperates with FFA and its metabolites to maintain lipid homeostasis by regulating heterodimer PPAR/RXR activation (Villarroya et al. 2004). However, alcohol reduces PPARα activity and RXRα protein levels as well as the ability of PPARα/RXRα heterodimers to bind to DNA (Fischer et al. 2003; Galli et al. 2001; Mello et al. 2009), resulting in impaired FFA catabolism, which promotes the development of alcoholic fatty liver. This effect of alcohol is abolished by alcohol dehydrogenase inhibitor 4-methylpyrazole and augmented by the aldehyde dehydrogenase inhibitor cyanamide, indicating that acetaldehyde is responsible for the action of alcohol (Galli et al. 2001).

RXRα is also involved in many other aspects of the development of ALD, ranging from alcohol metabolism and inflammatory responses to mitogenesis, and therefore, its loss may play a crucial role in the induction of severe alcoholic hepatic injury and cancer. RXRα occupies such unique position, based upon its ability to form obligate heterodimers with a variety of physiologically important partners, such as PPARs, β-catenin, and others (Altucci et al. 2007). For example, targeted deletion of RXRα gene in hepatocytes leads to the dysfunction of enzymes participating in cholesterol, FFA, steroids, and xenobiotics metabolism (Wan et al. 2000). Mice with RXRα-deficient hepatocytes fed a high-fat diet showed upregulation of adipogenic (Cebpb, Srebf1), apoptotic (Gzmb, Bcl_2), and proinflammatory (NFκB, TNFα) gene expression, while angiogenic (Nos3, Kdr) gene expression was downregulated (Razny et al. 2009; Wan et al. 2003). While the molecular mechanisms of gene regulation by RXRα remain to be established, experiments with RXRs knockout mice fed alcohol-containing diet demonstrate its unique modulatory and integrative roles across multiple metabolic and pathophysiological pathways in liver diseases. First, RXRα controls alcohol oxidation. Hepatocyte RXRα deficiency in mice leads to the induction of alcohol dehydrogenase activity and to the reduction of aldehyde dehydrogenase, resulting in acetaldehyde accumulation and the sensitizing of the mice to alcohol-induced damage (Gyamfi et al. 2006). Since RXRα regulates the expression of many xenochemical enzymes of the cytochrome P450 family and the synthesis of universal methyl donor *S*-adenosylmethionine (SAMe) and antioxidant glutathione (GSH), RXRα downregulation by alcohol reduces the production of key hepatoprotective agents against lipid peroxidation and oxidative stress, and also induces aberrant DNA methylation patterns frequently encountered in cancers (Dai et al. 2003; Lieber 2000). In addition, deficiency in RXRα results in the elevation of proinflammatory cytokines production that further predisposes the liver to chronic inflammation, which is a risk factor for cancer development (Gyamfi et al. 2008). Hepatocytes from alcohol-fed RXRα-deficient mice show increased NFκB activation and a robust induction of hepatic mRNA levels of IL-6, IL-1β, TNFα, and macrophage inflammatory protein (MIP)-2. Interestingly, the loss of RXRα represents a common mechanism that persists in early pathologic changes, precarcinogenic growth, and cancer. Consequently, decreased RXRα gene expression was found in the early stages of hepatocarcinogenesis in both precancerous lesions of HCC, preneoplastic foci and nodules, as well as in adenoma and HCC (Nagao et al. 1998; Ando et al. 2007). It has been suggested that downregulation of the retinoid receptors causes an increase in the free levels of their heterodimeric partner β-catenin, activates the β-catenin/Wnt signaling, overexpresses the cyclin D1 protein, and thus contributes to liver carcinogenesis.

Fibrogenesis and innate immunity. Alcohol ultimately induces tissue injury that simultaneously activates the innate immune system, tissue repair, and remodeling responses, the highly balanced contributions of which are necessary to restore organ integrity and function. Liver repair and regeneration following hepatic tissue injury can normally restore organ homeostasis. However, alcohol is known to impair liver regeneration by inhibiting insulin signaling, inducing fibrogenic response through activating HSC, and compromising innate immune reaction through the inhibition and reduction of the natural killer (NK) cells (de la Monte et al. 2008; Ohata et al. 1997; Radaeva et al. 2006). Retinoids play an important role in hepatic stromal tissue homeostasis/remodeling through their effects on HSC. The loss of cellular vitamin A in HSC correlates with their activation and transdifferentiation into myofibroblasts, which results in fibrosis. In vitro or in vivo administration of retinoids prevents the morphological transition of HSC into myofibroblasts and inhibits the progression of experimentally induced hepatic fibrosis (Hellemans et al. 1999). Moreover, several lines of evidence suggest that RA might be an important endogenous mechanism that controls dynamic reciprocal interactions among different cells responsible for consequences in normal tissue homeostasis or excessive scarring (Blomhoff and Wake 1991; Okuno et al. 1999; Friedman et al. 2007). Specifically, RA, endogenously produced by HSC during early stages of activation, induces these cells to express of the NK cell ligand retinoic acid early transcript 1 (Raet1), which subsequently initiates NK cell-mediated cytotoxicity against these cells in vitro and in vivo (Radaeva et al. 2007). By contrast, chronically activated HSC or myofibroblasts (that lost their cytoplasmic retinol and cannot produce RA) became nonresponsive to RA and resistant to NK cells killing. This RA-driven mechanism can affect the rate of tissue repair and the degree of fibrosis. At initial stages of tissue injury, endogenous RA signaling in repair-mediating cells through selective upregulation of Raet1 stimulates the innate immune system to control inflammation and promote cellular repair, while in later stages RA signaling downregulation may contribute to the progression to chronic disease and fibrosis. Indeed, in rats with low hepatic retinoid levels, CCl_4-induced liver fibrosis was more pronounced than in rats with sufficient hepatic retinoid levels (Seifert et al. 1994).

Cirrhosis and HCC. Hepatic retinoid level reduction by alcohol can lead to enhanced fibrogenesis that, in turn, may eventually constitute an irreversible process with regenerative diffuse parenchymal nodular transformation, cirrhosis, and HCC. Alcohol-related HCCs are associated with cirrhosis in a majority of cases, indicating that the pathological events leading to cirrhosis precede those causing cancer, or that the structural alterations of cirrhosis favor hepatocyte dedifferentiation (Stickel et al. 2002). Since dedifferentiation is ultimately associated with increased proliferation rate, the dedifferentiation hypothesis fits perfectly with findings that low hepatic RA concentration due to alcohol leads to an upregulation of AP-1 (c-jun and c-fos) gene expression that may promote proliferation and malignant transformation of hepatocytes by alcohol (Wang et al. 1998; Wang 2005). Supplementation of animals with ATRA to normal RA levels dramatically decreases c-Jun gene expression and AP-1 DNA-binding activities as well as normalizing hepatocyte proliferation (Chung et al. 2001).

Liver stem cells and HCC. Interestingly, alcohol-induced RA-dependent hepatocyte hyperproliferation may not only lead to the neoplastic transformation of preexisting hepatocytes but also compromise organ regeneration by liver stem cells. The activation of liver stem cells requires a uniform inhibition of parenchymal proliferation (Fausto and Campbell 2003), and their differentiation depends on RA. In contrast to its antiproliferative effect on fully differentiated hepatocytes, RA exerts two apparently opposing effects, namely, differentiation and proapoptotic effects, in fetal hepatocytes, the precursors of adult liver stem cells (Shiojiri et al. 1991). These effects are linked to the inhibition of cyclin D1-cdk4 and to the reduction of both c-myc and Bcl-2 (Alisi et al. 2003). The electron-microscopic studies suggest that RA plays an important role in regulating terminal hepatic differentiation. The appearance of specific morphological features of hepatocytes, including smooth endoplasmic reticulum, glycogen particles, and bile canaliculi, coincides with peak RA levels (Makita et al. 2005) and RA-dependent erythropoiesis in the fetal mouse liver. It is interesting to note that liver stem cells are highly responsive to vitamin A deprivation (Hu et al. 1994) and always appear in close proximity to activated HSC, suggesting a possible involvement of RA in control of their behavior. Deficiency of RA in alcoholic livers blocks differentiation and apoptosis in the progeny of liver stem cells, while promoting their proliferation. This may explain the development of anaplastic poorly differentiated HCCs without preexisting cirrhosis, which are also observed in alcoholics, albeit rarely (Kuper et al. 2001; Fattovich et al. 2004).

The presence of several retinoid-containing cell types that apparently possess a cell-specific mode of RA action in the liver, as well as the existence of a local gradient in RA availability due to the opposite distribution of catabolic and synthetic enzymes throughout the liver lobule, add further complexity to RA-signaling. In addition, investigation of cross talks between retinoid signaling and other factors known to elicit hepatocarcinogenesis and alcohol-related pathogenesis will provide further insight into the mechanism of ALD progression to chronicity and cancer.

Retinoic acid and organ interactions in alcohol-induced pathogenesis. Hepatic retinoid metabolism is closely intergrated with that in peripheral tissue through rapid inter-organ transfer and recycling. Alcohol-induced depletion of retinoids in the liver affects retinoids partitioning and disturbs whole-body retinoid homeostasis. This could provide important mechanisms by which alcohol-induced pathology in one organ influences the functioning of other organs, leading to the multiple organ dysfunctions often observed in alcohol abuse. For example, it has been shown that cirrhotic rats develop numerous degenerative changes and hyperproliferation in the interstinal mucosa compared to control animals (Ramachandran et al. 2002; Natarajan et al. 2006). These changes were due to altered retinoid metabolism in the intestine of cirrhotic rats. A decrease in the levels of retinal, retinoic acid, and retinol was evident in the intestine by 3 months, when liver cirrhosis was evident histologically, and these remained low until 6 months. A decrease in the activities of retinaldehyde oxidase, retinaldehyde reductase, and retinol dehydrogenase was also seen in intestine from cirrhotic rats (Natarajan et al. 2009).

Although much has been learned about the interactions between RA and receptors at transcriptional regulatory sites, knowledge of downstream dynamic changes leading cells to cancer is limited. Understanding the effects of RA in the presence of alcohol represents an even greater challenge, because of their overlap at many levels of regulation when many intermediate molecules are involved. Investigations incorporating advanced technologies of genomics, proteomics, and computational biology would help to understand the role of RA in alcohol-induced malignancy.

References

Albrechtsson E, Ohlsson B, Axelson J (2002) The expression of retinoic acid receptors and the effects in vitro by retinoids in human pancreatic cancer cell lines. Pancreas 25:49–56.

Alisi A, Leoni S, Piacentani A, Conti Devirgiliis L (2003) Retinoic acid modulates the cell-cycle in fetal rat hepatocytes and HepG2 cells by regulating cyclin-cdk activities. Liver Int 23:179–86.

Altucci L, Leibowitz MD, Ogilvie KM, de Lera AR, Gronemeyer H (2007) RAR and RXR modulation in cancer and metabolic disease. Nat Rev Drug Discov 6:793–810.

Ando N, Shimizu M, Okuno M, Matsushima-Nishiwaki R, Tsurumi H, Tanaka T, Moriwaki H (2007) Expression of retinoid X receptor alpha is decreased in 3′-methyl-4-dimethylaminoazobenzene-induced hepatocellular carcinoma in rats. Oncol Rep 18:879–84.

Balmer JE, Blomhoff R (2002) Gene expression regulation by retinoic acid. J Lipid Res 43:1773–808.

Bastien J, Adam-Stitah S, Riedl T, Egly JM, Chambon P, Rochette-Egly C (2000) TFIIH interacts with the retinoic acid receptor gamma and phosphorylates its AF-1-activating domain through cdk7. J Biol Chem 275:21896–904.

Blomhoff R, Blomhoff HK (2006) Overview of retinoid metabolism and function. J Neurobiol 66:606–30.

Blomhoff R, Wake K (1991) Perisinusoidal stellate cells of the liver: important roles in retinol metabolism and fibrosis. FASEB J 5:271–7.
Bogos K, Renyi-Vamos F, Kovacs G, Tovari J, Dome B (2008) Role of retinoic receptors in lung carcinogenesis. J Exp Clin Cancer Res 27:18.
Boyle JO (2001) Retinoid mechanisms and cyclins. Curr Oncol Rep 3:301–5.
Brabender J, Danenberg KD, Metzger R, Schneider PM, Lord RV, Groshen S, Tsao-Wei DD, Park J, Salonga D, Hölscher AH, Danenberg PV (2002) The role of retinoid X receptor messenger RNA expression in curatively resected non-small cell lung cancer. Clin Cancer Res 8:438–43.
Brabender J, Lord RV, Metzger R, Park J, Salonga D, Danenberg KD, Hölscher AH, Danenberg PV, Schneider PM (2004) Role of retinoid X receptor mRNA expression in Barrett's esophagus. J Gastrointest Surg 8:413–22.
Breitkopf K, Nagy LE, Beier JI, Mueller S, Weng H, Dooley S (2009) Current experimental perspectives on the clinical progression of alcoholic liver disease. Alcohol Clin Exp Res 33:1647–55.
Brembeck FH, Kaiser A, Detjen K, Hotz H, Foitzik T, Buhr HJ, Riecken EO, Rosewicz S (1998) Retinoic acid receptor alpha mediates growth inhibition by retinoids in rat pancreatic carcinoma DSL-6A/C1 cells. Br J Cancer 78:1288–95.
Buletic Z, Soprano KJ, Soprano DR (2006) Retinoid targets for the treatment of cancer. Crit Rev Eukaryot Gene Expr 16:193–210.
Chakraborty S, Senyuk V, Nucifora G (2001) Genetic lesions and perturbation of chromatin architecture: a road to cell transformation. J Cell Biochem 82:310–25.
Cheer SM, Foster RH (2000) Alitretinoin. Am J Clin Dermatol 1:307–14.
Christov K (2009) To kill tumor cells or permanently paralyze them in senescence? J BUON 14:189–96.
Chung J, Liu C, Smith DE, Seitz HK, Russell RM, Wang XD (2001) Restoration of retinoic acid concentration suppresses ethanol-enhanced c-Jun expression and hepatocyte proliferation in rat liver. Carcinogenesis. 22:1213–9.
Collins SJ (2008) Retinoic acid receptors, hematopoiesis and leukemogenesis. Curr Opin Hematol 15:346–51.
Crabb DW, Pinairs J, Hasanadka R, Fang M, Leo MA, Lieber CS, Tsukamoto H, Motomura K, Miyahara T, Ohata M, Bosron W, Sanghani S, Kedishvili N, Shiraishi H, Yokoyama H, Miyagi M, Ishii H, Bergheim I, Menzl I, Parlesak A, Bode C (2001) Alcohol and retinoids. Alcohol Clin Exp Res 25:207S-217S.
Dai T, Wu Y, Leng AS, Ao Y, Robel RC, Lu SC, French SW, Wan YJ (2003) RXRalpha-regulated liver SAMe and GSH levels influence susceptibility to alcohol-induced hepatotoxicity. Exp Mol Pathol 75:194–200.
Dan Z, Popov Y, Patsenker E, Preimel D, Liu C, Wang XD, Seitz HK, Schuppan D, Stickel F (2005) Hepatotoxicity of alcohol-induced polar retinol metabolites involves apoptosis via loss of mitochondrial membrane potential. FASEB J 19:845–7.
de la Monte SM, Yeon JE, Tong M, Longato L, Chaudhry R, Pang MY, Duan K, Wands JR (2008) Insulin resistance in experimental alcohol-induced liver disease. J Gastroenterol Hepatol 23:e477-86.
De Luca LM, Brugh M, Silverman-Jones CS (1984) Retinyl palmitate, retinyl phosphate, and dolichyl phosphate of postnuclear membrane fraction from hepatoma, host liver, and regenerating liver: marginal vitamin A status of hepatoma tissue. Cancer Res 44:224–32.
De Luca LM, Tarone R, Huynh M, Jones CS, Chen LC (1996) Dietary retinoic acid inhibits mouse skin carcinogenesis irrespective of age at initiation. Nutr Cancer 25:249–57.
Debier C, Larondelle Y (2005) Vitamins A and E: metabolism, roles and transfer to offspring. Br J Nutr 93:153–74.
Dimberg A, Bahram F, Karlberg I, Larsson LG, Nilsson K, Oberg F (2002) Retinoic acid-induced cell cycle arrest of human myeloid cell lines is associated with sequential down-regulation of c-Myc and cyclin E and posttranscriptional up-regulation of p27(Kip1). Blood 99:2199–206.
Duester G (2008) Retinoic acid synthesis and signaling during early organogenesis. Cell 134:921–31.

Eisinger AL, Nadauld LD, Shelton DN, Prescott SM, Stafforini DM, Jones DA (2007) Retinoic acid inhibits beta-catenin through suppression of Cox-2: a role for truncated adenomatous polyposis coli. J Biol Chem 282:29394–400.
El-Metwally TH, Pour PM (2007) The retinoid induced pancreatic cancer redifferentiation-apoptosis sequence and the mitochondria: a suggested obligatory sequence of events. JOP 8:268–78.
Esteller M, Guo M, Moreno V, Peinado MA, Capella G, Galm O, Baylin SB, Herman JG (2002) Hypermethylation-associated Inactivation of the Cellular Retinol-Binding-Protein 1 Gene in Human Cancer. Cancer Res 62:5902–5.
Evron E, Dooley WC, Umbricht CB, Rosenthal D, Sacchi N, Gabrielson E, Soito AB, Hung DT, Ljung B, Davidson NE, Sukumar S (2001) Detection of breast cancer cells in ductal lavage fluid by methylation-specific PCR. Lancet 357:1335–6.
Fattovich G, Stroffolini T, Zagni I, Donato F (2004) Hepatocellular carcinoma in cirrhosis: incidence and risk factors. Gastroenterology 127:S35-50.
Fausto N, Campbell JS (2003) The role of hepatocytes and oval cells in liver regeneration and repopulation. Mech Dev 120:117–30.
Fischer M, You M, Matsumoto M, Crabb DW (2003) Peroxisome proliferator-activated receptor alpha (PPARalpha) agonist treatment reverses PPARalpha dysfunction and abnormalities in hepatic lipid metabolism in ethanol-fed mice. J Biol Chem 278:27997–8004.
Freemantle SJ, Spinella MJ, Dmitrovsky E (2003) Retinoids in cancer therapy and chemoprevention: promise meets resistance. Oncogene 22:7305–15.
Friedman SL, Rockey DC, Bissell DM (2007) Hepatic fibrosis 2006: report of the Third AASLD Single Topic Conference. Hepatology 45:242–9.
Galli A, Pinaire J, Fischer M, Dorris R, Crabb DW (2001) The transcriptional and DNA binding activity of peroxisome proliferator-activated receptor alpha is inhibited by ethanol metabolism. A novel mechanism for the development of ethanol-induced fatty liver. J Biol Chem 276:68–75.
Graham S, Marshall J, Haughey B, Brasure J, Freudenheim J, Zielezny M, Wilkinson G, Nolan J (1990) Nutritional epidemiology of cancer of the esophagus. Am J Epidemiol 131:454–67.
Gudas LJ (1992) Retinoids, retinoid-responsive genes, cell differentiation, and cancer. Cell Growth Differ 3:655–62.
Guo X, Knudsen BS, Peehl DM, Ruiz A, Bok D, Rando RR, Rhim JS, Nanus DM, Gudas LJ (2002) Retinol metabolism and lecithin:retinol acyltransferase levels are reduced in cultured human prostate cancer cells and tissue specimens. Cancer Res 62:1654–61.
Guo X, Nanus DM, Ruiz A, Rando RR, Bok D, Gudas LJ (2001) Reduced levels of retinyl esters and vitamin A in human renal cancers. Cancer Res 61:2774–81.
Gyamfi MA, He L, French SW, Damjanov I, Wan YJ (2008) Hepatocyte retinoid X receptor alpha-dependent regulation of lipid homeostasis and inflammatory cytokine expression contributes to alcohol-induced liver injury. J Pharmacol Exp Ther 324:443–53.
Gyamfi MA, Kocsis MG, He L, Dai G, Mendy AJ, Wan YJ (2006) The role of retinoid X receptor alpha in regulating alcohol metabolism. J Pharmacol Exp Ther 319:360–8.
Harisiadis L, Miller RC, Hall EJ, Borek C (1978) A vitamin A analogue inhibits radiation-induced oncogenic transformation. Nature 274:486–7.
Harris H (2004) Tumour suppression: putting on the brakes. Nature 427:201.
Haugen BR, Larson LL, Pugazhenthi U, Hays WR, Klopper JP, Kramer CA, Sharma V (2004) Retinoic acid and retinoid X receptors are differentially expressed in thyroid cancer and thyroid carcinoma cell lines and predict response to treatment with retinoids. J Clin Endocrinol Metab 89:272–80.
Hayden LJ, Satre MA (2002) Alterations in cellular retinol metabolism contribute to differential retinoid responsiveness in normal human mammary epithelial cells versus breast cancer cells. Breast Cancer Res Treat 72:95–105.
Hellemans K, Grinko I, Rombouts K, Schuppan D, Geerts A (1999) All-trans and 9-cis retinoic acid alter rat hepatic stellate cell phenotype differentially. Gut 45:134–42.
Higuchi E, Chandraratna RA, Hong WK, Lotan R (2003) Induction of TIG3, a putative class II tumor suppressor gene, by retinoic acid in head and neck and lung carcinoma cells and its association with suppression of the transformed phenotype. Oncogene 22:4627–35.

Hong WK, Sporn MB (1997) Recent advances in chemoprevention of cancer. Science 278:1073–7.
Hu Z, Fujio K, Marsden ER, Thorgeirsson SS, Evarts RP (1994) Hepatic regeneration in vitamin A-deficient rats: changes in the expression of transforming growth factor alpha/epidermal growth factor receptor and retinoic acid receptors alpha and beta. Cell Growth Differ 5:503–8.
Jaster R, Hilgendorf I, Fitzner B, Brock P, Sparmann G, Emmrich J, Liebe S (2003) Regulation of pancreatic stellate cell function in vitro: biological and molecular effects of all-trans retinoic acid. Biochem Pharmacol 66:633–41.
Kane MA, Folias AE, Wang C, Napoli JL (2010) Ethanol elevates physiological all-trans-retinoic acid levels in select loci through altering retinoid metabolism in multiple loci: a potential mechanism of ethanol toxicity. FASEB J 24:823–32.
Karamouzis MV, Papavassiliou AG (2005) Retinoid receptor cross-talk in respiratory epithelium cancer chemoprevention. Trends Mol Med 11:10–6.
Kedishvili NY, Gough WH, Chernoff EA, Hurley TD, Stone CL, Bowman KD, Popov KM, Bosron WF, Li TK (1997) cDNA sequence and catalytic properties of a chick embryo alcohol dehydrogenase that oxidizes retinol and 3beta,5alpha-hydroxysteroids. J Biol Chem 272:7494–500.
Kim H, Lapointe J, Kaygusuz G, Ong DE, Li C, van de Rijn M, Brooks JD, Pollack JR (2005) The retinoic acid synthesis gene ALDH1a2 is a candidate tumor suppressor in prostate cancer. Cancer Res 65:8118–24.
Kumar A, Singh CK, DiPette DD, Singh US (2010) Ethanol impairs activation of retinoic acid receptors in cerebellar granule cells in a rodent model of fetal alcohol spectrum disorders. Alcohol Clin Exp Res 34(5):928–37.
Kuper H, Ye W, Broomé U, Romelsjö A, Mucci LA, Ekbom A, Adami HO, Trichopoulos D, Nyrén O (2001) The risk of liver and bile duct cancer in patients with chronic viral hepatitis, alcoholism, or cirrhosis. Hepatology 34:714–8.
Kurebayashi J, Tanaka K, Otsuki T, Moriya T, Kunisue H, Uno M, Sonoo H (2000) All-trans-retinoic acid modulates expression levels of thyroglobulin and cytokines in a new human poorly differentiated papillary thyroid carcinoma cell line, KTC-1. J Clin Endocrinol Metab 85:2889–96.
Kurlandsky SB, Gamble MV, Ramakrishnan R, Blaner WS (1995) Plasma delivery of retinoic acid to tissues in the rat. J Biol Chem 270:17850–7.
Langenfeld J, Kiyokawa H, Sekula D, Boyle J, Dmitrovsky E (1997) Posttranslational regulation of cyclin D1 by retinoic acid: a chemoprevention mechanism. Proc Natl Acad Sci U S A 94:12070–4.
Lasnitzki I (1955) The influence of A hypervitaminosis on the effect of 20-methylcholanthrene on mouse prostate glands grown in vitro. Br J Cancer 9:434–41.
Leo MA, Lieber CS (1999) Alcohol, vitamin A, and beta-carotene: adverse interactions, including hepatotoxicity and carcinogenicity. Am J Clin Nutr 69:1071–85.
Leo MA, Seitz HK, Maier H, Lieber CS (1995) Carotenoid, retinoid and vitamin E status of the oropharyngeal mucosa in the alcoholic. Alcohol Alcohol 30:163–70.
Lieber CS (2000) Alcoholic liver disease: new insights in pathogenesis lead to new treatments. J Hepatol 32:113–28.
Lieber CS (2003) Relationships between nutrition, alcohol use, and liver disease. Alcohol Res Health 27:220–31.
Lin M, Zhang M, Abraham M, Smith SM, Napoli JL (2003) Mouse retinal dehydrogenase 4 (RALDH4), molecular cloning, cellular expression, and activity in 9-cis-retinoic acid biosynthesis in intact cells. J Biol Chem 278:9856–61.
Liu M, Iavarone A, Freedman LP (1996) Transcriptional activation of the human p21(WAF1/CIP1) gene by retinoic acid receptor. Correlation with retinoid induction of U937 cell differentiation. J Biol Chem 271:31723–8.
Liu C, Russell RM, Seitz HK, Wang XD (2001) Ethanol enhances retinoic acid metabolism into polar metabolites in rat liver via induction of cytochrome P4502E1. Gastroenterology 120:179–89.
Lotan R (1996) Retinoids in cancer chemoprevention. FASEB J 10:1031–9.

Lotan Y, Xu XC, Shalev M, Lotan R, Williams R, Wheeler TM, Thompson TC, Kadmon D (2000) Differential expression of nuclear retinoid receptors in normal and malignant prostates. J Clin Oncol 18:116–21.

Love JM, Gudas LJ (1994) Vitamin A, differentiation and cancer. Curr Opin Cell Biol 6:825–31.

Makita T, Duncan SA, Sucov HM (2005) Retinoic acid, hypoxia, and GATA factors cooperatively control the onset of fetal liver erythropoietin expression and erythropoietic differentiation. Dev Biol 280:59–72.

Manor D, Shmidt EN, Budhu A, Flesken-Nikitin A, Zgola M, Page R, Nikitin AY, Noy N (2003) Mammary carcinoma suppression by cellular retinoic acid binding protein-II. Cancer Res 63:4426–33.

Marrs JA, Clendenon SG, Ratcliffe DR, Fielding SM, Liu Q, Bosron WF (2010) Zebrafish fetal alcohol syndrome model: effects of ethanol are rescued by retinoic acid supplement. Alcohol 44(7–8):707–15.

Martinet N, Alla F, Farré G, Labib T, Drouot H, Vidili R, Picard E, Gaube MP, Le Faou D, Siat J, Borelly J, Vermylen P, Bazarbachi T, Vignaud JM, Martinet Y (2000) Retinoic acid receptor and retinoid X receptor alterations in lung cancer precursor lesions. Cancer Res 60:2869–75.

McCormick DL, Burns FJ, Albert RE (1981) Inhibition of benz[a]pyrene-induced mammary carcinogenesis by retinyl acetate. J Natl Cancer Inst 66:559–64.

Mello T, Polvani S, Galli A (2009) Peroxisome proliferator-activated receptor and retinoic x receptor in alcoholic liver disease. PPAR Res 2009:748174.

Miano JM, Berk BC (2000) Retinoids: versatile biological response modifiers of vascular smooth muscle phenotype. Circ Res 87:355–62.

Michalik L, Wahli W (2007) Guiding ligands to nuclear receptors. Cell 129:649–51

Minucci S, Pelicci PG (1999) Retinoid receptors in health and disease: co-regulators and the chromatin connection. Semin Cell Dev Biol 10:215–25.

Mobarhan S, Seitz HK, Russell RM, Mehta R, Hupert J, Friedman H, Layden TJ, Meydani M, Langenberg P (1991) Age-related effects of chronic ethanol intake on vitamin A status in Fisher 344 rats. J Nutr 121:510–7.

Mongan NP, Gudas LJ (2007) Diverse actions of retinoid receptors in cancer prevention and treatment. Differentiation 75:853–70.

Nadauld LD, Phelps R, Moore BC, Eisinger A, Sandoval IT, Chidester S, Peterson PW, Manos EJ, Sklow B, Burt RW, Jones DA (2006) Adenomatous polyposis coli control of C-terminal binding protein-1 stability regulates expression of intestinal retinol dehydrogenases. J Biol Chem 281:37828–35.

Nadauld LD, Shelton DN, Chidester S, Yost HJ, Jones DA (2005) The zebrafish retinol dehydrogenase, rdh1l, is essential for intestinal development and is regulated by the tumor suppressor adenomatous polyposis coli. J Biol Chem 280:30490–5.

Nagao Y, French BA, Cai Y, French SW, Wan YJ (1998) Inhibition of PPAR alpha/RXR alpha-mediated direct hyperplasia pathways during griseofulvin-induced hepatocarcinogenesis. J Cell Biochem 69:189–200.

Napoli JL (1996) Retinoic acid biosynthesis and metabolism. FASEB J 10:993–1001.

Napoli JL, Boerman MH, Chai X, Zhai Y, Fiorella PD (1995) Enzymes and binding proteins affecting retinoic acid concentrations. J Steroid Biochem Mol Biol 53:497–502.

Natarajan SK, Amirtharaj GJ, Ramachandran A, Pulimood AB, Balasubramanian KA (2009) Retinoid metabolism in the small intestine during development of liver cirrhosis. J Gastroenterol Hepatol 24:821–9.

Natarajan SK, Ramamoorthy P, Thomas S, Basivireddy J, Kang G, Ramachandran A, Pulimood AB, Balasubramanian KA (2006) Intestinal mucosal alterations in rats with carbon tetrachloride-induced cirrhosis: changes in glycosylation and luminal bacteria. Hepatology 43:837–46.

Naves MM, Silveira ER, Dagli ML, Moreno FS (2001) Effects of beta-carotene and vitamin A on oval cell proliferation and connexin 43 expression during hepatic differentiation in the rat(1). J Nutr Biochem 12:685–692.

Niles RM (2004) Signaling pathways in retinoid chemoprevention and treatment of cancer. Mutat Res 555:81–96.
Ochoa WF, Torrecillas A, Fita I, Verdaguer N, Corbalán-García S, Gomez-Fernandez JC (2003) Retinoic acid binds to the C2-domain of protein kinase C(alpha). Biochemistry 42: 8774–9.
Ohata M, Lin M, Satre M, Tsukamoto H (1997) Diminished retinoic acid signaling in hepatic stellate cells in cholestatic liver fibrosis. Am J Physiol 272:G589-96.
Okuno M, Kojima S, Matsushima-Nishiwaki R, Tsurumi H, Muto Y, Friedman SL, Moriwaki H (2004) Retinoids in cancer chemoprevention. Curr Cancer Drug Targets 4:285–98.
Okuno M, Sato T, Kitamoto T, Imai S, Kawada N, Suzuki Y, Yoshimura H, Moriwaki H, Onuki K, Masushige S, Muto Y, Friedman SL, Kato S, Kojima S (1999) Increased 9,13-di-cis-retinoic acid in rat hepatic fibrosis: implication for a potential link between retinoid loss and TGF-beta mediated fibrogenesis in vivo. J Hepatol 30:1073–80.
Pang M, de la Monte SM, Longato L, Tong M, He J, Chaudhry R, Duan K, Ouh J, Wands JR (2009) PPARdelta agonist attenuates alcohol-induced hepatic insulin resistance and improves liver injury and repair. J Hepatol 50:1192–201.
Parlesak A, Menzl I, Feuchter A, Bode JC, Bode C (2000) Inhibition of retinol oxidation by ethanol in the rat liver and colon. Gut 47:825–31.
Patek AJ, Haig C (1939) The occurrence of abnormal dark adaptation and its relation to vitamin A metabolism in patients with cirrhosis of the liver. J Clin Invest 18:609–16.
Picard E, Seguin C, Monhoven N, Rochette-Egly C, Siat J, Borrelly J, Martinet Y, Martinet N, Vignaud JM (1999) Expression of retinoid receptor genes and proteins in non-small-cell lung cancer. J Natl Cancer Inst 91:1059–66.
Poulain S, Evenou F, Carré MC, Corbel S, Vignaud JM, Martinet N (2009) Vitamin A/retinoids signalling in the human lung. Lung Cancer 66:1–7.
Radaeva S, Sun R, Jaruga B, Nguyen VT, Tian Z, Gao B (2006) Natural killer cells ameliorate liver fibrosis by killing activated stellate cells in NKG2D-dependent and tumor necrosis factor-related apoptosis-inducing ligand-dependent manners. Gastroenterology 130:435–52.
Radaeva S, Wang L, Radaev S, Jeong WI, Park O, Gao B (2007) Retinoic acid signaling sensitizes hepatic stellate cells to NK cell killing via upregulation of NK cell activating ligand RAE1. Am J Physiol Gastrointest Liver Physiol 293:G809-16.
Ramachandran A, Prabhu R, Thomas S, Reddy JB, Pulimood A, Balasubramanian KA (2002) Intestinal mucosal alterations in experimental cirrhosis in the rat: role of oxygen free radicals. Hepatology 35:622–9.
Razny U, Wator L, Polus A, Wan YJ, Dyduch G, Tomaszewska R, Dembinska-Kiec A (2009) Hepatocyte RXR alpha deletion in mice leads to inhibition of angiogenesis. Genes Nutr 4:69–72.
Reynolds CP, Lemons RS (2001) Retinoid therapy of childhood cancer. Hematol Oncol Clin North Am 15:867–910.
Roberts RA, Kimber I (1999) Cytokines in non-genotoxic hepatocarcinogenesis. Carcinogenesis 20:1397–401.
Rosales FJ, Ritter SJ, Zolfaghari R, Smith JE, Ross AC (1996) Effects of acute inflammation on plasma retinol, retinol-binding protein, and its mRNA in the liver and kidneys of vitamin A-sufficient rats. J Lipid Res 37:962–71.
Ross AC, Zolfaghari R (2004) Regulation of hepatic retinol metabolism: perspectives from studies on vitamin A status. J Nutr 134:269S-275S.
Sano T, Kagawa M, Okuno M, Ishibashi N, Hashimoto M, Yamamoto M, Suzuki R, Kohno H, Matsushima-Nishiwaki R, Takano Y, Tsurumi H, Kojima S, Friedman SL, Moriwaki H, Tanaka T (2005) Prevention of rat hepatocarcinogenesis by acyclic retinoid is accompanied by reduction in emergence of both TGF-alpha-expressing oval-like cells and activated hepatic stellate cells. Nutr Cancer 51:197–206.
Satake K, Takagi E, Ishii A, Kato Y, Imagawa Y, Kimura Y, Tsukuda M (2003) Anti-tumor effect of vitamin A and D on head and neck squamous cell carcinoma. Auris Nasus Larynx 30:403–12.

Schug TT, Berry DC, Shaw NS, Travis SN, Noy N (2007) Opposing effects of retinoic acid on cell growth result from alternate activation of two different nuclear receptors. Cell 129:723–33.
Schug TT, Berry DC, Toshkov IA, Cheng L, Nikitin AY, Noy N (2008) Overcoming retinoic acid-resistance of mammary carcinomas by diverting retinoic acid from PPARbeta/delta to RAR. Proc Natl Acad Sci U S A 105:7546–51.
Seifert WF, Bosma A, Brouwer A, Hendriks HF, Roholl PJ, van Leeuwen RE, van Thiel-de Ruiter GC, Seifert-Bock I, Knook DL (1994) Vitamin A deficiency potentiates carbon tetrachloride-induced liver fibrosis in rats. Hepatology 19:193–201.
Seitz HK (2000) Alcohol and retinoid metabolism. Gut 47:748–50.
Seitz HK, Stickel F (2006) Risk factors and mechanisms of hepatocarcinogenesis with special emphasis on alcohol and oxidative stress. Biol Chem 387:349–60.
Seitz HK, Cho CH (2009) Contribution of alcohol and tobacco use in gastrointestinal cancer development. Methods Mol Biol 472:217–41.
Shelton DN, Sandoval IT, Eisinger A, Chidester S, Ratnayake A, Ireland CM, Jones DA (2006) Up-regulation of CYP26A1 in adenomatous polyposis coli-deficient vertebrates via a WNT-dependent mechanism: implications for intestinal cell differentiation and colon tumor development. Cancer Res 66:7571–7.
Sheren-Manoff M, Shin SJ, Su D, Bok D, Rando RR, Gudas LJ (2006) Reduced lecithin:retinol acyltransferase expression in human breast cancer. Int J Oncol 29:1193–9.
Shiojiri N, Lemire JM, Fausto N (1991) Cell lineages and oval cell progenitors in rat liver development. Cancer Res 51:2611–20.
Shiraishi-Yokoyama H, Yokoyama H, Matsumoto M, Imaeda H, Hibi T (2006) Acetaldehyde inhibits the formation of retinoic acid from retinal in the rat esophagus. Scand J Gastroenterol 41:80–6.
Shukla SD, Aroor AR (2006) Epigenetic effects of ethanol on liver and gastrointestinal injury. World J Gastroenterol 12:5265–71.
Shukla SD, Velazquez J, French SW, Lu SC, Ticku MK, Zakhari S (2008) Emerging role of epigenetics in the actions of alcohol. Alcohol Clin Exp Res 32:1525–34.
Simanowski UA, Homann N, Knühl M, Arce L, Waldherr R, Conradt C, Bosch FX, Seitz HK (2001) Increased rectal cell proliferation following alcohol abuse. Gut 49:418–22.
Shin DJ, Odom DP, Scribner KB, Ghoshal S, McGrane MM (2002) Retinoid regulation of the phosphoenolpyruvate carboxykinase gene in liver. Mol Cell Endocrinol 195(1–2):39–54.
Soprano DR, Qin P, Soprano KJ (2004) Retinoic acid receptors and cancers. Annu Rev Nutr 24:201–21.
Stickel F, Schuppan D, Hahn EG, Seitz HK (2002) Cocarcinogenic effects of alcohol in hepatocarcinogenesis. Gut 51:132–9.
Sun SY, Lotan R (2002) Retinoids and their receptors in cancer development and chemoprevention. Crit Rev Oncol Hematol 41:41–55.
Taimi M, Helvig C, Wisniewski J, Ramshaw H, White J, Amad M, Korczak B, Petkovich M (2004) A novel human cytochrome P450, CYP26C1, involved in metabolism of 9-cis and all-trans isomers of retinoic acid. J Biol Chem 279:77–85.
Tallman MS, Wiernik PH (1992) Retinoids in cancer treatment. J Clin Pharmacol 32:868–88.
Thatcher JE, Isoherranen N (2009) The role of CYP26 enzymes in retinoic acid clearance. Expert Opin Drug Metab Toxicol 5:875–86.
Vigushin DM, Coombes RC (2004) Targeted histone deacetylase inhibition for cancer therapy. Curr Cancer Drug Targets 4:205–18.
Villarroya F, Iglesias R, Giralt M (2004) Retinoids and retinoid receptors in the control of energy balance: novel pharmacological strategies in obesity and diabetes. Curr Med Chem 11:795–805.
von Wangenheim KH, Peterson HP (2008) The role of cell differentiation in controlling cell multiplication and cancer. J Cancer Res Clin Oncol 134:725–41.
Wald N, Idle M, Boreham J, Bailey A (1980) Low serum-vitamin-A and subsequent risk of cancer. Preliminary results of a prospective study. Lancet 2:813–5.

Wan YJ, An D, Cai Y, Repa JJ, Hung-Po Chen T, Flores M, Postic C, Magnuson MA, Chen J, Chien KR, French S, Mangelsdorf DJ, Sucov HM (2000) Hepatocyte-specific mutation establishes retinoid X receptor alpha as a heterodimeric integrator of multiple physiological processes in the liver. Mol Cell Biol 20:4436–44.

Wan YJ, Han G, Cai Y, Dai T, Konishi T, Leng AS (2003) Hepatocyte retinoid X receptor-alpha-deficient mice have reduced food intake, increased body weight, and improved glucose tolerance. Endocrinology 144:605–11.

Wang J, Saunthararajah Y, Redner RL, Liu JM (1999) Inhibitors of histone deacetylase relieve ETO-mediated repression and induce differentiation of AML1-ETO leukemia cells. Cancer Res 59:2766–9.

Wang XD, Liu C, Chung J, Stickel F, Seitz HK, Russell RM (1998) Chronic alcohol intake reduces retinoic acid concentration and enhances AP-1 (c-Jun and c-Fos) expression in rat liver. Hepatology 28:744–50.

Wang XD (2005) Alcohol, vitamin A, and cancer. Alcohol 35:251–8.

Westerbacka J, Kolak M, Kiviluoto T, Arkkila P, Sirén J, Hamsten A, Fisher RM, Yki-Järvinen H (2007) Genes involved in fatty acid partitioning and binding, lipolysis, monocyte/macrophage recruitment, and inflammation are overexpressed in the human fatty liver of insulin-resistant subjects. Diabetes 56:2759–65.

Wojcik E, Dvorak C, Chianale J, Traber PG, Keren D, Gumucio JJ (1988) Demonstration by in situ hybridization of the zonal modulation of rat liver cytochrome P-450b and P-450e gene expression after phenobarbital. J Clin Invest 82(2):658–66.

Wolbach SB, Howe PR (1925) Tissue changes following deprivation of fat-soluble a vitamin. J Exp Med 42:753–777.

Yang Q, Sakurai T, Kakudo K (2002) Retinoid, retinoic acid receptor beta and breast cancer. Breast Cancer Res Treat 76:167–73.

Yelin R, Kot H, Yelin D, Fainsod A (2007) Early molecular effects of ethanol during vertebrate embryogenesis. Differentiation 75:393–403.

Zancai P, Cariati R, Rizzo S, Boiocchi M, Dolcetti R (1998) Retinoic acid-mediated growth arrest of EBV-immortalized B lymphocytes is associated with multiple changes in G1 regulatory proteins: p27Kip1 up-regulation is a relevant early event. Oncogene 17:1827–36.

Zhai Y, Sperkova Z, Napoli JL (2001) Cellular expression of retinal dehydrogenase types 1 and 2: effects of vitamin A status on testis mRNA. J Cell Physiol 186(2):220–32.

Zhan HC, Gudas LJ, Bok D, Rando R, Nanus DM, Tickoo SK (2003) Differential expression of the enzyme that esterifies retinol, lecithin:retinol acyltransferase, in subtypes of human renal cancer and normal kidney. Clin Cancer Res 9:4897–905.

Zhang W, Rashid A, Wu H, Xu XC (2001) Differential expression of retinoic acid receptors and p53 protein in normal, premalignant, and malignant esophageal tissues. J Cancer Res Clin Oncol 127:237–42.

Chapter 8
Alcohol, Altered Protein Homeostasis, and Cancer

András Orosz

Abbreviations

AKRB10	Aldo-keto reductase 1B10
ALD	Alcoholic liver disease
Apaf-1	Apoptotic peptidase activating factor 1
APC/C	Anaphase Promoting Complex C
CRC	Colorectal cancer
DBD	DNA binding domain
DNA-PK	DNA damage response kinase
ESCC	Esophageal squamous cell carcinoma
FAH	Fumarylacetoacetate hydrolase
GR	Glucocorticiod receptor
HCC	Hepatocellular carcinoma
HDAC	Histone deacetylase
HRGβ1	Heregulin β1
HSE	Heat shock element
HSF	Heat shock factor
HSP	Heat shock protein
HSR	Heat shock response
HT1	Hereditary tyrosinemia type 1
IL-1β	Interleukin 1 beta
PDC	Programmed cell death
PDIA3	Protein disulfide isomerase-associated 3
PN	Proteostasis network
ROS	Reactive oxygen species

A. Orosz (✉)
Division of Metabolism and Health Effects, National Institute on Alcohol Abuse and Alcoholism, National Institutes of Health, Bethesda, MD, USA
e-mail: orosza@mail.nih.gov

S. Zakhari et al. (eds.), *Alcohol and Cancer*, DOI 10.1007/978-1-4614-0040-0_8,
© Springer Science+Business Media, LLC 2011

TNFα	Tumor necrosis factor alpha
uPA	Urokinase plasminogen activator
UPR	Unfolded protein response

Guardians of the Proteome: The Emerging Role of HSF1 and HSPs in Cancer

The HSF Family of Transcriptional Regulators

In Eukaryotes the Heat Shock Response is regulated by the evolutionally conserved transcription factor known as Heat Shock Factor. While single cell eukaryotes (*Saccharomyces cerevisiae, Kluyveromyces lactis and Schizosaccharomyces pombe*) and *Drosophila* have only one general HSF, multiple members of the HSF family exist in plants, mammals and other vertebrates, but the ubiquitously expressed HSF1 is the only true stress-inducible homologue of the general HSF present in lower eukaryotes (Wu 1995). HSF1 disruption in mice leads to the complete loss of thermotolerance and profound increase in heat induced apoptosis. However, HSF1 also mediates other cellular functions unrelated to its role in cell survival. *hsf1* loss induces placental defects, decreased embryo survival, growth retardation, female infertility and disruption of developmental programs leading to pleiotropic pathological outcomes in different organ systems (Xiao et al. 1999). Many HSF1 pathways play pivotal roles in cell growth, cell proliferation and cell death processes placing HSF1 at the hub of cancer regulatory networks.

Transcriptional Regulation of the Stress Response

Transcriptional regulation of the HSR is mediated mainly by a preexisting transcriptional activator, HSF, which binds to heat shock element (HSE) present in all heat shock gene promoters and characterized as inverse reiterations of the pentanucleotide sequence 5′-nGAAn-3′ (Xiao et al. 1991); (Wu 1995). HSF consists of the highly conserved N-terminal DNA binding domain (DBD), followed by the trimerization domain (HR-A/B) containing hydrophobic heptad repeats, and the C-terminal array of conserved hydrophobic region (HR-C).Under normal conditions HSF is present as a latent monomer that binds DNA with low affinity. Upon heat stress HSF is reversibly converted to a trimeric state and acquires high DNA binding affinity (Fig. 8.2). Maintenance of the HSF monomers is dependent on the hydrophobic heptad repeats located at the amino and the carboxy-terminal regions that suppress trimerization and high affinity DNA binding via intramolecular hydrophobic interaction (Westwood et al. 1991; Baler et al. 1993; Rabindran et al. 1993; Wu 1995; Zuo et al. 1995).

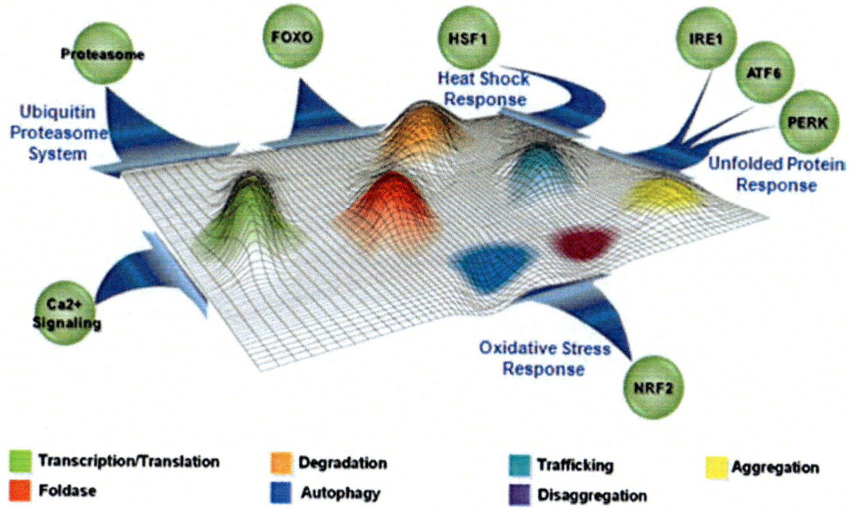

Fig. 8.1 The Proteostasis Network (PN): The PN in the cells regulates a complex array of interacting biological processes to maintain protein homeostasis or proteostasis. Functions of the PN include protein folding, degradation of misfolded proteins and their transport to appropriate destination in the cell. Proteostasis regulators are designed to rebalance the network to a therapeutic state that is sufficient to control or delay progression of disease. (From Proteostasis Therapeutics, http://www.proteostasis.com)

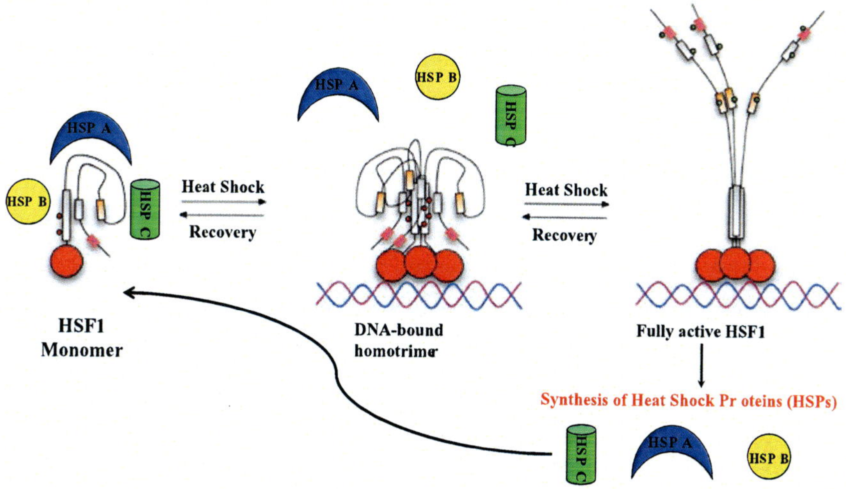

Fig. 8.2 Feedback regulation of the Heat Shock Response. (Modified from Wu 1995)

Molecular chaperones, downstream targets of HSF play a key role keeping HSF in inactive conformation by shifting the equilibrium toward the monomeric inert state. For example, complexes between HSP70 and HSF have been detected during the recovery phase of heat shock (Abravaya et al. 1992; Baler et al. 1992; Shi et al. 1998), suggesting an autoregulatory role of chaperones in heat shock response. Other chaperones such as HSP90 and HDJ-1/HSP40 have also been shown to negatively regulate HSF (Mosser et al. 1993; Ali et al. 1998; Shi et al. 1998; Zou et al. 1998). Under non-stress conditions, transcriptionally inactive HSF1 is maintained in a large protein complex, containing HSP90 and immunophilins CYP40, FKBP1, FKBP2 and P23. Heat stress dissociates this complex leading to HSP90 sequestration to denatured proteins, while allowing HSF1 trimerization and subsequent DNA binding at HSE elements in the HSP promoters.

Although the significance of cytoplasmic-nuclear relocalization of HSF during stress remains controversial, in certain cells and organisms HSF is predominantly nuclear (*Drosophila, Xenopus*) before and after heat shock, while in others (e.g. human or mouse tissue culture cells) cytoplasmic-nuclear relocalization may play considerable role in the regulation of stress response (Westwood et al. 1991; Zuo et al. 1995; Orosz et al. 1996).

The Role of Signal Transduction Pathways and HSF1 Phosphorylation in Cancer

Following heat shock HSF becomes hyperphosphorylated, although the role of phosphorylation in HSF activation or deactivation remains elusive. Phosphorylation predominantly earmarks serine residues both on the latent and on the transcriptionally active HSF1 molecule. HSF1 contains multiple phosphorylation sites both with activating (T142, S195, S230, S326) and inhibitory (S121, S303, S307, S363) capacity that permits an intricate regulatory response to heat stress, metabolic status, and pathophysiological conditions (Fig. 8.3). Recent studies implicated the role of S121 phosphorylation in HSP90 binding and HSF1 inhibition (Wang et al. 2006). Phosphorylation of serine 303 and 307 by GSK3 and ERK1 leads to inhibition that is, at least partially, mediated by the phosphoserine binding protein 14-3-3ε, which exports HSF1 to the cytoplasm rendering it unavailable for DNA binding and transcriptional activation (Wang et al. 2003). The T146 within and S230 and beyond the HR-A/C domain are positive regulators and required for transcriptional activation (Holmberg et al. 2001; Soncin et al. 2003). Polo-like kinase 1 also phosphorylates HSF1 enhancing its nuclear localization (Kim et al. 2005), while S326 has been implicated in stress induced transactivation (Guettouche et al. 2005). **Stress-specific activation is initiated by upstream tyrosine kinases that** do not directly phosphorylate HSF1 (Chu et al. 1996), indicating their indirect effect in HSP transcription regulation. Emerging work provides a compelling demonstration that malignant cell transformation can hijack several stress signaling pathways to activate HSF1 and elevate HSP expression under non-stress condition promoting tumorigenesis and rapid somatic evolution (Khaleque et al. 2005; Ciocca et al. 2006).

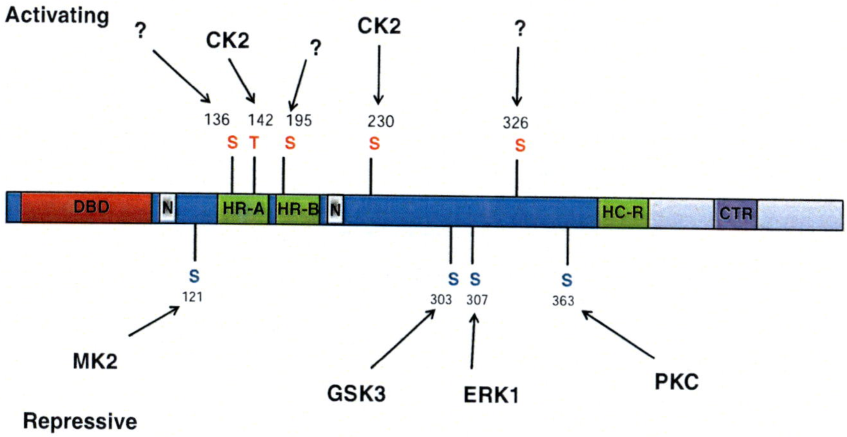

Fig. 8.3 Regulatory phosphorylation sites of HSF1. *DBD* DNA binding domain, *N* nuclear localization signal, *HR* hydrophobic repeat, *CTR* C-terminal repeat, *S* phosphorylated Serine, *T* Phosphorylated Threonine residues. (Modified from Voellmy R, Boellmann F: Adv. Exp. Med. Biol. 594:89–99, 2007)

The Unorthodox Role of HSF1 in Tumorigenesis: Repression of Non-HSP Genes

Contrary to its major role as powerful transcriptional activator of the HSPs, HSF1 also has the surprising ability to repress many unconventional target genes. Several of these genes encode inducible, inflammatory cytokines including interleukin 1 beta (IL-1β) and tumor necrosis factor alpha (TNFα) (Cahill et al. 1996, 1997; Singh et al. 2000, 2002; Xie et al. 2002a, b), while others are proto-oncogenes, including c-*fms*, c-*fos*, or serine proteases (urokinase plasminogen activator, uPA) (Chen et al. 1997). Earlier studies from *Drosophila* demonstrated that the repressor function of HSF is an evolutionarily conserved (Westwood et al. 1991), but unique property of HSF1 among the mammalian HSF family members (Chen et al. 1997; Xie et al. 2002a).

Mechanistic studies with histone deacetylase (HDAC) inhibitor trichostatin A suggest a role of HDACs in IL-1β promoter repression via HSF1 specific recruitment (Chen et al. 1997; Xie et al. 2002a). A current hypothesis of short term gene repression emphasizes the importance of histone modifications and nucleosome structure over the target promoters (Davis and Brackmann 2003). Specifically, the modification of histone H3 and H4 tails by acetylation, methylation, or phosphorylation regulates transcription by two distinct mechanisms: (1) altering histone association with the DNA to either relax (acetylation, phosphorylation) or compact (methylation) the chromatin and (2) provide a unique binding platform for proteins via the distinct pattern of modifications, also known as the histone code (Marmorstein 2001). Short range nucleosome structure is also morphed by ATP-dependent chromatin remodeling complexes, which often associate with specific DNA binding transcription factors and facilitate RNA Pol II movement on chromatin template (Vignali et al. 2000). A recent proteomic screen of HSF1 associated co-repressor molecules identified MTA1 that is in tight association with HSF1 (Khaleque et al. 2008). MTA1 is in a unique co-repressor complex that contains both ATP-dependent chromatin remodeling protein Mi2 and histone deacetylases HDAC1 and HDAC2. These studies show that the HSF1-MTA1 complex binds to the target genes and represses them in a manner that is dependent on the HDAC activities of the repressor complex (Khaleque et al. 2008). Thus, HSF1 activated by different environmental cues and signaling pathways recruits co-repressor complexes to promoters where they, by histone deacetylation and/or ATP-dependent chromatin remodeling, create a compacted chromatin structure conducive of gene repression. This general gene repressing mechanism may promote tumorigenesis by inhibiting the expression of tumor suppressors and inflammatory cytokines TNFα and IL-1β creating a favorable environment for cancer. These findings support the notion that both histone modifications and chromatin remodeling are important for efficient heat shock gene transcription. Consequently, interaction of HSF1 with histone modifying enzymes and chromatin remodeling complexes may play a significant role in cancer. Because of its delicate control mechanisms, HSF1 is particularly prone to loss of regulation that leads to misregulated expression of HSPs and other non orthodox HSF1 targets observed in cancer.

HSF1, Cell Cycle and Cancer

Besides its well characterized transcriptional regulatory properties, HSF1 has additional cellular roles that promote malignancy. During mitosis HSF1 gains activation through trimerization equal to heat stress, however this activation does not lead to *hsp* transcription or elevated level of HSPs synthesis (Bruce et al. 1999). The first observation linking HSF1 to malignancy came from differential gene expression analysis of nonmetastatic PC-3 human prostate carcinoma cells versus their isogenic metastatic variant PC-3M that identified HSF1 as an overexpressed gene product in PC-3M cells (Hoang et al. 2000). Using the same experimental model Wang and colleagues found that HSF1 overexpression increases cellular DNA content, while a dominant negative HSF1 protein restores normal polyploidy (Wang et al. 2004), hence these studies identified HSF1 as a mitotic spindle checkpoint regulator. This checkpoint links DNA replication to the successful completion of anaphase through the regulation of cell cycle genes including securin and Cyclin B1. Cyclin B1 degradation is essential to exit from mitosis; and while elevated levels of HSF1 block this process, dominant negative HSF1 promotes it (Wang et al. 2004). Cyclin B1 degradation is regulated by APC/C (Anaphase Promoting Complex C), an ubiquitine E3 ligase that directly ubiquitinates Cyclin B1 and other substrates to promote their destruction by the 26S proteasome (Peters 2006). Recent studies provided further understanding the role HSF1 plays in genomic instability: the regulatory domain of HSF1 (AA 212–380) was found to interact directly with Cdc20. This binding in turn inhibited interaction between Cdc20 and Cdc27, phosphorylation of Cdc27 and the ubiquitination activity of APC (Lee et al. 2008). These findings imply a novel function of HSF1 frequently overexpressed in cancers to inhibit APC/C activity via the interaction of Cdc20 leading to aneuploidy and genomic instability.

HSF1 is involved in resistance to cell death pathways, in particular apoptosis. DNA damage response kinase (DNA-PK) has been shown to be tightly bound to HSF1 that will increase its kinase activity leading to apoptosis resistance (Nueda et al. 1999), however, the mechanism of tumorigenesis through this pathway remains to be elucidated. Recent large-scale screening for genes that support anti-cancer drug resistance identified HSF1 as a potent inducer of multidrug resistance phenotype (Tchenio et al. 2006) and a powerful promoter of cancer.

HSF1 Activation During Malignant Transformation

Although HSF1 level is elevated in many types of cancers and its activation promotes oncogenesis (Hoang et al. 2000), this function is independent of the stress of pro-malignant stimuli (e.g., hypoxia due to deteriorating tumor milieu). Recent studies show that heregulin β1 (HRGβ1) is an important inducer of HSF1 in mammary tissue. HRGβ1 is released in the tumor environment, binds to its receptors on neighboring cells and induces signal transduction cascades that mediate the complete malignant program in female breast (Khaleque et al. 2008). HRGβ1 acts through a novel HSF1-dependent pathway to induce anchorage independent growth, resistance to apoptosis presumably via the elevation of HSP levels in cancer. HRGβ1 induces HSP60, HSP70 and HSP90 expression in cancer cells through HSF1 activation that is accomplished by inhibition of the constitutive HSF1 repressor kinase GSK3 that represses HSF1 by phosphorylation. GSK3 repression involves upstream signaling events brought about by HRGβ1 receptor binding that initiates sequential activation of c-*erb*B-1, PI-3K and AKT. GSK3 is a powerful repressor of HSF1 by constitutive phosphorylation in the regulatory domain that inhibits trans-activation under normal conditions, but this suppression is relieved during heat shock or other stress conditions (Green et al. 1995; Chu et al. 1996; Newton et al. 1996). The ERK cascade is also activated by HRGβ1, which leads to the phosphorylation of HSF1 on Ser307 and subsequent repression (Chu et al. 1996; Wang et al. 2003). Recent studies provide indications how HRGβ1 circumvent ERK inhibition: according to this model ERK binds to HSF1 and phosphorylates it on Ser307, which in concert with a secondary phosphorylation event on Ser303 by GSK3 will lead to 14-3-3ε recruitment and repression by subsequent cytoplasmic sequestration. High affinity binding of 14-3-3ε requires the presence of dual phosphorylation marks at positions Ser 303 and Ser307 to provide a binding platform for 14-3-3ε allowing export of HSF1 to the cytoplasm (Wang et al. 2003). HRGβ1 activation of the PI-3K/AKT pathway overrides ERK repression of HSF1 by phosphorylation induced inactivation of GSK3 that in turn leads to HSF1 Ser303 dephosphorylation and preservation of transcriptional activity of HSF1 that is analogous to heat shock signaling cascades (Wang et al. 2004).

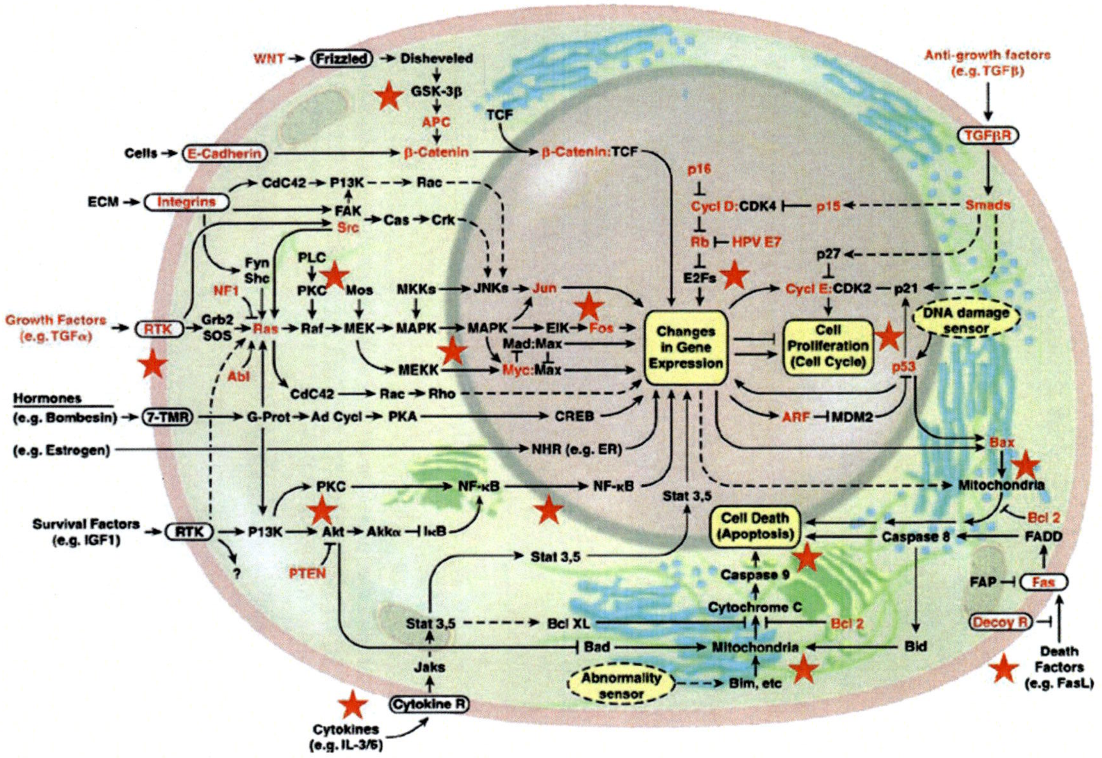

Fig. 8.4 Circuit of cell signaling pathways in normal and cancer cells. In addition to the prototypical growth signaling circuit centered around Ras and coupled to a spectrum of extracellular cues, other component circuits transmit antigrowth and differentiation signals or mediate commands to live or die by apoptosis. **Genetic reprogramming in cancer cells occurs through functionally altered genes highlighted in red, generally identified as oncogenes or tumor suppressor** genes. HSF1 and HSPs, marked with stars, modulate many important nodes of the signaling circuit emphasizing their importance in oncogenic transformation. (From Hanahan and Weinberg 2000)

In addition, since HSP genes have been demonstrated to be repressed by the p53 pathway, loss of function mutations in p53 or p63 also contribute to HSP accumulation in cancer (Agoff et al. 1993; Madden et al. 1997; Jung et al. 2001). Signal transduction pathways with connections to HSF1 and HSPs in oncogenic transformation are shown on Fig. 8.4.

Modulation of Oncogenesis by HSF1 and HSPs

Most tumors emerge in a sequential progression of cells from transformed, but minimally altered state that can grow and form nodules to a multiply deviated state with unlimited growth capability, manipulation of tumor microenvironment, invasion of surrounding tissues and escape in the circulation to form metastatic colonies at distant locations. This progression includes diverse molecular and morphological changes that have been classified by Hanahan and Weinberg (2000) into six essential alterations of cell physiology: (1) self sufficiency of growth signals; (2) insensitivity to growth inhibition; (3) evasion of programmed cell death (PDC); (4) limitless replicative potential; (5) sustained angiogenesis, and (6) tissue invasion and metastasis (see Chap. 1). In contrast to their widely appreciated beneficial effects in survival and longevity, HSF1 and several HSPs, chiefly HSP90, 70 and 27, support malignant transformation to the detriment of the organism through the modification of all hallmarks traits of cancer (Fig. 8.5).

The principal role of HSP90, in concert with other molecular chaperones, is to stabilize the delicate structure of cell surface receptors, protein kinases and transcription factors that support normal cellular growth (Neckers and Ivy 2003). The high molecular weight HSP90 chaperone complexes are also required to maintain the active conformation of signaling molecules rapidly triggered by growth signals. Transformed proteins such as v-Src, BCR-ABL and p53 achieve stable conformation owing to HSP90 chaperoning function. Thus, oncogenic programs subvert HSP90 chaperone machinery to support the autonomous function of unstable growth signaling molecules, as well as to biochemically "buffer" the growing pool of mutant proteins.

HSP90 inhibits programmed cell death through direct binding to Apoptotic peptidase-activating factor 1 (Apaf-1) and inhibiting its oligomerization, procaspase 9 recruitment and apoptosis (Pandey et al. 2000). HSP90 also interacts with the phosphorylated form of serine/threonine kinase AKT/PKB that generates a survival signal in response to growth factor stimulation. AKT phosphorylation of the BCL-2 family protein BAD and caspase-9 leads to their inactivation and inhibition of apoptosis (Cardone et al. 1998). Additionally, AKT can inhibit NF-κB mediated PCD via phosphorylation of IκB kinase (Ozes et al. 1999). Alternative mechanisms of NF-κB inhibition by HSP90 include stabilization of the receptor interacting protein (RIP) (Lewis et al. 2000) or interactions within the IκB kinase (IKK) complex, which include HSP90 and Cdc37 as structural components. There is convincing evidence that increased expression of HSP70 or HSP27 inhibits caspase dependent apoptosis (Beere 2001). Prominent molecular targets for HSP70 and HSP27 in the caspase

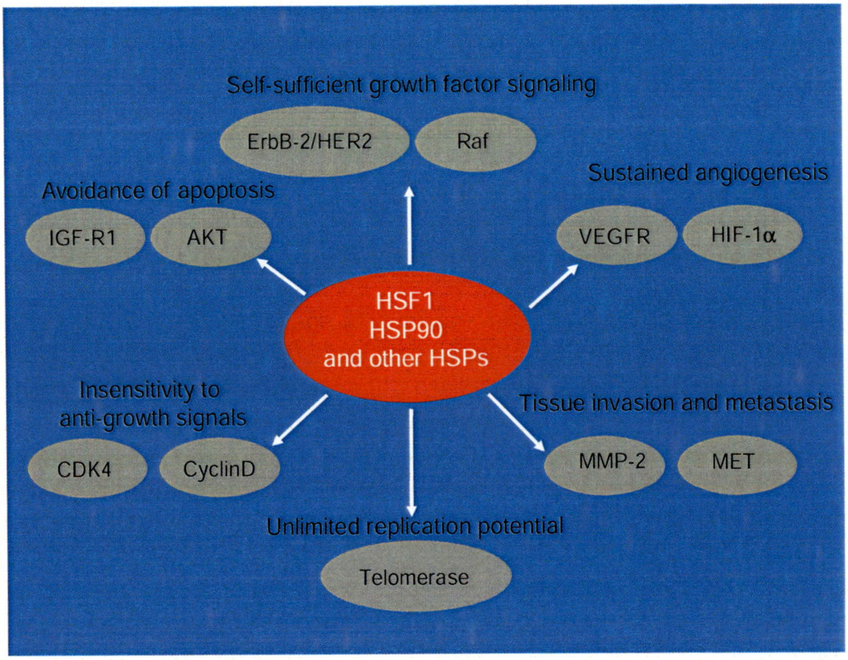

Fig. 8.5 Schematic illustration of the central role of HSF1, HSP90 and other HSPs in supporting all of the hallmark traits of cancer cells by chaperoning the various client proteins shown, as well as others. (Modified from Karapanagiotou et al. 2009)

dependent apoptotic pathway are c-JUN kinase, Apaf-1 and caspase-8. HSP70 also inhibits the PCD pathway involving digestion by lysosome derived cathepsins (Nylandsted et al. 2004) through inhibition of lysosomal membrane permeabilization. Loss of function studies established that HSF1 is an essential inhibitor of apoptosis after stress (McMillan et al. 1998), but the details of this regulation beyond and above its transcriptional activator function require further investigations.

Activation of HSF1 and elevated expression HSPs has been implicated in increased longevity in several species, suggesting a role in resistance to cellular senescence (Hsu et al. 2003). In all somatic cells replicative checkpoints place a limit on the permitted number of cell divisions, and when that limit is achieved cells enter the pathway of cellular senescence (Nelson and White 2004; Campisi 2005). To escape senescence and undergo unlimited growth, cancer cells must evade the "crisis" point at which telomeres shortened enough to prevent successful future cell divisions (Campisi 2005). HSP90 is essential for telomerase stability, while the non-stress inducible HSP70.2, and the mitochondrial HSP75 are antagonizing both p53 dependent and independent senescence pathways, underscoring the importance of HSPs in cellular transformation (Workman 2004).

Since diffusion distance of oxygen in tissues (100 μm) restrict unlimited growth, tumors must create an assembly of microcirculation by de novo angiogenesis

(Folkman 2002).This process is regulated at the level of protein stability by the primary sensor of tumor cell hypoxia, transcription factor HIF1α, and elevated levels of HSP90 and HSP70 are needed to mediate HIF1α accumulation and stability (Zhou et al. 2004). HIF1α has several downstream targets to regulate proliferation and mobility of vascular endothelial cells and at least two of them, vascular endothelial growth factor (VEGF) and nitric oxide synthase, require HSP90 to sustain their induction and stability (Neckers and Ivy 2003; Sun and Liao 2004; Pfosser et al. 2005). The essential role of HSP90 in tumor angiogenesis is demonstrated by the findings that overexpression of HSP90 enhance, while cancer therapy HSP90 inhibitors diminish tumor angiogenesis (Sun and Liao 2004; Pfosser et al. 2005).

Invasion and metastasis are the trademark features of advance stage cancers. Cancer cells overexpressing HSF1 and HSPs are more prone to invade their microenvironment and spread to distant organs, although the molecular underpinnings involved are not fully understood (Hoang et al. 2000; Dai et al. 2007). Additional evidence of *hsf1* role in metastasis has emerged from studies of heregulin stimulation of anchorage independence growth of tumor cells that required the *hsf1* gene (Hoang et al. 2000). Clinical studies provide further indication of the positive correlation between exaggerated expression of HSF1 and its downstream products HSP27 and HSP70 in the invasive and metastatic ability of tumors (Ciocca and Calderwood 2005). Recent work unraveled an important extracellular role for HSP90 in the invasion step of metastasis by its binding to matrix metalloprotein 2, a key player in invasion (Eustace and Jay 2004). Additional mechanisms of invasion and metastasis that are supported by HSPs comprise (1) increased survival of tumor cells in the bloodstream due to PCD inhibitory properties of HSP70 and HSP27; (2) emergence and licensing of genetic changes favoring invasion and metastasis due to stabilization of mutant proteins by HSP90; (3) altered inflammatory properties of tumor microenvironment at least partially due to HSP70 release from necrotic cells (Ciocca and Calderwood 2005). Clearly, HSF1 and HSPs have widespread and multifaceted contributions to the development of advanced metastatic cancers that may be exploited to develop future therapeutic interventions.

HSF1 and HSP Drugs as Novel Anticancer Therapy

There is solid, experimental evidence for the existence of non-oncogenic drug targets that can be effectively exploited in cancer treatment. In a tumorigenic pathway not every protein can be activated by overexpression or point mutation to drive tumorigenesis, while they can still represent a potential rate limiting step as well as an effective cancer drug target. This phenomenon is termed 'non-oncogenic addiction' to describe the profound dependence of cancer cells on the regular cellular function of certain genes, which themselves are not categorized as oncogenes (Solimini et al. 2007). One of the largest group of genes fulfilling these criteria comprise a slew of stress inducible HSPs and their transcriptional master regulator HSF1. One plausible

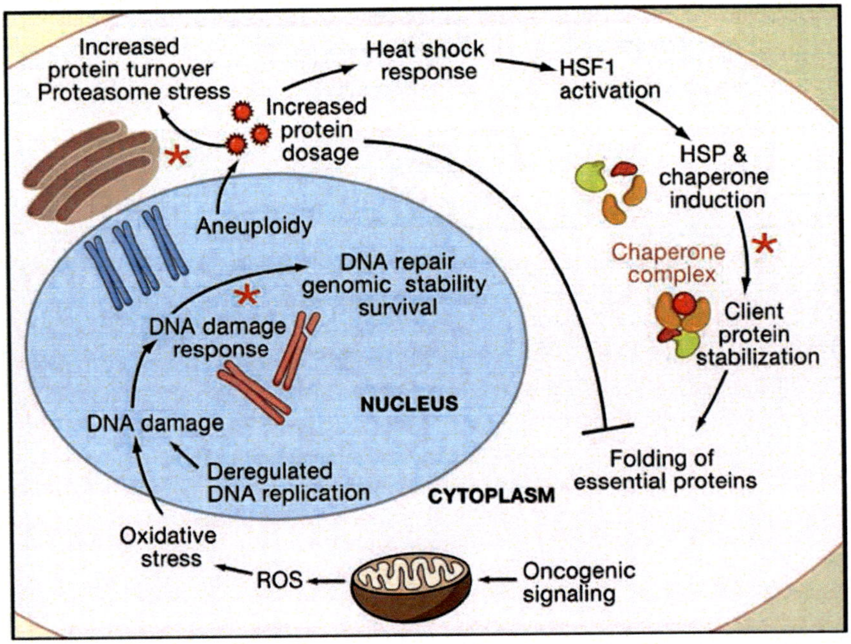

Fig. 8.6 Cellular stress pathway activation in cancer cells leads to non-oncogenic addiction. Cancer cells exhibit increased dependence on several stress response pathways including those for oxidative damage, DNA damage, and heat-shock. *Asterisks* (*) denotes sites of therapeutic intervention in these pathways where inhibitors of non-oncogenic such as HSP90 (geldanamycin) exploit these dependencies of cancer cells to achieve their therapeutic efficacy. From (Solimini et al. 2007)

explanation of HSF1 function in this process is the induction of HSP90, often described as the cancer chaperone, which has been widely associated with the tumorigenesis pathway and is overexpressed in many different types of cancers (Whitesell and Lindquist 2005) Geldanamycine inhibits HSP90 activity by interacting with its ATP-binding pocket leading to destabilization and destruction of its client proteins by the proteasome pathway. Reduction of client kinases have been proposed to convey the anticancer effects of geldanamycine (Dai et al. 2007), but destruction of diverse HSP90 substrate proteins required for tumor growth in different phases of malignant transformation also play a role. Cancer cells exhibit high levels of proteotoxic stress, reactive oxygen species, spontaneous DNA rearrangements and aneuploidy, each of them accounting for certain form of cellular stress. Hence, cancer cells are highly dependent upon the general stress response machinery that can be effectively targeted in cancer therapy. Although only HSP90 have been successfully targeted in clinical cancer therapy, it is likely that because of their prevalent anti-apoptotic roles HSF1, HSP27 and HSP70 and other tissue specific HSP family members may soon follow suit. Potential therapeutic intervention sites in oncogenic stress response pathways are illustrated in Fig. 8.6.

The Role of HSF1 and HSPs in Ethanol-Induced Tumorigenesis

Although the role of HSF1 and HSPs in the development of ethanol-induced cancers is relatively unknown, numerous current publications indicate possible contribution of molecular chaperones in alcohol-related tumorigenesis.

Teramoto and colleagues recently reported the protein expression profile characteristics in hepatocellular carcinoma (HCC) (Teramoto et al. 2008), one of the most aggressive human cancers with several major risk factors including excessive alcohol drinking. They found that heat shock proteins HSP90α, HSP70 4, 5, 8 and 9B, protein disulfide isomerase-associated 3 (PDIA3) and aldo-keto reductase 1B10 (AKRB10) were overexpressed in HCC. Two of these proteins were identified as potential biomarkers: AKR1B10 corresponds to well differentiated HCC and PDIA3 reflects the histological grade and α-fetoprotein level of the tumor. GRP78, an HSP70 family member localized in the endoplasmic reticulum was also up-regulated. The authors hypothesize that elevated level of GRP78 may support aggressive growth and the suppression of tumor rejection in HCC, while abundantly expressed HSP70 9B (mortalin) has been associated with metastasis and early recurrence These results shed light on the molecular understanding of the role of HSPs in HCC pathogenesis and provide clues to effective therapeutic options.

Heavy alcohol consumption can contribute to DNA, protein, cell and organ damage partly through reactive oxygen species (ROS) production and mitochondrial dysfunction. Despite the well established role of ROS in ethanol induced tissue injury, the proteins that are selectively oxidized by ROS are poorly characterized. In their recent studies, Suh and colleagues identified the oxidized mitochondrial proteins in alcohol treated human hepatoma cells and mouse livers (Suh et al. 2004). They showed that molecular chaperone proteins GRP78, GRP75, HSP70, HSP60, protein disulphate isomerase, and prohibitin were selectively oxidized by CYP2E1-generated ROS. They hypothesize that oxidation of these proteins may lead to the inhibition of their cellular function and altered cellular physiology. How mitochondrial HSP oxidation alters cellular functions leading to pathological signaling, cell death or oncogenic transformation requires further investigations.

Vogel and colleagues (2004) analyzed the relationship between chronic liver disease and in vivo programmed cell death in a murine model of hereditary tyrosinemia type 1 (HT1). HT1 is an autosomal recessive disorder caused by the deficiency of fumarylacetoacetate hydrolase (FAH) that leads to gradual liver disease frequently progressing to hepatocarcinoma (HCC). Unexpectedly, $fah^{-/-}$ animals with preexisting liver injury due to interrupted drug treatment of HT1 were resistant to Fas ligand-induced apoptosis and acetaminophen-induced necrosis-like cell death. Molecular analysis identified prominent up-regulation of anti-apoptotic HSPs 27, 32 and 70, and c-Jun expression in stressed mice. In contrast, the p38 and JNK stress activated kinase pathways were markedly impaired in apoptosis resistant livers. In conclusion, these results present evidence that chronic liver disease can provide paradoxical cell death resistance in vivo. These findings may have more general ramifications for chronic liver diseases associated with oxidative stress including chronic and excessive alcohol consumption. Hence, stress induced malfunction of the cell death machinery may play a role in alcoholic liver disease (ALD) and may significantly contribute to the risk of developing HCC.

Kubish and colleagues examined the role of long term alcohol consumption on pancreatic gene expression in rats and their potential associations to pancreatic injury (Kubisch et al. 2006). Their large scale studies concluded that alcohol has a profound effect on pancreatic gene expression profile that may contribute to pancreatic tissue damage. Among the most highly induced genes by ethanol are the ER stress regulated transcription factor ATF3 and two of the most abundant cytoplasmic heat shock proteins HSP70 and HSP27. Although generally protective, these HSPs may contribute to the development of chronic pancreatitis in heavy alcohol consumption. Specifically, elevated expression of HSP70 mRNA stabilizes cytokine and proto-oncogene mRNAs by the sequestration of AUF1, an AU rich element binding protein that under normal conditions facilitates the decay of these prooncogenes. While the strong anti-apoptotic effects of HSP27 may initially be protective in pancreatitis, high HSP27 expression may pave the way to more severe injury after repeated insults by blocking programmed cell death. Since chronic pancreatitis is a major risk factor for the development of pancreatic cancer, dysregulated HSPs and HSF1 may significantly contribute to this devastating disease, the fourth leading cause of cancer-related deaths in humans.

In Western countries upper esophageal squamous cell carcinoma (ESCC) is a relatively infrequent malignancy with extremely bleak prognosis. In Europe and North America, ESCC have been ascribed to alcohol and tobacco abuse, while in Asian countries spicy food, hot drinks, opium smoking and human papillomavirus infections are the most significant risk factors. Lambot and colleagues (2000) examined whether changes in stress inducible HSP27 expression can be demonstrated during oesophageal carcinogenesis. They found that in human oesophagus alcohol and various other stresses generate focal perturbations in the epithelial stress response. Their data indicate that HSP27 expression progressively increases from normal oesophageal squamous epithelium, to dysplasia, in situ carcinoma and invasive carcinoma, and in ESCC HSP27 expression increases in proportion to the anaplasia of the tumor. The prognostic value of this finding and the molecular underpinnings of alcohol induced HSP27 expression and ESCC require further investigations. Others (Yagui-Beltran et al. 2001) demonstrated that the human oesopageal squamous epithelium exhibits a novel type of stress response where some of the canonical HSPs, including HSP70 are down-regulated, while other cell type specific HSPs take their place. Whether this distinctive phenomenon of tissue specific HSP expression will prove to be a protective or predisposing condition in oesophageal carcinogenesis remains to be investigated.

Finally, induction of HSF1 and its target genes including HSP27, HSP90 and iNOS expression has been demonstrated in sporadic colorectal cancer (CRC) (Cen et al. 2004). These studies suggest that induction of the heat shock response has been actively driving the development of CRC instead of being a passive bystander. The authors hypothesize that contribution of the stress response to CRC coincides with the fact that the colon as an open system can retain chronic stress substances including alcohol, meat and others for a long period of time. Prolonged exposure of stress substances upregulates the HSR and other proteostasis pathways and predisposes the colon to tumorigenic transformation by the enhancement of the functions of oncogenic proteins and blocking apoptosis. The exact details of the derailed HSR pathways in CRC development need to be delineated.

Conclusions

Growing evidence from different experimental models and human studies support the notion that the heat shock response may play an important and decisive role in alcohol-induced carcinogenesis. HSF1 is under tight and elaborate regulation in unstressed normal tissues, but in cancer these controls are bypassed leading to elevated HSF1 expression, constitutive activation and upregulated expression of target HSPs. Exaggerated levels of HSF1 and HSPs play essential, facilitating roles in cancer by permitting autonomous growth and allowing accumulation of overexpressed and mutated oncogenes and preventing programmed cell death pathways, thus switching gene expression pathways towards more metastatic phenotype. However, the abundance and pleiotropic functions of these evolutionally conserved stress pathways also afford unprecedented and unforeseen therapeutic opportunities that can be exploited in the treatment of alcohol induced and other malignancies of different etiology that are currently emerging.

References

Abravaya K, Myers MP, Murphy SP, Morimoto RI (1992) The human heat shock protein hsp70 interacts with HSF, the transcription factor that regulates heat shock gene expression. Genes Dev 6:1153–1164.

Agoff SN, Hou J, Linzer DI, Wu B (1993) Regulation of the human hsp70 promoter by p53. Science 259:84–87.

Ali A, Bharadwaj S, O'Carroll R, Ovsenek N (1998) HSP90 interacts with and regulates the activity of heat shock factor 1 in Xenopus oocytes. Mol Cell Biol 18:4949–4960.

Baler R, Dahl G, Voellmy R (1993) Activation of human heat shock genes is accompanied by oligomerization, modification, and rapid translocation of heat shock transcription factor HSF1. Mol Cell Biol 13:2486–2496.

Baler R, Welch WJ, Voellmy R (1992) Heat shock gene regulation by nascent polypeptides and denatured proteins: hsp70 as a potential autoregulatory factor. J Cell Biol 117:1151–1159.

Beere HM (2001) Stressed to death: regulation of apoptotic signaling pathways by the heat shock proteins. Sci STKE 2001:re1.

Bruce JL, Chen C, Xie Y, Zhong R, Wang YQ, Stevenson MA, Calderwood SK (1999) Activation of heat shock transcription factor 1 to a DNA binding form during the G(1)phase of the cell cycle. Cell Stress Chaperones 4:36–45.

Cahill CM, Lin HS, Price BD, Bruce JL, Calderwood SK (1997) Potential role of heat shock transcription factor in the expression of inflammatory cytokines. Adv Exp Med Biol 400B:625–630.

Cahill CM, Waterman WR, Xie Y, Auron PE, Calderwood SK (1996) Transcriptional repression of the prointerleukin 1beta gene by heat shock factor 1. J Biol Chem 271:24874–24879.

Campisi J (2005) Senescent cells, tumor suppression, and organismal aging: good citizens, bad neighbors. Cell 120:513–522.
Cardone MH, Roy N, Stennicke HR, Salvesen GS, Franke TF, Stanbridge E, Frisch S, Reed JC (1998) Regulation of cell death protease caspase-9 by phosphorylation. Science 282:1318–1321.
Cen H, Zheng S, Fang YM, Tang XP, Dong Q (2004) Induction of HSF1 expression is associated with sporadic colorectal cancer. World J Gastroenterol 10:3122–3126.
Chen C, Xie Y, Stevenson MA, Auron PE, Calderwood SK (1997) Heat shock factor 1 represses Ras-induced transcriptional activation of the c-fos gene. J Biol Chem 272:26803–26806.
Chu B, Soncin F, Price BD, Stevenson MA, Calderwood SK (1996) Sequential phosphorylation by mitogen-activated protein kinase and glycogen synthase kinase 3 represses transcriptional activation by heat shock factor-1. J Biol Chem 271:30847–30857.
Ciocca DR, Calderwood SK (2005) Heat shock proteins in cancer: diagnostic, prognostic, predictive, and treatment implications. Cell Stress Chaperones 10:86–103.
Ciocca DR, Gago FE, Fanelli MA, Calderwood SK (2006) Co-expression of steroid receptors (estrogen receptor alpha and/or progesterone receptors) and Her-2/neu: Clinical implications. J Steroid Biochem Mol Biol 102:32–40.
Dai C, Whitesell L, Rogers AB, Lindquist S (2007) Heat shock factor 1 is a powerful multifaceted modifier of carcinogenesis. Cell 130:1005–1018.
Davis PK, Brackmann RK (2003) Chromatin remodeling and cancer. Cancer Biol Ther 2:22–29.
Eustace BK, Jay DG (2004) Extracellular roles for the molecular chaperone, hsp90. Cell Cycle 3:1098–1100.
Folkman J (2002) Role of angiogenesis in tumor growth and metastasis. Semin Oncol 29:15–18.
Green M, Schuetz TJ, Sullivan EK, Kingston RE (1995) A heat shock-responsive domain of human HSF1 that regulates transcription activation domain function. Mol Cell Biol 15:3354–3362.
Guettouche T, Boellmann F, Lane WS, Voellmy R (2005) Analysis of phosphorylation of human heat shock factor 1 in cells experiencing a stress. BMC Biochem 6:4.
Hanahan D, Weinberg RA (2000) The hallmarks of cancer. Cell 100:57–70.
Hoang AT, Huang J, Rudra-Ganguly N, Zheng J, Powell WC, Rabindran SK, Wu C, Roy-Burman P (2000) A novel association between the human heat shock transcription factor 1 (HSF1) and prostate adenocarcinoma. Am J Pathol 156:857–864.
Holmberg CI, Hietakangas V, Mikhailov A, Rantanen JO, Kallio M, Meinander A, Hellman J, Morrice N, MacKintosh C, Morimoto RI, Eriksson JE, Sistonen L (2001) Phosphorylation of serine 230 promotes inducible transcriptional activity of heat shock factor 1. EMBO J 20:3800–3810.
Hsu AL, Murphy CT, Kenyon C (2003) Regulation of aging and age-related disease by DAF-16 and heat-shock factor. Science 300:1142–1145.
Jung MS, Yun J, Chae HD, Kim JM, Kim SC, Choi TS, Shin DY (2001) p53 and its homologues, p63 and p73, induce a replicative senescence through inactivation of NF-Y transcription factor. Oncogene 20:5818–5825.
Karapanagiotou EM, Syrigos K, Saif MW (2009) Heat shock protein inhibitors and vaccines as new agents in cancer treatment. Expert Opin Investig Drugs 18(2):161–174.
Khaleque MA, Bharti A, Gong J, Gray PJ, Sachdev V, Ciocca DR, Stati A, Fanelli M, Calderwood SK (2008) Heat shock factor 1 represses estrogen-dependent transcription through association with MTA1. Oncogene 27:1886–1893.
Khaleque MA, Bharti A, Sawyer D, Gong J, Benjamin IJ, Stevenson MA, Calderwood SK (2005) Induction of heat shock proteins by heregulin beta1 leads to protection from apoptosis and anchorage-independent growth. Oncogene 24:6564–6573.
Kim SA, Yoon JH, Lee SH, Ahn SG (2005) Polo-like kinase 1 phosphorylates heat shock transcription factor 1 and mediates its nuclear translocation during heat stress. J Biol Chem 280:12653–12657.
Kubisch CH, Gukovsky I, Lugea A, Pandol SJ, Kuick R, Misek DE, Hanash SM, Logsdon CD (2006) Long-term ethanol consumption alters pancreatic gene expression in rats: a possible connection to pancreatic injury. Pancreas 33:68–76.

Lambot MA, Peny MO, Fayt I, Haot J, Noel JC (2000) Overexpression of 27-kDa heat shock protein relates to poor histological differentiation in human oesophageal squamous cell carcinoma. Histopathology 36:326–330.
Lee YJ, Lee HJ, Lee JS, Jeoung D, Kang CM, Bae S, Lee SJ, Kwon SH, Kang D, Lee YS (2008) A novel function for HSF1-induced mitotic exit failure and genomic instability through direct interaction between HSF1 and Cdc20. Oncogene 27:2999–3009.
Lewis J, Devin A, Miller A, Lin Y, Rodriguez Y, Neckers L, Liu ZG (2000) Disruption of hsp90 function results in degradation of the death domain kinase, receptor-interacting protein (RIP), and blockage of tumor necrosis factor-induced nuclear factor-kappaB activation. J Biol Chem 275:10519–10526.
Madden SL, Galella EA, Zhu J, Bertelsen AH, Beaudry GA (1997) SAGE transcript profiles for p53-dependent growth regulation. Oncogene 15:1079–1085.
Marmorstein R (2001) Protein modules that manipulate histone tails for chromatin regulation. Nat Rev Mol Cell Biol 2:422–432.
McMillan DR, Xiao X, Shao L, Graves K, Benjamin IJ (1998) Targeted disruption of heat shock transcription factor 1 abolishes thermotolerance and protection against heat-inducible apoptosis. J Biol Chem 273:7523–7528.
Mosser DD, Duchaine J, Massie B (1993) The DNA-binding activity of the human heat shock transcription factor is regulated in vivo by hsp70. Mol Cell Biol 13:5427–5438.
Neckers L, Ivy SP (2003) Heat shock protein 90. Curr Opin Oncol 15:419–424.
Nelson DA, White E (2004) Exploiting different ways to die. Genes Dev 18:1223–1226.
Newton EM, Knauf U, Green M, Kingston RE (1996) The regulatory domain of human heat shock factor 1 is sufficient to sense heat stress. Mol Cell Biol 16:839–846.
Nueda A, Hudson F, Mivechi NF, Dynan WS (1999) DNA-dependent protein kinase protects against heat-induced apoptosis. J Biol Chem 274:14988–14996.
Nylandsted J, Gyrd-Hansen M, Danielewicz A, Fehrenbacher N, Lademann U, Hoyer-Hansen M, Weber E, Multhoff G, Rohde M, Jaattela M (2004) Heat shock protein 70 promotes cell survival by inhibiting lysosomal membrane permeabilization. J Exp Med 200:425–435.
Orosz A, Wisniewski J, Wu C (1996) Regulation of Drosophila heat shock factor trimerization: global sequence requirements and independence of nuclear localization. Mol Cell Biol 16:7018–7030.
Ozes ON, Mayo LD, Gustin JA, Pfeffer SR, Pfeffer LM, Donner DB (1999) NF-kappaB activation by tumour necrosis factor requires the Akt serine-threonine kinase. Nature 401:82–85.
Pandey P, Saleh A, Nakazawa A, Kumar S, Srinivasula SM, Kumar V, Weichselbaum R, Nalin C, Alnemri ES, Kufe D, Kharbanda S (2000) Negative regulation of cytochrome c-mediated oligomerization of Apaf-1 and activation of procaspase-9 by heat shock protein 90. EMBO J 19:4310–4322.
Peters JM (2006) The anaphase promoting complex/cyclosome: a machine designed to destroy. Nat Rev Mol Cell Biol 7:644–656.
Pfosser A, Thalgott M, Buttner K, Brouet A, Feron O, Boekstegers P, Kupatt C (2005) Liposomal Hsp90 cDNA induces neovascularization via nitric oxide in chronic ischemia. Cardiovasc Res 65:728–736.
Rabindran SK, Haroun RI, Clos J, Wisniewski J, Wu C (1993) Regulation of heat shock factor trimer formation: role of a conserved leucine zipper. Science 259:230–234.
Shi Y, Mosser DD, Morimoto RI (1998) Molecular chaperones as HSF1-specific transcriptional repressors. Genes Dev 12:654–666.
Singh IS, He JR, Calderwood S, Hasday JD (2002) A high affinity HSF-1 binding site in the 5′-untranslated region of the murine tumor necrosis factor-alpha gene is a transcriptional repressor. J Biol Chem 277:4981–4988.
Singh IS, Viscardi RM, Kalvakolanu I, Calderwood S, Hasday JD (2000) Inhibition of tumor necrosis factor-alpha transcription in macrophages exposed to febrile range temperature. A possible role for heat shock factor-1 as a negative transcriptional regulator. J Biol Chem 275:9841–9848.

Solimini NL, Luo J, Elledge SJ (2007) Non-oncogene addiction and the stress phenotype of cancer cells. Cell 130:986–988.

Soncin F, Zhang X, Chu B, Wang X, Asea A, Ann Stevenson M, Sacks DB, Calderwood SK (2003) Transcriptional activity and DNA binding of heat shock factor-1 involve phosphorylation on threonine 142 by CK2. Biochem Biophys Res Commun 303:700–706.

Suh SK, Hood BL, Kim BJ, Conrads TP, Veenstra TD, Song BJ (2004) Identification of oxidized mitochondrial proteins in alcohol-exposed human hepatoma cells and mouse liver. Proteomics 4:3401–3412.

Sun J, Liao JK (2004) Induction of angiogenesis by heat shock protein 90 mediated by protein kinase Akt and endothelial nitric oxide synthase. Arterioscler Thromb Vasc Biol 24:2238–2244.

Tchenio T, Havard M, Martinez LA, Dautry F (2006) Heat shock-independent induction of multidrug resistance by heat shock factor 1. Mol Cell Biol 26:580–591.

Teramoto R, Minagawa H, Honda M, Miyazaki K, Tabuse Y, Kamijo K, Ueda T, Kaneko S (2008) Protein expression profile characteristic to hepatocellular carcinoma revealed by 2D-DIGE with supervised learning. Biochim Biophys Acta 1784:764–772.

Vignali M, Hassan AH, Neely KE, Workman JL (2000) ATP-dependent chromatin-remodeling complexes. Mol Cell Biol 20:1899–1910.

Vogel A, van Den Berg IE, Al-Dhalimy M, Groopman J, Ou CN, Ryabinina O, Iordanov MS, Finegold M, Grompe M (2004) Chronic liver disease in murine hereditary tyrosinemia type 1 induces resistance to cell death. Hepatology 39:433–443.

Wang X, Grammatikakis N, Siganou A, Calderwood SK (2003) Regulation of molecular chaperone gene transcription involves the serine phosphorylation, 14-3-3 epsilon binding, and cytoplasmic sequestration of heat shock factor 1. Mol Cell Biol 23:6013–6026.

Wang X, Khaleque MA, Zhao MJ, Zhong R, Gaestel M, Calderwood SK (2006) Phosphorylation of HSF1 by MAPK-activated protein kinase 2 on serine 121, inhibits transcriptional activity and promotes HSP90 binding. J Biol Chem 281:782–791.

Wang Y, Theriault JR, He H, Gong J, Calderwood SK (2004) Expression of a dominant negative heat shock factor-1 construct inhibits aneuploidy in prostate carcinoma cells. J Biol Chem 279:32651–32659.

Westwood JT, Clos J, Wu C (1991) Stress-induced oligomerization and chromosomal relocalization of heat-shock factor. Nature 353:822–827.

Whitesell L, Lindquist SL (2005) HSP90 and the chaperoning of cancer. Nat Rev Cancer 5:761–772.

Workman P (2004) Altered states: selectively drugging the Hsp90 cancer chaperone. Trends Mol Med 10:47–51.

Wu C (1995) Heat shock transcription factors: structure and regulation. Annu Rev Cell Dev Biol 11:441–469.

Xiao H, Perisic O, Lis JT (1991) Cooperative binding of Drosophila heat shock factor to arrays of a conserved 5 bp unit. Cell 64:585–593.

Xiao X, Zuo X, Davis AA, McMillan DR, Curry BB, Richardson JA, Benjamin IJ (1999) HSF1 is required for extra-embryonic development, postnatal growth and protection during inflammatory responses in mice. EMBO J 18:5943–5952.

Xie Y, Chen C, Stevenson MA, Auron PE, Calderwood SK (2002a). Heat shock factor 1 represses transcription of the IL-1beta gene through physical interaction with the nuclear factor of interleukin 6. J Biol Chem 277:11802–11810.

Xie Y, Chen C, Stevenson MA, Hume DA, Auron PE, Calderwood SK (2002b). NF-IL6 and HSF1 have mutually antagonistic effects on transcription in monocytic cells. Biochem Biophys Res Commun 291:1071–1080.

Yagui-Beltran A, Craig AL, Lawrie L, Thompson D, Pospisilova S, Johnston D, Kernohan N, Hopwood D, Dillon JF, Hupp TR (2001) The human oesophageal squamous epithelium exhibits a novel type of heat shock protein response. Eur J Biochem 268:5343–5355.

Zhou J, Schmid T, Frank R, Brune B (2004) PI3K/Akt is required for heat shock proteins to protect hypoxia-inducible factor 1alpha from pVHL-independent degradation. J Biol Chem 279: 13506–13513.
Zou J, Guo Y, Guettouche T, Smith DF, Voellmy R (1998) Repression of heat shock transcription factor HSF1 activation by HSP90 (HSP90 complex) that forms a stress-sensitive complex with HSF1. Cell 94:471–480.
Zuo J, Rungger D, Voellmy R (1995) Multiple layers of regulation of human heat shock transcription factor 1. Mol Cell Biol 15:4319–4330.

Chapter 9
Alcohol and the Inflammatory Function of Immune Cells in Cancer Development

H. Joe Wang

Abbreviations

AID	Activation-induced cytidine deaminase
COX2	Cyclooxygenase 2
CSF-1	Colony-stimulating factor
CYP2E1	Cytochrome P450 2E1
DEN	Diethylnitrosamine
DRRs	Danger recognition receptors
EGF	Epidermal growth factor
EMT	Epithelial–mesenchymal transition
HBV	Hepatitis B virus
HCC	Hepatocellular carcinoma
HCV	Hepatitis C virus
HIF1	Hypoxia-inducible factor 1
Ig	Immunoglobulin
IKKb	I-kappa-b kinase 1
IL	Interleukin
LPS	Lipopolysaccharide
MDSC	Myeloid-derived suppressor cell
NADH	Nicotinamide adenine dinucleotide hydrate
NADPH	Nicotinamide adenine dinucleotide phosphate
NF-κB	Nuclear factor κB

H.J. Wang (✉)
Division of Metabolism and Health Effects, National Institute on Alcohol Abuse and Alcoholism, National Institutes of Health, Bethesda, MD, USA
e-mail: Wangh4@mail.nih.gov

S. Zakhari et al. (eds.), *Alcohol and Cancer*, DOI 10.1007/978-1-4614-0040-0_9,
© Springer Science+Business Media, LLC 2011

NK	Nature killer (cell)
PGE2	Prostaglandin E2
PRR	Pattern recognition receptors
PTEN	Phosphatase and tensin homologue deleted on chromosome 10
ROS	Reactive oxygen species
STAT3	Signal transducer and activator of transcription 3
TAM	Tumor-associated macrophage
TAN	Tumor-associated neutrophil
TGFβ	Transforming growth factor-β
Th	T helper cell
TLRs	Toll-like receptors
TNFα	Tumor necrosis factor alpha
VEGF	Vascular endothelial growth factor

Introduction

The concept that inflammation promotes carcinogenesis was first proposed by Rudolf Virchow in 1863 based on the observation that neoplastic tissues were enriched with leukocytes (reviewed in Balkwill and Mantovani 2001). It has since been supported by a large amount of evidence from epidemiological, clinical, and, more recently, molecular genetic studies (Mantovani et al. 2008). Chronic inflammation, mostly resulting from chronic infections, is an underlying condition for up to 15% of all cancers (Table 9.1; Coussens and Werb 2002; Grivennikov et al. 2010). Long-term use of nonsteroidal anti-inflammatory drugs reduces the risk of developing colon and other cancers. In experimental settings, many key inflammatory cells and factors have been shown to play indispensible roles in various steps of cancer development. Last but not the least, numerous oncogenic/epigenetic changes in human cancers have been functionally linked to their abilities to activate the inflammatory program and/or attract inflammatory cells to the cancer microenvironment.

Alcohol abuse is often associated with local and systemic inflammatory conditions. An elevated level of proinflammatory cytokines has been found in different organs and in circulation in alcoholics and alcohol-fed animals with or without liver diseases (McClain et al. 1999; Latvala et al. 2005; Qin et al. 2008). Furthermore, genetic studies have established in animal models that the proinflammatory cytokine, TNFα, and its receptor are causally linked to alcohol-mediated liver injury. As described in this chapter, alcohol-related chronic inflammation has a number of features similar to that found in the cancer microenvironment. Consistently, genetic variations in several inflammatory genes are associated with increased risks of liver and lung cancers in humans who abuse alcohol (Sakamoto et al. 2008; Kiyohara et al. 2010). Clinical studies also show that alcohol synergistically interacts with

Table 9.1 Chronic inflammatory conditions associated with neoplastic pathologies[a]

Pathologic condition	Associated neoplasm(s)	Etiologic agent
Asbestosis, silicosis	Mesothelioma, lung carcinoma	Asbestos fibers, silica particles
Bronchitis	Lung carcinoma	Silica, asbestos, smoking (nitrosamines, peroxides)
Cystitis, bladder inflammation	Bladder carcinoma	Chronic indwelling, urinary catheters
Gingivitis, *lichen planus*	Oral squamous cell carcinoma	
Inflammatory bowel disease, Crohn's disease, chronic ulcerative colitis	Colorectal carcinoma	
Lichen sclerosis	Vulvar squamous cell carcinoma	
Chronic pancreatitis, hereditary pancreatitis	Pancreatic carcinoma	Alcoholism, mutation in trypsinogen gene
Reflux esophagitis, Barrett's esophagus	Esophageal carcinoma	Gastric acids
Sialadenitis	Salivary gland carcinoma	
Sjögren syndrome, Hashimoto's thyroiditis	MALT[b] lymphoma	
Prostatitis	Prostate carcinoma	
Cancers associated with infectious agents		
Opisthorchis, cholangitis	Cholangiosarcoma, colon carcinoma	Liver flukes (*Opisthorchis viverrini*), bile acids
Chronic cholecystitis	Gall bladder cancer	Bacteria, gall bladder stones
Gastritis/ulcers	Gastric adenocarcinoma, MALT	*Helicobacter pylori*
Hepatitis	Hepatocellular carcinoma	Hepatitis B and/or C virus
Mononucleosis	B-cell non-Hodgkin's lymphoma, Burkitts lymphoma	Epstein-Barr virus
AIDS	Non-Hodgkin's lymphoma, squamous cell carcinoma, Kaposi's sarcoma	Human immunodeficiency virus, human herpesvirus type 8
Osteomyelitis	Carcinoma in draining sinuses	Bacterial infection
Pelvic inflammatory disease, chronic cervicitis	Ovarian carcinoma, cervical/anal carcinoma	Gonnorrhea, chlamydia, human papillomavirus
Chronic cystitis	Bladder, liver, rectal carcinoma, follicular lymphoma of the spleen	Schistosomiasis

[a]From Tlsty and Coussens (2006)
[b]*MALT* mucosa-associated lymphoid tissue

viral hepatitis to increase the inflammatory response and incidence of liver cancer (Singal and Anand 2007; Hassan et al. 2002). A recent study links the bacterial product lipopolysaccharide (LPS) in alcohol-fed animals to an increased incidence of liver cancer, further supporting the idea that alcohol-related inflammation can play a significant role in cancer development (Machida et al. 2009).

Major Components of an Inflammatory Response

NF-κB and STAT3

Nuclear factor κB (NF-κB) has a dual role as a signal integrator for transducing cytoplasmic signaling from a variety of infections and stress conditions, and as a core nuclear transcription factor for controlling the expression of a large array of genes. NF-κB targets include genes coding for immune mediators and factors with diverse functions in tissue repair and remodeling, such as cell proliferation and survival (antiapoptosis), angiogenesis, and cell migration (Pahl 1999; Pasparakis 2009). Activation of NF-κB can be induced by different types of inflammation inducers and sustained by a feed-foward loop via the autocrine or paracrine action of NF-κB target gene products (e.g., cytokines TNFα and IL-1β).

Signal transducer and activator of transcription 3 (STAT3) is another key transcription regulator of the inflammatory response and is functionally related to NF-κB. STAT3 also performs a dual function in transducing cytoplasmic signals from extracellular stimuli (cytokines and growth factors, in particular IL-6) and in regulating the expression of a selected set of genes coding for immune mediators, growth factors, and angiogenesis factors (Alvarez and Frank 2004). STAT3 regulated immune mediators play a key role in establishing a polarized tumor promoting inflammatory environment by stimulating the differentiation of naïve $CD4^+$ T cells into Th2, Th17, Treg, and by suppressing Th1 (see discussion below). Activation of STAT3 is sustained by a feed-forward loop by its target gene products, e.g., IL-6 and IL-10, as well as by epidermal growth factor (EGF).

Proinflammatory and Anti-inflammatory Mediators

Cytokines TNFα, IL-1β, and IL-6 are the primary proinflammatory cytokines that are induced during the early stage of an acute inflammatory response. Analogous to inflammation inducers, these cytokines can activate NF-κB (by TNFα, IL-1β) and STAT3 (by IL-6) through their cognate cell surface receptors. Production of these cytokines is further induced by the activated NF-κB and STAT3. Thus, these cytokines provide the host the positive feed-forward stimuli to rapidly amplify and sustain the production of the same cytokines and secondary immune mediators. Their ability to amplify and sustain inflammation explains why these cytokines can induce an inflammatory response in the absence of any exogenous or endogenous inducer. By activating NF-κB and STAT3, these cytokines also support various tissue repair activities including cell proliferation and survival, angiogenesis, and migration of diverse immune cells.

Other cytokines, such as IL-10 and TGFβ, have anti-inflammatory activities important for controlling excessive inflammatory response. IL-10 exerts its anti-inflammatory effect by inhibiting TNFα and IL-6 production from macrophages. In addition, IL-10, alone and in combination with other cytokines, plays an important role in the differentiation of adaptive T-cell immunity and suppression of proinflammatory Th1 T-cell immunity (Couper et al. 2008). TGFβ is an important negative regulator of cell proliferation and plays an important role in tissue remodeling and the differentiation of adaptive immune cells (Massagué 2008).

Inflammatory Immune Cells

The most common innate immune cells found at the sites of inflammation are neutrophils, macrophages, and NK cells (Medzhitov 2008). Neutrophils are recruited early in an acute inflammation and are responsible for microbe killing by phagocytosis and production of reactive oxygen species (ROS, via the respiratory burst). Macrophages, such as Kupffer cells in the liver, play an important role in resolving inflammation through phagocytic activity that removes cell debris. Different adaptive immune cells can also play important roles in chronic inflammation.

Acute inflammation is initiated by danger signals in exogenous microbial products (pathogenic factors) or endogenous molecules (from damaged cells). These signals are detected by macrophages via membrane-bound pathogen pattern recognition receptors (PRR) for exogenous inducers or danger recognition receptors (DRRs) for endogenous inducers. The best known PRRs are toll-like receptors (TLRs), which recognize molecular features in bacterial and viral products such as lipopolysaccharides (by TLR4), peptidoglycan (by TLR2), and single-stranded RNA (by TLR7). The receptor–ligand binding activates intracellular signaling pathways, which in turn activate several key transcription regulators including NF-κB and STAT3. These regulators then drive the expression of a large array of genes coding for inflammatory mediators including cytokines, chemokines, acute-phase response proteins, and the enzyme cyclooxygenase 2 (COX2) that synthesizes prostaglandins. These immune mediators carry out diverse functions of altering endothelial permeability, attracting and activating more immune cells to kill and clear infected and damaged cells. They also provide paracrine stimuli for cell proliferation, angiogenesis, tissue repair and remodeling, and ultimately, the resolution of inflammation.

During prolonged inflammation, innate immune cells and their cytokines also play a crucial role in developing the adaptive immune response. Macrophages and dendritic cells, via antigen presentation, help drive the differentiation of different branches of T-cell-mediated cellular, or B cell-mediated humoral, adaptive immunity. These adaptive immune cells can function as inflammation amplifiers by secreting additional cytokines and chemokines (Murphy et al. 2007).

Chronic Inflammation and Its Immune Cell Environment

Chronic inflammation develops when acute inflammation fails to eliminate an infectious agent or results from autoimmune or autoinflammatory diseases. The cellular and cytokine milieu generated by chronic inflammation vary significantly with the inflammation inducing agents and the involvement of distinct types of innate and adaptive immune cells. For example, psoriasis is a chronic inflammatory disease mediated by Th1cells characterized by accumulation of neutrophils and monocytes in the skin (Nickoloff et al. 2005). By contrast, in chronic inflammation associated with *Schistosoma mansoni* infection, the predominant cells involved are the Th2 type which activates B cells to produce high level of IgE (Murphy et al. 2007). The predominance of either the Th1 or Th2 phenotype in different cases is known as the polarized immune response. It has been reported that different types of TLR ligands might affect this polarization (Johansson et al. 2008). In addition to the initial influence from an inflammatory or infectious agent, this polarization can be further strengthened by a cytokine-based reciprocal inhibition of the development of Th1 or Th2 (Murphy et al. 2007).

The immune cells and cytokine milieu of a given chronic inflammation are also influenced by cellular and/or organismic feedback control mechanisms. For example, release of cortisol in the circulation is a neuroendocrine response to systemic and local inflammation. Cortisol can significantly suppress the production of TNFα from macrophages and monocytes but has no effect on IL-10, an anti-inflammatory cytokine involved in activating the Th2 response (Richards et al. 2000). Repeated exposure of dendritic cells to LPS also leads to an increased production of IL-10, which inhibits the production of primary proinflammatory cytokines TNFα and IL-6 (Yanagawa and Onoé 2007). Chronic inflammation also leads to the accumulation of myeloid-derived suppressor cells (MDSCs), which have been known to suppress the antitumor immune response (Ostrand-Rosenberg and Sinha 2009).

Mechanisms Underlying Cancer-Related Inflammation

Cellular Characteristics of Pro- and Anti-tumorigenic Inflammation

Histopathological studies have established that macrophages are the most common immune cells in cancer (tumor-associated macrophages, TAMs) and their presence is mostly associated with a poor patient prognosis (Qian and Pollard 2010). TAMs in human cancers appear to share a common phenotype, known as "alternatively activated" or M2, that has a low expression of TNFα and IL-6 and high expression of IL-10 and TGFβ. TNFα and IL-6 are known protumorigenic growth factors and IL-10 and TGFβ are believed to play roles in suppressing antitumor immunity (Mantovani et al. 2008). Genetic studies of the macrophage's function in experimental cancer models have largely supported a protumorigenic role for macrophages. For example, reduced macrophage density in cancer via ablation of macrophage growth factor (CSF-1) slows the rate of tumor progression. Consistently, overexpressing CSF-1 is associated with accelerated tumor progression. Several other immune cells, including mast cells and neutrophils (tumor associated neutrophil, TAN), can also have protumorigenic functions. Together, these innate inflammatory cells contribute to the formation of a protumorigenic inflammatory environment (de Visser et al. 2006).

By contrast, infiltration by lymphocytes (cytotoxic T cells and Th1 cells) in cancerous tissue is less common and their presence is associated with a better prognosis. Specifically, cytotoxic T cells or a Th1 inflammatory response is considered antitumorigenic. Other antitumorigenic cells include cytotoxic NK cells and dendritic cells (which play a role in activating Th1 CD4+ T cells) (de Visser et al. 2006).

Genetic and Epigenetic Activation of Protumorigenic Inflammation in Cancer Cells

The ability to activate an inflammatory program has been found in a number of oncogenes. For example, RET/PTC1 is a protein tyrosine kinase that induces the expression of inflammation mediator genes including the cytokine IL-1β, COX2, chemokines, growth factors, and extracellular matrix-degrading enzymes (Borrello et al. 2005). Oncogenic mutations in the epidermal growth factor (EGF) receptor and tyrosine kinase, another protein commonly associated with lung and breast cancers and glioblastoma, activate the expression of COX2, which in turn induces the inflammation mediator prostaglandin E2 (PGE2) (Xu and Shu 2007). Ras and Myc are among the most prevalent oncogenes in human cancers, and their activation induces IL-1β expression (Mantovani et al. 2008). The Ras oncogene also induces the expression of IL-6 and chemokine CXCL8 (IL-8), both of which are believed to promote angiogenesis by recruiting leukocytes to the cancer microenvironment (Ancrile et al. 2007; Sparmann and Bar-Sagi 2004). Inflammatory mediator expression has also been linked to genetic changes of tumor suppressor genes, such as those coding for TGFβ and the phosphatase and tensin homologue deleted on chromosome 10 (PTEN) (Mantovani et al. 2008).

Activation of key regulators of the inflammatory response, NF-κB and/or STAT3, is a frequent oncogenic/epigenetic event in tumorigenesis (Naugler and Karin 2008). Inhibition of NF-κB in these cancers is associated with increased apoptosis. Thus, the primary protumorigenic role of NF-κB in these cancer cells appears to be antiapoptotic. NF-κB has also been implicated in epithelial–mesenchymal transition (EMT)-mediated cancer cell development (Chua et al. 2007).

An IL-6-STAT3 feed-forward signaling loop is a common mechanism in different cancers, activation of which is considered an epigenetic event because it is mostly independent of genetic changes in cancer cells (Yu et al. 2009). As described earlier, STAT3 signaling, which is activated by IL-6 and also stimulates IL-6 production, is protumorigenic because it stimulates the expression of genes supporting cell proliferation, survival, and angiogenesis. In cultured mammary epithelial cells, the IL-6–STAT3 feed-forward loop can be activated via transient expression of a STAT3 upstream gene, Src, a protooncogenic tyrosine kinase and is sufficient for cell transformation, which is characterized by increased motility and invasive ability, and tumor formation in nude mice. This transformation can also be achieved by transient exposure of the normal cells in culture to IL-6 (Iliopoulos et al. 2009).

Indispensible Role of Immune Cells in Cancer Development

Activation of an inflammatory program in precancer cells by itself is often insufficient for cancer development. For example, although an oncogenic change in Kras, a protein coded by a rat sarcoma viral gene homolog, can induce IL-1β production, it is insufficient to induce pancreatic cancer. Rather, the combination of the mutated Kras and a mild chronic pancreatitis is necessary for the induction of pancreatic ductal adenocarcinoma in a mouse model (Guerra et al. 2007). Consistently, in many cases, activation of NF-κB and STAT3 in cancer cells is not dependent on oncogenic changes, but rather on stimuli derived from cancer-surrounding immune cells (Grivennikov and Karin 2010). Recent studies have shown that in many animal models, activation of these inflammation regulators in the immune cells is indispensible for tumorigenesis and tumor progression (reviewed in Grivennikov and Karin 2010).

In mouse models of hepatocellular carcinoma (HCC), immune cell-generated cytokines are critical for cancer development. In a mouse model with an multiple drug resistance 2 P-glycoprotein (Mdr2) deletion, HCC development was preceded by hepatocyte hyperplasia, portal inflammation, and immune cell infiltration (Pikarsky et al. 2004). In these hyperproliferative hepatocytes, NF-κB was activated and its activation was prevented by treatment with ibuprofen (a nonsteroidal anti-inflammatory drug). Importantly, hepatocyte NF-κB activation was dependent on the paracrine action of TNFα supplied by endothelial and inflammatory immune cells. Furthermore, depletion of TNFα by antibody increased hepatocyte apoptosis and reduced HCC incidence (Pikarsky et al. 2004). Therefore, the protumorigenic role of immune cells, via TNFα, is to support cancer cell survival. In another model, mice exposed to the tumorigenic agent diethylnitrosamine (DEN) developed HCC following DEN-mediated hepatocyte cell death. The DEN-induced HCC is dependent on NF-κB activation and IL-6 production in the Kupffer cells (Maeda et al. 2005; Naugler et al. 2007). Deletion of NF-κB-activating kinase IKKb gene in myeloid cells (progenitors of Kupffer cells and other innate immune cells), or knockout of the IL-6 gene, reduced the incidence of HCC. It was suggested that IL-6 from Kupffer cells serves as a growth stimulating signal for a compensatory hepatocyte proliferation, eventually leading to hyperproliferation, in the presence of DEN-induced cell injury. A protumorigenic role of NF-κB in myeloid cells has also been demonstrated in a mouse model of colitis-associated colon cancers (Greten et al. 2004).

Tumor-associated macrophages (TAM) are the best-studied cells among tumor-infiltrating inflammatory cells. Their role in cancer development has been demonstrated in a breast cancer mouse model (Lin et al. 2001). The absence of macrophages as a result of gene deletion of macrophage colony-stimulating factor (CSF-1) delayed the development of the tumors into metastatic carcinomas without affecting the incidence and growth of the tumors. Coculture of cancer cells with monocyte-derived macrophages increased the invasiveness of cancer cells (Hagemann et al. 2005). The increase of cancer cell invasiveness is dependent on TNFα from macrophages and TNFα-induced NF-κB activation in the cancer cells. In addition to innate immune cells, adaptive immune B cells have a protumorigenic role, and deposition of antibody by

B cells on immune cells in the cancer microenvironment has been proposed to mediate the release of protumorigenic inflammatory mediators (de Visser et al. 2005).

Although beyond the scope of this discussion, a protumorigenic role for different inflammatory cells and mediators has been demonstrated or implicated in almost all substages of cancer development including tumorigenesis, tumor promotion, angiogenesis, and metastasis (reviewed in Grivennikov et al. 2010).

Inflammation-Based Evasion of Antitumor Immunity and Cancer Inhibitory Inflammation

In cancer patients, myeloid-derived suppressor cells (MDSCs) are often enriched in the cancer microenvironment and in circulation (Ostrand-Rosenberg and Sinha 2009). These cells have characteristics of immature myeloid cells that are precursors of dendritic cells, macrophages, and/or granulocytes. MDSCs suppress the function of antitumor immune cells that include natural killer (NK) cells, macrophages, and $CD4^+$ and $CD8^+$ T cells (see Chap. 10). Cytokines derived from cancer cells, such as granulocyte-macrophage colony-stimulating factor (GM-CSF), have been linked to the development of MDSCs (Marigo et al. 2008). Interestingly, MDSCs also accumulate in the periphery in response to bacterial infection and autoimmune conditions. The inflammatory cytokines IL-1β, IL-6 and the mediator prostaglandin E2 have been shown to induce MDSC development (Ostrand-Rosenberg and Sinha 2009).

A key factor in cancer inflammatory cell-mediated evasion of antitumor immune response appears to be STAT3. Its ablation in hematopoietic cells in a mouse tumor model triggers an inhibition of tumor growth and metastasis by both innate and adaptive immune cells (Kortylewski et al. 2005). The action of STAT3 in the evasion of antitumor immunity seems to be closely related to its role in the induction of IL-10, which inhibits the development of antitumor immunity, especially Th1 cytotoxic T cells. Therefore, in addition to its role in promoting cancer cell growth, STAT3 plays a significant role in restraining or limiting antitumor immunity (Yu et al. 2009).

Chronic Inflammation-Driven Carcinogenesis

The best known examples of cancer that are originated from preexisting inflammatory environments include *Helicobacter pylori* induced gastritis, HCV- or HBV-induced hepatitis, and microflora-linked inflammatory bowel diseases. In all these cases, the risk for cancer development correlates with the extent and severity of inflammatory conditions in patients. Consistently, STAT3 activation is a common feature in these cancers (Yu et al. 2009). Furthermore, studies of gene polymorphisms also implicate inflammation in cancer development. In the case of *H. pylori* infection, polymorphisms associated with elevated expression of inflammatory cytokine genes IL-1β and TNFα increase the risk of gastric cancer (Polk and Peek 2010).

Overexpressing IL-1β in mice in stomach epithelial (parietal) cells stimulates carcinoma development when infected with a related mouse-adapted Helicobacter species, *H. felis*. As discussed earlier in an animal model of colitis-associated colon cancer, TNFα as well as IL-6 are required for cancer development. Recent studies have also found that polymorphisms of TNFα and IL-1β genes correlate with increased risk of colitis-associated colorectal cancer (reviewed in Feagins et al. 2009). Given that TNFα, IL-1β, IL-6 are primary inflammatory mediators that have pleiotropic and target cell type-specific functions, the specific mechanisms leading to cancer development are likely to be complex.

Alcohol-Induced Inflammation and Cancer Development

Chronic Inflammatory Conditions Caused by Alcohol Use

The best studied inflammatory condition associated with alcohol use is alcoholic liver disease. Patients with alcoholic liver disease (hepatitis or cirrhosis) often show symptoms of systemic inflammation including fever, anorexia, and elevation of circulating proinflammatory cytokines (McClain et al. 1999). Furthermore, an increase in circulating cytokines has also been observed in alcoholics without liver disease (Table 9.2; Fig. 9.1).

As discussed below, chronic alcohol abuse promotes systemic and local inflammation via three broad and interconnected mechanisms: (1) increasing the translocation of exogenous inflammatory inducers, such as LPS, from gut microflora, (2) modulating immune cells and their response to inflammatory inducers, and (3) increasing reactive oxygen species (ROS) and tissue injury due to alcohol metabolism and alcohol-related nutritional abnormalities (reviewed in Wang et al. 2010). In addition, alcohol-related inflammatory conditions can be exacerbated by interacting with other chronic medical conditions including viral hepatitis.

Table 9.2 Features of alcohol-related chronic inflammatory conditions

Features	Known function
Liver and circulating cytokines[a] (TNFα & IL-6)	Inflammation amplifiers; growth factors
Endotoxemia (circulating LPS)[b]	Inducer of cytokine production via TLR4
Liver & circulating chemokine[a] (IL-8)	Chemoattractant for neutrophils; angiogenic factor
Immune cells	
Neutrophils[c]	Cytotoxicity (ROS, RNS)
Th17 T cells[d]	Amplifier of inflammation
MDSCs (myeloid-derived suppressor cells)[e]	Immune suppressor; angiogenic factor

[a]McClain et al. (1999), Latvala et al. (2005)
[b]Fukui (2005)
[c]Jaeschke (2002)
[d]Lemmers et al. (2009)
[e]Zhang and Meadows (2010)

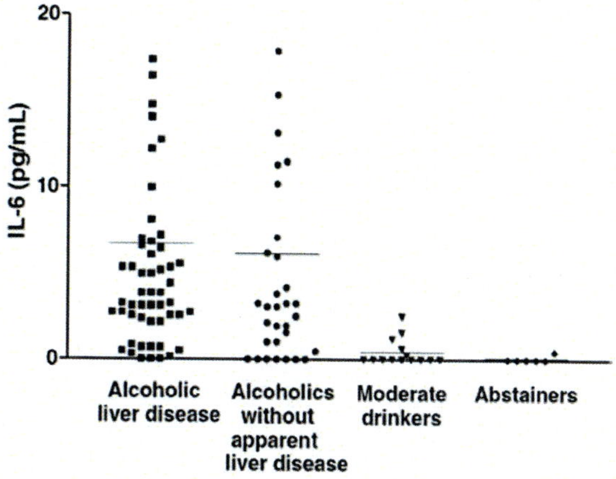

Fig. 9.1 Plasma IL-6 level in alcoholics. Reprinted by permission from Macmillan Publishers Ltd: [the American Journal of Gastroenterology] (Latvala et al. 2005), copyright (2005)

Alcohol use stimulates the translocation of microbial products, especially LPS, into circulation, a phenomenon reported extensively in animal models and humans (Wang et al. 2010). LPS, a major cell-wall component of Gram-negative bacteria, is a potent inducer of the inflammatory response. This response is mediated by the cell surface receptor TLR4 that is highly expressed in innate immune cells. Mechanistically, alcohol exposure can cause a significant influx of gut microflora products by altering gut epithelial cell permeability and leakiness, as well as gut microflora composition. The continued presence of circulating LPS in alcohol abusers directly contributes to the elevation of circulating inflammatory cytokines.

Chronic alcohol exposure is also known to modulate the response of immune cells to inflammation inducers such as LPS (Wang et al. 2010). Alcohol feeding in mice for up to 7 weeks potentiated the LPS-induced production of proinflammatory cytokines from monocytes. Monocytes from alcoholics with liver diseases spontaneously produce TNFα and overproduce it in response to LPS exposure (McClain et al. 2002). Chronic alcohol consumption also adversely affects the number and function of NK cells and is associated with a reduced basal level of neuroendocrine activities that regulate the inflammatory responses. Finally, since the liver plays a critical role in detoxification of microbial products, alcohol-related liver damage also inadvertently prolongs the bioactivity of microbial products in circulation.

Furthermore, tissue injury caused by alcohol abuse and metabolism, especially in the liver, might play an important role in the amplification and maintenance of chronic inflammatory conditions. Factors released from damaged/dead cells, known as "danger signals", provide endogenous inducers of inflammatory responses. Alcohol-induced tissue injury is believed to be mediated by multiple mechanisms that involve the accumulation of ROS, mitochondrial defects and cell death, hypoxia, and autoimmune responses (reviewed in Albano 2008). As a key feature of alcohol-induced injury, increased ROS is a by-product of alcohol metabolism via CYP2E1 enzyme, the mitochondrial respiratory chain, and respiratory burst via the activation of Kupffer cells and infiltrating neutrophils. The potency of ROS in tissue damage is further increased by alcohol abuse-associated iron overload. In addition to its potential role in DNA damage and mutagenesis, mitochondrial dysfunction, and cell death, ROS itself is an activator of the inflammatory regulator NF-κB in some cells (Gloire et al. 2006).

Alcohol-induced tissue injury is characterized by mitochondrial damage, apoptosis and necrosis in hepatocytes. For example, by blocking methionine synthesis, alcohol interferes with glutathione (GSH) synthesis and causes homocysteine accumulation. The latter effect has been linked to ER stress. ER stress in turn stimulates a Ca^{2+} release-dependent mitochondrial permeability transition (MPT), a key event that triggers apoptosis. Increased ROS, produced from mitochondria driven by alcohol metabolism, might also contribute to GSH depletion, which is known to sensitize hepatocytes to TNFα-induced killing. As discussed earlier, TNFα level is elevated by alcohol use through activation of Kupffer cells by LPS. Alcohol metabolism is also associated with hypoxia, which can cause both cellular injury and induction of inflammation-related transcription regulator HIF-1 (Arteel et al. 1996).

Acetaldehyde, a key alcohol metabolite, and a number of products generated from it can form adducts that induce the adaptive immune response, which correlates with the severity of liver damage, increased IgG loading, and increased proinflammatory Th17 T cells (Rolla et al. 2000; Duryee et al. 2007; Lemmers et al. 2009). Thus, alcohol use can activate multiple processes that might interact additively or synergistically in causing tissue injury and the inflammatory response.

Epidemiological studies suggest that alcohol use promotes HCC development by synergistically interacting with chronic HCV infection, diabetes, or obesity (Hassan et al. 2002; Hart et al. 2010). A common feature shared by all these conditions is chronic inflammation. For example, alcohol abuse, chronic HCV infection, and obesity are all associated with increasing levels of circulating LPS (Caradonna et al. 2002; Cani et al. 2007; Wang et al. 2010). Alcohol abuse, obesity, and diabetes are also associated with elevated levels of proinflammatory cytokines (Hotamisligil et al. 1993; Pickup et al. 1997; Wang et al. 2010). In addition, the inflammatory condition associated with alcohol and HCV could also be enhanced by their separate ability to induce ROS production. It was demonstrated in cultured cells expressing HCV core protein that alcohol exposure can further increase the level of ROS and cell death (Otani et al. 2005).

Protumorigenic Potential of Alcohol-Related Inflammation

Significantly, alcohol-induced inflammatory conditions have a number of features that had been implicated in cancer promotion in non-alcohol use settings. First, alcoholics have liver and systemic elevation of protumorigenic inflammatory mediators, in particular, IL-6 (Nicolaou et al. 2004; Latvala et al. 2005, Fig. 9.1). By activating STAT3, IL-6 can play a role not only in cell proliferation but also in cell survival, angiogenesis, and damage protection. Consistent with the elevated IL-6, STAT3 is activated in hepatocytes in patients with alcoholic hepatitis and this activation is associated with elevated expression of cell survival genes (Larrea et al. 2006;

Horiguchi et al. 2007). STAT3 activation is also observed in hepatocytes in patients with HCV and HCV/alcohol (Horiguchi et al. 2007). Elevated IL-6 has been implicated in the development of different types of cancer including high-fat-diet-induced HCC in mice and has been proposed to be the best predictor of HCC development in patients with HBV infection (Park et al. 2010; Grivennikov et al. 2010). IL-6 is also an autocrine/paracrine growth factor for multiple myeloma, liver, and breast cancer (Kawano et al. 1988; Studebaker et al. 2008).

Second, alcohol abuse alters the number and functions of innate and adaptive inflammatory cells and these alterations also have the potential to be protumorigenic (Murugaiyan and Saha 2009; Lemmers et al. 2009). Alcoholics with liver disease have a significant increase in their plasma IgA and IgG, some of which had specificity to adducts derived from alcohol metabolites, suggesting increases of B cell functions (Lee 1965; Clot et al. 1996). An increase of IL-17 secreting cells and neutrophils in the liver and in circulation appears to be a unique feature of patients with alcoholic liver diseases (Lemmers et al. 2009). Both B cell and IL-17 producing Th17 cells have been implicated in tumor promoting inflammation, whereas neutrophils have been linked to increased angiogenesis in cancer settings (de Visser et al. 2005; Grivennikov et al. 2010). In addition, chronic alcohol use is associated with NK cell dysfunction (Jeong et al. 2008) and accumulation of MDSCs (Zhang and Meadows 2010), changes that have also been found in cancer patients.

Third, as discussed earlier, chronic alcohol abuse can cause perpetual cell injuries (esp. in the liver), which not only sustain the inflammation but also drive compensatory cell proliferation. The cell proliferation in turn provides increased opportunities for carcinogenesis in a potentially protumorigenic environment. Chronic alcohol-use-related tissue injury is characterized by apoptosis and necrosis, especially in the liver and pancreas (Feldstein and Gores 2004; Papachristou et al. 2006). Many factors including alcohol metabolism-induced hypoxia, infiltrating neutrophils, Ig loading, oxidative stress, iron overload, homocysteine accumulation, and circulating LPS and cytokines could contribute to the injury and stimulate compensatory proliferation (Albano 2008).

Lastly, alcohol abuse leads to the elevation of circulating LPS, which might have numerous of protumorigenic roles. For example, alcohol-induced elevation of LPS has been suggested to be important in stimulating ROS production in macrophages via a respiratory burst catalyzed by membrane bound NADPH oxidase (Kono et al. 2000). ROS are capable of inducing nonspecific DNA damage, resulting in oncogenic mutations. LPS also induces the expression of activation-induced cytidine deaminase (AID), an enzyme known to contribute to gastric and liver cancer by inducing somatic mutations (reviewed in Grivennikov et al. 2010). Elevated LPS is also expected to play a key role, via activating TLR4 on variety of immune cells, in the production of the aforementioned cytokine IL-6 as a tumor promoting growth stimulus. Furthermore, LPS and TLR4 signaling have been linked to other growth-stimulating pathways implicated in HCC development (Berasain et al. 2009). Last but not the least, in animal models, LPS itself caused increased progression of cancer metastasis, a phenomenon dependent on NF-κB signaling (Naugler and Karin 2008).

Clinical and Experimental Evidence Supporting Alcohol-Induced Inflammation in Cancer Development

Based on case controlled studies of Japanese HCC and lung cancer patients, variations in the inflammatory mediator genes for IL-1β have been found to confer a significant risk for lung and liver cancers in alcoholics (Sakamoto et al. 2008; Kiyohara et al. 2010). Variations of TLR4 and IL-10 genes have been found to be associated with the risk of alcoholic liver disease and fibrosis (Wilfred de Alwis and Day 2007; Huang et al. 2007). Such findings are relevant, since alcoholic liver disease, especially cirrhosis, is a strong predictor of HCC (Voigt 2005).

Although experimental studies of the effect of chronic alcohol use on cancer development are limited, research findings support the hypothesis that chronic alcohol promotes cancer via its association with inflammation. In a transplant melanoma mouse model, Tan et al. (2007) found that chronic alcohol was associated with an increase in angiogenic cytokine VEGF expression and a twofold increase in tumor weight. Alcohol abuse in conjunction with HCV was demonstrated to synergistically accelerate the progression of liver diseases and HCC (Hassan et al. 2002). Another study in a mouse model suggests that alcohol-mediated LPS translocation could play a significant role in HCC development in the context of HCV infection (Machida et al. 2009) and that the increase in the incidence of hepatoma due to chronic alcohol feeding in mice expressing HCV NS5A is dependent on the LPS receptor TLR4 (Machida et al. 2009).

Future Perspectives

Clinical and experimental evidence supports the premise that alcohol-related inflammation has the capacity to promote cancer development, especially in the liver. However, functional study of inflammatory cells and mediators in developing alcohol-related cancer in the liver and other organs is lacking. For example, IL-6 has been implicated in promoting the development of many types of cancers, and its level is significantly elevated in alcoholics. Its role in developing alcohol-related liver cancer could be examined in animal models, e.g., by a gene knockout approach. In the longer term, a comprehensive examination of inflammatory cells and mediators in the microenvironment of alcohol-related cancers using high-throughput and/or systems biology approaches is needed. Such research will provide a close-up look into the influence of alcohol-related inflammation on cancer that might be critical for setting future research directions. Lastly, since inflammation is a pathological condition shared by alcohol and comorbid conditions (smoking, viral hepatitis, and obesity), the role of alcohol-related inflammation in cancer development should be examined under comorbid conditions.

References

Albano E. (2008) New concepts in the pathogenesis of alcoholic liver disease. Expert Rev Gastroenterol Hepatol. 2:749–59.

Alvarez JV, Frank DA. (2004) Genome-wide analysis of STAT target genes: elucidating the mechanism of STAT-mediated oncogenesis. Cancer Biol Ther. 3:1045–50.

Ancrile B, Lim KH, Counter CM. (2007) Oncogenic Ras-induced secretion of IL6 is required for tumorigenesis. Genes Dev. 21:1714–9.

Arteel GE, Raleigh JA, Bradford BU, Thurman RG. (1996) Acute alcohol produces hypoxia directly in rat liver tissue in vivo: role of Kupffer cells. Am J Physiol. 271(3 Pt 1):G494-500.

Balkwill F, Mantovani A. (2001) Inflammation and cancer: back to Virchow? Lancet. 357:539–45.

Berasain C, Castillo J, Perugorria MJ, Latasa MU, Prieto J, Avila MA. (2009) Inflammation and liver cancer: new molecular links. Ann N Y Acad Sci. 1155:206–21.

Borrello MG, Alberti L, Fischer A, et al., (2005) Induction of a proinflammatory program in normal human thyrocytes by the RET/PTC1 oncogene. Proc Natl Acad Sci USA. 102:14825–30.

Cani PD, Amar J, Iglesias MA, Poggi M, Knauf C, et al., (2007) Metabolic endotoxemia initiates obesity and insulin resistance. Diabetes. 56:1761–72.

Caradonna L, Mastronardi ML, Magrone T, Cozzolongo R, Cuppone R, Manghisi OG, Caccavo D, Pellegrino NM, Amoroso A, Jirillo E, Amati L. (2002) Biological and clinical significance of endotoxemia in the course of hepatitis C virus infection. Curr Pharm Des. 8:995–1005.

Chua HL, Bhat-Nakshatri P, Clare SE, et al. (2007) NF-kappaB represses E-cadherin expression and enhances epithelial to mesenchymal transition of mammary epithelial cells: potential involvement of ZEB-1 and ZEB-2. Oncogene. 26:711–24.

Clot P, Albano E, Eliasson E, Tabone M, Aricò S, Israel Y, Moncada C, Ingelman-Sundberg M. (1996) Cytochrome P4502E1 hydroxyethyl radical adducts as the major antigen in autoantibody formation among alcoholics. Gastroenterology. 111:206–16.

Couper KN, Blount DG, Riley EM. (2008) IL-10: the master regulator of immunity to infection. J Immunol. 180:5771–7.

Coussens LM, Werb Z. (2002) Inflammation and cancer. Nature. 420:860–7.

de Visser KE, Eichten A, Coussens LM. (2006) Paradoxical roles of the immune system during cancer development. Nat Rev Cancer. 6:24–37.

de Visser KE, Korets LV, Coussens LM. (2005) De novo carcinogenesis promoted by chronic inflammation is B lymphocyte dependent. Cancer Cell. 7:411–23.

Duryee MJ, Klassen LW, Thiele GM. (2007) Immunological response in alcoholic liver disease. World J Gastroenterol. 13:4938–46.

Feagins LA, Souza RF, Spechler SJ. (2009) Carcinogenesis in IBD: potential targets for the prevention of colorectal cancer. Nat Rev Gastroenterol Hepatol. 6:297–305.

Feldstein A, Gores GJ. (2004) Steatohepatitis and apoptosis: therapeutic implications. Am J Gastroenterol. 99:1718–9.

Fukui H. (2005) Relation of endotoxin, endotoxin binding proteins and macrophages to severe alcoholic liver injury and multiple organ failure. Alcohol Clin Exp Res 29:172S-179S

Gloire G, Legrand-Poels S, Piette J. (2006) NF-kappaB activation by reactive oxygen species: fifteen years later. Biochem Pharmacol. 72:1493–505.

Greten FR, Eckmann L, Greten TF, et al. (2004) IKKbeta links inflammation and tumorigenesis in a mouse model of colitis-associated cancer. Cell. 118:285–96.

Grivennikov SI, Greten FR, Karin M. (2010) Immunity, inflammation, and cancer. Cell. 140:883–99.

Grivennikov SI, Karin M. (2010) Dangerous liaisons: STAT3 and NF-kappaB collaboration and crosstalk in cancer. Cytokine Growth Factor Rev. 21:11–19.

Guerra C, Schuhmacher AJ, Cañamero M, et al. (2007) Chronic pancreatitis is essential for induction of pancreatic ductal adenocarcinoma by K-Ras oncogenes in adult mice. Cancer Cell. 11:291–302.

Hagemann T, Wilson J, Kulbe H, et al. (2005) Macrophages induce invasiveness of epithelial cancer cells via NF-kappa B and JNK. J Immunol. 175:1197–205.
Hart CL, Morrison DS, Batty GD, Mitchell RJ, Davey Smith G. (2010) Effect of body mass index and alcohol consumption on liver disease: analysis of data from two prospective cohort studies. BMJ. 340:c1240.
Hassan MM, Hwang LY, Hatten CJ, et al. (2002) Risk factors for hepatocellular carcinoma: synergism of alcohol with viral hepatitis and diabetes mellitus. Hepatology. 36:1206–13.
Horiguchi N, Ishac EJ, Gao B. (2007) Liver regeneration is suppressed in alcoholic cirrhosis: correlation with decreased STAT3 activation. Alcohol. 41:271–80.
Hotamisligil GS, Shargill NS, Spiegelman BM. (1993) Adipose expression of tumor necrosis factor-alpha: direct role in obesity-linked insulin resistance. Science. 259:87–91.
Huang H, Shiffman ML, Friedman S, et al. (2007) A 7 gene signature identifies the risk of developing cirrhosis in patients with chronic hepatitis C. Hepatology. 46:297–306.
Iliopoulos D, Hirsch HA, Struhl K. (2009) An epigenetic switch involving NF-kappaB, Lin28, Let-7 MicroRNA, and IL6 links inflammation to cell transformation. Cell. 139:693–706.
Jaeschke H. (2002) Neutrophil-mediated tissue injury in alcoholic hepatitis. Alcohol. 27:23–7.
Jeong WI, Park O, Gao B. (2008) Abrogation of the antifibrotic effects of natural killer cells/interferon-gamma contributes to alcohol acceleration of liver fibrosis. Gastroenterology. 134:248–58.
Johansson M, Denardo DG, Coussens LM. (2008) Polarized immune responses differentially regulate cancer development. Immunol Rev. 222:145–54.
Kawano M, Hirano T, Matsuda T, Taga T, Horii Y, Iwato K, Asaoku H, Tang B, Tanabe O, Tanaka H, et al. (1988) Autocrine generation and requirement of BSF-2/IL-6 for human multiple myelomas. Nature. 332:83–5.
Kiyohara C, Horiuchi T, Takayama K, Nakanishi Y. (2010) IL1B rs1143634 polymorphism, cigarette smoking, alcohol use, and lung cancer risk in a Japanese population. J Thorac Oncol. 5:299–304.
Kono H, Rusyn I, Yin M, Gäbele E, Yamashina S, Dikalova A, Kadiiska MB, Connor HD, Mason RP, Segal BH, Bradford BU, Holland SM, Thurman RG. (2000) NADPH oxidase-derived free radicals are key oxidants in alcohol-induced liver disease. J Clin Invest. 106:867–72.
Kortylewski M, Kujawski M, Wang T, et al. (2005) Inhibiting Stat3 signaling in the hematopoietic system elicits multicomponent antitumor immunity. Nat Med. 11:1314–21.
Larrea E, Aldabe R, Molano E, et al. (2006) Altered expression and activation of signal transducers and activators of transcription (STATs) in hepatitis C virus infection: in vivo and in vitro studies. Gut. 55:1188–96.
Latvala J, Hietala J, Koivisto H, Järvi K, Anttila P, Niemelä O. (2005) Immune Responses to Ethanol Metabolites and Cytokine Profiles Differentiate Alcoholics with or without Liver Disease. Am J Gastroenterol. 100:1303–10.
Lee FI. (1965) Immunoglobulins in viral hepatitis and active alcoholic liver-disease. Lancet. 2:1043–6.
Lemmers A, Moreno C, Gustot T, et al. (2009) The interleukin-17 pathway is involved in human alcoholic liver disease. Hepatology. 49:646–57.
Lin EY, Nguyen AV, Russell RG, Pollard JW. (2001) Colony-stimulating factor 1 promotes progression of mammary tumors to malignancy. J Exp Med. 193:727–40.
Machida K, Tsukamoto H, Mkrtchyan H, et al. (2009) Toll-like receptor 4 mediates synergism between alcohol and HCV in hepatic oncogenesis involving stem cell marker Nanog. Proc Natl Acad Sci U S A. 106:1548–53.
Maeda S, Kamata H, Luo JL, Leffert H, Karin M. (2005) IKKbeta couples hepatocyte death to cytokine-driven compensatory proliferation that promotes chemical hepatocarcinogenesis. Cell. 121:977–90.
Mantovani A, Allavena P, Sica A, Balkwill F. (2008) Cancer-related inflammation. Nature. 454:436–44.
Marigo I, Dolcetti L, Serafini P, Zanovello P, Bronte V. (2008) Tumor-induced tolerance and immune suppression by myeloid derived suppressor cells. Immunol Rev. 222:162–79.

Massagué J. (2008) TGFbeta in Cancer. Cell. 134:215–30.
McClain CJ, Barve S, Deaciuc I, Kugelmas M, Hill D. (1999) Cytokines in alcoholic liver disease. Semin Liver Dis. 19:205–19.
McClain CJ, Hill DB, Song Z, Deaciuc I, Barve S. (2002) Monocyte activation in alcoholic liver disease. Alcohol. 27:53–61.
Medzhitov R. (2008) Origin and physiological roles of inflammation. Nature. 454:428–35.
Murphy KP, Travers P, Walport M, Janeway C. (2007) Immunobiology (7th ed). Garland Science, New York, New York.
Murugaiyan G, Saha B. (2009) Protumor vs antitumor functions of IL-17. J Immunol. 183:4169–75.
Naugler WE, Karin M. (2008) NF-kappaB and cancer-identifying targets and mechanisms. Curr Opin Genet Dev18:19–26.
Naugler WE, Sakurai T, Kim S, Maeda S, Kim K, Elsharkawy AM, Karin M. (2007) Gender disparity in liver cancer due to sex differences in MyD88-dependent IL-6 production. Science. 317:121–4.
Nickoloff B. J., Ben-Neriah, Y. & Pikarsky, E. (2005) Inflammation and cancer: is the link as simple as we think? J. Invest. Dermatol. 124, x-xiv.
Nicolaou C, Chatzipanagiotou S, Tzivos D, et al. (2004) Serum cytokine concentrations in alcohol-dependent individuals without liver disease. Alcohol. 32:243–7.
Ostrand-Rosenberg S, Sinha P. (2009) Myeloid-derived suppressor cells: linking inflammation and cancer. J Immunol. 182:4499–506.
Otani K, Korenaga M, Beard MR, et al. (2005) Hepatitis C virus core protein, cytochrome P450 2E1, and alcohol produce combined mitochondrial injury and cytotoxicity in hepatoma cells. Gastroenterology. 128:96–107.
Pahl HL. (1999) Activators and target genes of Rel/NF-kappaB transcription factors. Oncogene. 18:6853–66.
Papachristou GI, Papachristou DJ, Morinville VD, Slivka A, Whitcomb DC. (2006) Chronic alcohol consumption is a major risk factor for pancreatic necrosis in acute pancreatitis. Am J Gastroenterol. 101:2605–10.
Park EJ, Lee JH, Yu GY, et al. (2010) Dietary and genetic obesity promote liver inflammation and tumorigenesis by enhancing IL-6 and TNF expression. Cell. 140:197–208.
Pasparakis M. (2009) Regulation of tissue homeostasis by NF-kappaB signalling: implications for inflammatory diseases. Nat Rev Immunol. 9:778–88.
Pickup JC, Mattock MB, Chusney GD, Burt D. (1997) NIDDM as a disease of the innate immune system: association of acute-phase reactants and interleukin-6 with metabolic syndrome X. Diabetologia. 40:1286–92.
Pikarsky E, Porat RM, Stein I, et al. (2004) NF-kappaB functions as a tumour promoter in inflammation-associated cancer. Nature. 431:461–6.
Polk DB, Peek RM Jr. (2010) Helicobacter pylori: gastric cancer and beyond. Nat Rev Cancer. 10:403–14.
Qian BZ, Pollard JW. (2010) Macrophage diversity enhances tumor progression and metastasis. Cell. 141:39–51.
Qin L, He J, Hanes RN, Pluzarev O, Hong JS, Crews FT. (2008) Increased systemic and brain cytokine production and neuroinflammation by endotoxin following ethanol treatment. J Neuroinflammation. 5:10.
Richards DF, Fernandez M, Caulfield J, Hawrylowicz CM. (2000) Glucocorticoids drive human CD8(+) T cell differentiation towards a phenotype with high IL-10 and reduced IL-4, IL-5 and IL-13 production. Eur J Immunol. 30:2344–54.
Rolla R, Vay D, Mottaran E, Parodi M, Traverso N, Aricó S, Sartori M, Bellomo G, Klassen LW, Thiele GM, Tuma DJ, Albano E. (2000) Detection of circulating antibodies against malondialdehyde-acetaldehyde adducts in patients with alcohol-induced liver disease. Hepatology. 31:878–84.
Sakamoto T, Higaki Y, Hara M, et al. (2008) Interaction between interleukin-1beta -31T/C gene polymorphism and drinking and smoking habits on the risk of hepatocellular carcinoma among Japanese. Cancer Lett. 271:98–104.

Singal AK, Anand BS (2007) Mechanisms of synergy between alcohol and hepatitis C virus. J Clin Gastroenterol. 41:761–72.

Sparmann A, Bar-Sagi D. (2004) Ras-induced interleukin-8 expression plays a critical role in tumor growth and angiogenesis. Cancer Cell. 6:447–58.

Studebaker AW, Storci G, Werbeck JL, Sansone P, Sasser AK, Tavolari S, Huang T, Chan MW, Marini FC, Rosol TJ, Bonafé M, Hall BM. (2008) Fibroblasts isolated from common sites of breast cancer metastasis enhance cancer cell growth rates and invasiveness in an interleukin-6-dependent manner. Cancer Res. 68:9087–95.

Tan W, Bailey AP, Shparago M, Busby B, Covington J, Johnson JW, Young E, Gu JW. (2007) Chronic alcohol consumption stimulates VEGF expression, tumor angiogenesis and progression of melanoma in mice. Cancer Biol Ther. 6:1211–7.

Tlsty TD, Coussens LM. (2006) Tumor stroma and regulation of cancer development. Annu Rev Pathol. 1:119–50.

Voigt MD. (2005) Alcohol in hepatocellular cancer. Clin Liver Dis. 9:151–69.

Wang HJ, Zakhari S, Jung MK. (2010) Alcohol, inflammation, and gut-liver-brain interactions in tissue damage and disease development. World J Gastroenterol. 16:1304–13.

Wilfred de Alwis NM, Day CP. (2007) Genetics of alcoholic liver disease and nonalcoholic fatty liver disease. Semin Liver Dis. 27:44–54.

Xu K, Shu HK. (2007) EGFR activation results in enhanced cyclooxygenase-2 expression through p38 mitogen-activated protein kinase-dependent activation of the Sp1/Sp3 transcription factors in human gliomas. Cancer Res. 67:6121–9.

Yanagawa Y, Onoé K. (2007) Enhanced IL-10 production by TLR4- and TLR2-primed dendritic cells upon TLR restimulation. J Immunol. 178:6173–80.

Yu H, Pardoll D, Jove R. (2009) STATs in cancer inflammation and immunity: a leading role for STAT3. Nat Rev Cancer. 9:798–809.

Zhang H, Meadows GG. (2010) Chronic alcohol consumption enhances myeloid-derived suppressor cells in B16BL6 melanoma-bearing mice. Cancer Immunol Immunother. 59:1151–9.

Chapter 10
Immune Surveillance and Tumor Evasion

M. Katherine Jung

Abbreviations

B cell	Bone marrow-derived lymphocyte
IFN	Interferon
IL	Interleukin
MDSC	Myeloid-derived suppressor cells
MHC	Major histocompatibility complex
NFκB	Nuclear factor kappa-light-chain-enhancer of activated B cells
NK	Natural killer (cells)
NKT	Natural killer T (cells)
STAT	Signal transducer and activator of transcription
T cell	Thymus-derived lymphocyte
TAP	*T*ransporter *a*ssociated with antigen *p*rocessing
TGFβ	Transforming growth factor beta
Th1 and Th2	$CD4^+$ T helper cells
TNFα	Tumor necrosis factor alpha
Tregs	Regulatory T cells
VEGF	Vascular endothelial growth factor

M.K. Jung (✉)
Division of Metabolism and Health Effects, National Institute on Alcohol Abuse
and Alcoholism, National Institutes of Health, Bethesda, MD, USA
e-mail: jungma@mail.nih.gov

S. Zakhari et al. (eds.), *Alcohol and Cancer*, DOI 10.1007/978-1-4614-0040-0_10,
© Springer Science+Business Media, LLC 2011

Introduction

Tumors are composed of heterogeneous cell types, both diverse transformed cells of the tissue of origin and a variety of stromal cells. The tumor cells themselves differ in the degree of aneuploidy, the number and identity of mutations, the extent of genomic instability, the expression of surface antigens, and the capacity to express cytokines, growth factors, proteases, and angiogenic factors. The **stromal cells include fibroblasts, an assortment of leukocytes and lymphocytes,** and often cell types that make up blood vessels. Ongoing reciprocal interactions between tumor cells and stromal cells affect the establishment, progression, and maintenance of cancer, with immune cells in particular mediating antitumor surveillance (Fig. 10.1). This chapter explores the details of immune surveillance,

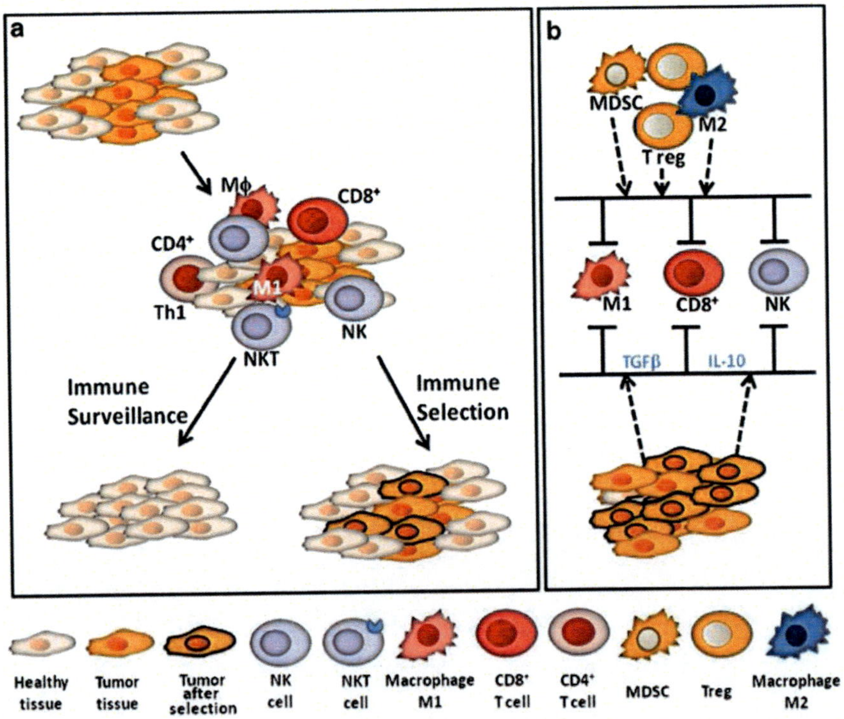

Fig. 10.1 Immune surveillance and tumor escape. (**a**) Immune cells recognize danger signals released from tumor tissue and activate host defense strategies. When immune surveillance prevails, the tumor is eradicated, but selection of the subset of the tumor cell population able to avoid immune destruction leads to a more successful tumor. (**b**) Tumor escape from immune surveillance depends on immune tolerance and immune suppression due to Tregs, MDSCs and tumor-associated macrophages (M2). Tumor cells themselves also produce immune-suppressing mediators

discusses the mechanisms by which tumors evade this surveillance, and explores the impact of alcohol on both.

The capacity of the immune system to recognize tumors as a threat to the host and eliminate them was suggested in the early twentieth century by Paul Ehrlich. Burnett and Thomas coined the term "cancer immunosurveillance" in the 1960s. The immune surveillance hypothesis has fallen in and out of favor over the years; however, accumulating evidence and recent advances in the understanding of tumor biology and immune function support the validity of the hypothesis.

Armed with the technology to knock out specific genes in mice, Mark Smyth revived interest in the field by demonstrating that mice lacking cytolytic function in lymphocytes and natural killer (NK) cells had a higher lifetime incidence of spontaneous B cell lymphoma (Smyth et al. 2000a). Both classes of cells were unable to lyse tumor cells due to deletion of the gene for perforin, a molecule that forms pores in the target cell. Concerns that the immune surveillance might be a characteristic unique to lymphoma were alleviated by the demonstration of a role for immune surveillance against other cancer types, including chemically induced fibrosarcomas (Smyth et al. 2000b), spontaneous adenocarcinomas (Street et al. 2002), and spontaneous uterine neoplasms (Hayashi and Faustman 2002). Immune surveillance of tumor initiation and metastasis (Cretney et al. 2002) in mice has been convincingly demonstrated. However, the picture in humans is less clear.

Immune Surveillance

Innate Antitumor Immunity

Innate defenses against tumors include natural killer (NK) cells, natural killer T (NKT) cells, macrophages, and dendritic cells, among others. NK cells are non-T, non-B-lymphocytes that recognize tumor cells and virus-infected cells without prior sensitization. Activation of NK cells is an innate and immediate response to danger signals (see Sidebar 1) produced by transformed host cells. One mechanism of NK cell cytotoxicity involves binding to the target cell, with the release of perforin, granzyme A, and granzyme B. Perforin forms pores in the membrane of the target cell, allowing the proteases granzyme A and B access to the cytoplasm. Granzyme B cleaves caspase 3, triggering apoptosis in the target cell. In addition to their innate cytolytic activity, NK cells regulate adaptive immunity by releasing cytokines that influence the maturation of dendritic cells (Zitvogel et al. 2006) and directly affect T cell homeostasis and activation (Zingoni et al. 2005).

Sidebar 1. The Danger Hypothesis

The classical theory of immune function held that the immune system distinguishes self from nonself. Nonhost foreign antigens were proposed to elicit both innate and adaptive immune responses, while host-derived antigens elicited tolerance by the immune system. However, many observations of immune function found the self–nonself theory lacking, so the danger hypothesis (Fuchs and Matzinger 1996; Matzinger 2002) arose as a better foundation for understanding the process. Accordingly, the immune system recognizes dangers to homeostasis, not only the presence of pathogens but also endogenous cells that are in distress. Cell changes that threaten the host release a distress signal. For example, necrotic tissue releases cellular components that send a danger signal and elicit an inflammatory response. By contrast, apoptotic cells in general do not elicit an inflammatory response. In the light of this hypothesis, cancer cells may send danger signals. Surveillance for danger signals and tumor antigens by the immune system is thought to combat the occurrence or growth of tumors.

Natural killer T (NKT) cells are distinguishable from NK cells by the presence of a T cell receptor. NKT cells do not recognize unique antigens as other T cells do; rather, they are activated by a class of glycolipids. Since the NKT response does not require priming by antigen presentation and cannot be boosted, the NKT cell response is considered an innate immune response. There are many functionally distinct NKT cell subsets, and NKT cell numbers vary widely among individuals (Godfrey et al. 2010). NKT cells express a broad range of cytokines within hours of activation. NKT cell function is highly immmunoregulatory, bridging innate and adaptive immunity. Cytokine release from NKT cells can polarize (see below) to a T helper 1 (Th1; proinflammatory) or Th2 (suppressing cell-mediated immunity) phenotype. They are thus capable of promoting antitumor immunity (Swann et al. 2009), but can suppress cell-mediated immunity in other cases. NKT cells also possess perforin-mediated and Fas-mediated cytolytic activity (Smyth et al. 2000b), so they also contribute directly to tumor cell destruction.

Immune cell tumor infiltrates can also include macrophages, neutrophils, $CD4^+$ T cells, $CD8^+$ T cells, regulatory T cells (Tregs), Th17 cells, and myeloid-derived suppressor cells (MDSC). Macrophages are key players in overall innate immunity, by being among the first cells to detect danger or infection and release cytokines to initiate the inflammatory response. Like dendritic cells, macrophages present antigen to lymphocytes to trigger adaptive immunity (See Sidebar 2), thus activating both arms of the immune response. In some cases, however, macrophages are alternatively activated, displaying an immunosuppressive M2 phenotype.

Adaptive Antitumor Immunity

Adaptive immunity also plays a role in tumor immune surveillance. $CD4^+$ and $CD8^+$ cell populations are enriched upon stimulation by tumor antigens. When $CD8^+$ T cells are stimulated by the presence of their cognate antigen, they proliferate and differentiate into cytolytic cells or memory cells. Memory T cells against colon cancer persist in mice even in the absence of antigen (Xiang et al. 1999), allowing primed $CD8^+$ T cells to reject subsequent tumor cell challenges. Cytolytic $CD8^+$ T cells execute perforin- and Fas-mediated apoptosis of the target cell. Activated $CD4^+$ cells, on the other hand, are not cytolytic; rather, they release cytokines that regulate other immune cell types. Antigen-specific $CD8^+$ cell differentiation requires costimulation by antigen-specific $CD4^+$ cells (Hung et al. 1998; Surman et al. 2000). Upon activation, $CD4^+$ cells polarize into Th1 or Th2 phenotypes. Th1 $CD4^+$ cells release the proinflammatory cytokines interferon γ (IFNγ) and tumor necrosis factor α (TNFα), which promote the destruction of cells that represent a threat to the host, while Th2 polarized cells release interleukin-4 (IL-4), IL-10, and transforming growth factor β (TGFβ), which are anti-inflammatory and immunosuppressive. Thus, polarization of $CD4^+$ helper cells to a Th2 phenotype in the tumor microenvironment suppresses cell-mediated antitumor activity. Naïve CD4 cells can also be stimulated to differentiate into T17 cells, which play a role in autoimmune disease due to a sustained inflammatory phenotype, or into regulatory T cells (Tregs). Tregs suppress antigen-specific responses by expressing IL-10 and TGFβ.

Sidebar 2. Antigen Presentation

Adaptive tumor immunity requires activation of $CD4^+$ and $CD8^+$ cells by specific antigens. When $CD8^+$ T cells are stimulated by the presence of their cognate antigen, they proliferate and differentiate into cytolytic cells and memory cells. Activated $CD4^+$ cells are not cytolytic; they release cytokines that stimulate or inhibit other immune cell types and promote $CD8^+$ proliferation. To be recognized by T cells, antigen must be cleaved into small peptides and then coupled to major histocompatibility complex (MHC) proteins by antigen-presenting cells. While all cells in the body express MHC proteins, the role of dendritic cells, as professional antigen-presenting cells, has especially equipped them to process antigen, couple it to MHC, and present it to naïve T cells. Impairment of dendritic cell function has a significant negative impact on the ability of the host to mount an immune response to specific antigens. Likewise, a deficiency in MHC molecules also impairs the adaptive response.

Immune Regulation

Polarized T cells influence and are influenced by macrophages and other components of innate immunity. For example, the proinflammatory cytokine IFNγ is produced by and stimulates both Th1 cells and classically activated macrophages, establishing and sustaining inflammation. Anti-inflammatory cytokines such as IL-10 and TGFβ reduce the activity of classically activate macrophages, with general reduction in inflammation. Intrinsic regulation of immune function involves complex communication, mediated by cytokines and other effector molecules, between innate and adaptive cells. Furthermore, immune regulation overall is very much influenced by extraimmune factors in the microenvironment, as is macrophage phenotype. Both immune and nonimmune cells send and receive cytokine and chemokine signals, so immune function is influenced by cross talk among multiple cell types, both systemically and within the tumor microenvironment. In addition, there is also a broader cross talk among immune, neural and endocrine systems that orchestrates the regulation of the immune response. The interactions among these systems may be differentially influenced by the tumor environment.

The opposing and competing phenotypes displayed by Th1 and Th2 cells are somewhat paralleled by the phenotypes of classically activated M1 macrophages (proinflammatory and phagocytic) and alternatively activated M2 macrophages (immune suppressive and tumor-supportive). The maturation of macrophages from myeloid precursors is influenced by the microenvironment, which includes locally expressed cytokines and effector molecules. Myeloid precursors have the potential to differentiate into monocytes, tissue-specific macrophages, dendritic cells, or to display MDSC characteristics. MDSCs inhibit the activation of tumor antigen-specific $CD4^+$ and $CD8^+$ cells (Serafini et al. 2004; Yang and Roden 2007). Tissue-specific macrophages can display a functional heterogeneity ranging on the continuum between the extreme M1 and M2 phenotypes (Fig. 10.2), encompassing the diverse roles that macrophages play in maintaining tissue homeostasis (Stout et al. 2009).

Tumors Evade Immune Surveillance

Despite the aforementioned host antitumor strategies, cancers do arise, and the relative success of the tumor is determined by the tumor microenvironment. Immune and nonimmune cells produce many of the same effector molecules and have receptors that make them responsive to signaling. Tumor cell-derived effector molecules and signaling support proliferation, angiogenesis and metastasis. In addition, genetic and epigenetic changes may allow tumor cells to evade immune surveillance by becoming less visible to detection or by interfering with immune regulation. In an immunosuppressive milieu, tumor proliferation will be favored (Fig. 10.1b).

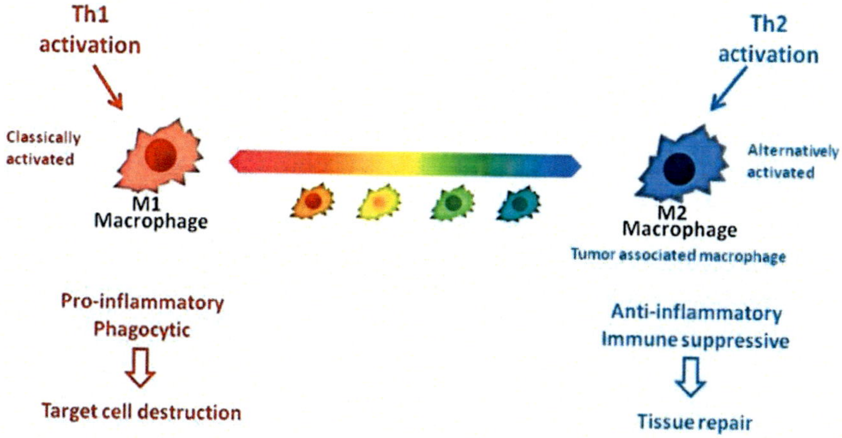

Fig. 10.2 Macrophage plasticity. The macrophage phenotype depends on signals received from the microenvironment. In a proinflammatory environment, macrophages are classically activated to destroy pathogens. However, in a generally Th2 environment, macrophages can be alternatively activated, as they are often found in tumors. M2 macrophages are immune suppressive and support tissue repair. In healthy tissue, macrophage phenotype and function span the range between M1 and M2

Tumors Avoid Immune Detection

Tumors can avoid immune detection by mutation of molecules required for the process of antigen presentation (Sidebar 2). In humans, loss of expression of MHC class I proteins (necessary for presenting tumor antigens to stimulate adaptive immunity) has been observed in several tumor types (Algarra et al. 1997; Khong and Restifo 2002), and reduced MHC class I expression is associated with invasive and metastatic cancers (Garrido et al. 1997). Loss of MHC class I expression is particularly prevalent in breast carcinoma (Cabrera et al. 1996). Similarly, down-regulation of TAP-1 and TAP-2, (*t*ransporter *a*ssociated with antigen *p*rocessing) has been observed in a variety of human carcinomas (Restifo et al. 1993; Korkolopoulou et al. 1996; Seliger et al. 1997).

Tumors can also avoid detection by direct mutation or elimination of the tumor antigens themselves. Since antigen expression within a tumor is heterogeneous, the portion of the tumor cell population that eliminates detectable antigens will avoid destruction, so will have the selective proliferative advantage to populate the tumor. Tumors arising in mouse strains lacking immune function are under no selective pressure, so when these tumors are transplanted into wild-type mice, they are highly immunogenic (Dunn et al. 2002). In humans, loss of expression of specific melanoma surface antigens correlates with increased disease severity (Hofbauer et al. 1998). Yet another tactic used to subvert immune attack involves mutations that interfere with the immune signaling that leads to tumor cell cytolysis (Shankaran et al. 2001). Selective pressure favors the subset of tumor cells that lack functional

IFNγ receptors. (Shankaran et al. 2001). Tumor escape occurs due to selection for tumor cell subpopulations that are not detected by immune surveillance.

Tumors Modify Immunoregulation

Another strategy by which tumors avoid immune destruction is suppression of immune function by co-opting intrinsic immunoregulatory signaling. Tumors release molecular factors capable of suppressing the immune system directly. Tumor-derived IL-10, IL-6, and vascular endothelial growth factor (VEGF) activate STAT3 in immune cells (Yu et al. 2007). In response to IL-10, STAT3 activates transcription of a specific set of genes whose products cause tumor-infiltrating immune cells to reduce immune surveillance (Wang et al. 2004). STAT3 is a negative regulator of Th1 (immune-stimulating) genes and is an activator of immunosuppressive genes (Wang et al. 2004). In addition, STAT3 target gene expression inhibits antigen-specific T cell differentiation, in part by inhibiting dendritic cell maturation (Wang et al. 2004). STAT3 mediates expression of IL-10 and TGFβ and is required for proper IL-10 receptor signaling (Yu et al. 2007). IL-10 and TGFβ in turn promote STAT3 activation, resulting in a feed-forward loop. In tumor-associated macrophages of the M2 phenotype, STAT3 activation inhibits proinflammatory cytokine expression (Yu et al. 2007), including IL-12, which is essential for induction of IFNγ (Trinchieri et al. 2003).

Just as cytokines of tumor origin modify the phenotype of immune cells, tumor or stromal cell-derived chemokines can dictate the distinct cell types recruited to the tumor microenvironment. Certain tumors express chemokines that recruit Tregs and MDSCs to the tumor microenvironment (Mantovani et al. 2008). Tregs suppress antigen specific $CD8^+$ cytotoxicity, partially by releasing IL-10 and TGFβ. MDSCs are recruited to the tumor by CC and CXC chemokines (Sawanobori et al. 2008; Yang et al. 2008; Mantovani et al. 2010). MDSCs supply the immunosuppressive chemokine TGFβ (Bierie and Moses 2010) and inhibit the expression of selectins by $CD4^+$ and $CD8^+$ cells, necessary for the homing of antigen-specific cells to the tumor (Hanson et al. 2009). Further, MDSCs may be responsible for the activation of the immune-quieting M2 phenotype in tumor-resident macrophages (Sinha et al. 2007). The abundance of IL-10 and TGFβ leads to a lack of expression of costimulatory molecules by tumor cells resulting in T cell anergy (Adkis and Blaser 2001; Yu et al. 2007) and suboptimal antitumor NK cell activation.

The lymphoid stroma of secondary lymph organs, such as lymph nodes or spleen, supports the activation of naïve T cells to effector cells, but also supports the development of tolerance and immune suppressive cells, such as Tregs and MDSCs. Tumors also have the capacity to recruit cell types that lead to the establishment of a tertiary lymphoid organ within the tumor stroma (Shields et al. 2010). This represents another means by which tumors escape or subvert local immune surveillance by directing the maturation or activation of Tregs, MDSCs, or M2 macrophages to support tumor growth.

Immune-Mediated Support of Tumor Survival

A remarkable component of stromal cell–tumor cell cross talk consists of the production by immune cells of growth factors and other molecules that stimulate tumor survival and spread. MDSCs enhance angiogenesis by expressing VEGF, promote immune tolerance by synthesizing TGFβ (Bierie and Moses 2010) and express matrix metalloproteases that assist in invasion and metastasis (Bierie and Moses 2010; Yang et al. 2008). Tumor-associated macrophages also express VEGF (Noonan et al. 2008) and other proangiogenic factors (Shojaei et al. 2007). In addition, tumor-associated macrophages express growth factors, including epidermal growth factor (Leek and Harris 2002).

Clinical Consequences

The nature of the tumor infiltrate establishes the balance between immune surveillance and tumor evasion and can predict clinical outcome. For example, in human colorectal cancer, the presence of cytotoxic $CD8^{+}$ T cells, memory T cells, and markers of Th1 polarization (favoring cell-mediated immunity) correlates with a low incidence of tumor recurrence, implicating cell-mediated tumor rejection (Galon et al. 2006). By contrast, tumor-specific Treg content in ovarian carcinoma is negatively correlated with survival (Curiel 2007). In general, Treg infiltrates predominate in late-stage tumors (Kortylewski et al. 2005).

Does Alcohol-Induced Immunosuppression Influence Cancer Incidence and Progression?

Alcohol consumption is associated with profound alterations of both innate and adaptive immunity (Cook 1998; Szabo 1999; Szabo and Mandrekar 2009) at multiple loci. Disruption of immune function by alcohol may contribute to the failure of immune surveillance that allows tumor escape. Alcohol-related modifications are likely to have complex consequences on the reciprocal interactions between tumor cells and immune and other stromal cells, ultimately favoring the establishment and growth of tumors.

Binge alcohol consumption suppresses immediate host defense, including the inflammatory response. By contrast, chronic alcohol consumption leads to chronic inflammation, yet paradoxically also suppresses immune function. The inflammation and increased oxidative burden caused by chronic alcohol consumption, while causing damage to host tissues, are associated with functional impairment of specific defense against infection and other threats to the host. Since the development of cancer proceeds over decades, it is likely that the effects of chronic alcohol consumption are of greater relevance than the effects of binge drinking on tumor success and survival.

Alcohol Alters Innate Immunity

Reports of alcohol's effects on NK cell number and function over the years have led to equivocal conclusions. For example, NK cell number in human alcoholics was not different from control populations (Cook et al. 1997; Irwin and Miller 2000) but NK cell activity was diminished in abstinent alcoholics compared to nondrinkers (Motivala et al. 2003). Comparison among the studies is difficult due to differences in duration and type of alcohol exposure, and the existence of distinct subtypes of NK cells. The latter is an important point, as increasing numbers of subtypes of NK cells with different signaling molecules and functions are discovered.

As discussed earlier, NK cells eliminate tumor cells by perforin- and granzyme-induced apoptosis. Ethanol consumption inhibits the expression of perforin, granzyme A, and granzyme B in NK cells due to reduced NFκB and AP-1 transcriptional activity (Spitzer and Meadows 1999; Zhou and Meadows 2003). Most of the studies of alcohol effects on NK cell function involved splenic NK cells rather than tumor-infiltrating NK cells. Since NK cell function can potentially be modified by the tumor microenvironment, the effect of alcohol on antitumor NK function remains uncertain. Origination and homing of NK cells may be significant. NK cells that originate in the thymus are functionally different from NK cells that originate in the bone marrow (Zhang and Meadows 2008). In a mouse model of chronic alcohol consumption, alcohol decreased the number of NK cells in the spleen, but did not alter the number of NK cells in the thymus (Zhang and Meadows 2008). In the bone marrow, alcohol interfered with the release of NK cells, leading to an alteration of the ratio of thymic to bone marrow-derived splenic NK cells (Zhang and Meadows 2008), with functional consequences. NK cells are known to influence dendritic cell function. When NK cell activity is negatively impacted, impairment of antigen presentation by dendritic cells (Zitvogel et al. 2006) and interference with the development of antigen-specific $CD8^+$ and $CD4^+$ cells may follow (Zingoni et al. 2005).

There are fewer reports of alcohol effects on NKT cells than on NK cells. Briefly, chronic alcohol exposure in rodents leads to an increase in the number of NKT cells in the liver (Minagawa et al. 2004). Since NKT cells bridge innate and adaptive immunity, promoting cell-mediated tumor immunity in some contexts and suppressing cell-mediated immunity in others, effects of alcohol on NKT cells may influence the balance between immune surveillance and tumor evasion.

Alcohol Affects Antigen Presentation

Alcohol affects several of the professional antigen-presenting cells. For example, after a single exposure to alcohol, monocyte antigen-presenting function is reduced (Szabo et al. 2004). Similarly, chronic alcohol reduces dendritic cell number, inhibits antigen-specific induction of T cell proliferation, and decreases the output of IL-12 from dendritic cells (Lau et al. 2006). Impairment of antigen presentation by dendritic cells and monocytes will interfere with the activation of antigen-specific $CD8^+$ and

CD4+ cells. Likewise, acute alcohol exposure leads to reduced dendritic cell IL-12 production, increased IL-10 production, and decreased expression of the costimulatory molecules CD80 and CD86 (Szabo et al. 2004). Furthermore, exposure of T cells to alcohol-treated dendritic cells results in T cell anergy (Mandrekar et al. 2004).

Alcohol Affects Adaptive Immunity

The generally immunosuppressive effects of chronic alcohol consumption on the adaptive immune response, especially cell-mediated immunity by CD8+ T cells, are likely to have a significant effect on tumor surveillance. In general, the weakened host defense of alcoholics is characterized by reduced numbers of T cells and alterations in their cytokine expression. Overall lymphocyte number is decreased in humans and rodents after chronic alcohol intake, including CD4+ T cells, CD8+ T cells, B cells, and NKT cells (Starkenburg et al. 2001; Song et al. 2002; Spies et al. 2004; Zhang and Meadows 2005). Paradoxically, persistent T cell activation and a heightened T cell response to nonspecific stimulation have been observed in alcoholics (Cook et al. 1991; Laso et al. 1999, 2010; Song et al. 2002). Activated subsets composed of CD8+ and NKT cells (Cook et al. 1991) or CD4+, CD8+ cells, and NKT cells (Laso et al. 2010) have been reported in the circulation of chronic alcoholics.

The subset of lymphocytes expressing the CD57 surface marker is enriched in alcoholics. In contrast to CD57− cells, which require T cell receptor (TCR) stimulation accompanied by a second signal to activate cytokine production, CD57+ cells are activated without a second signal and produce more INFγ and TNFα (Song et al. 2001) than CD57− cells. Thus, alcoholics have a larger proportion of a subset of T cells that increases a rapid cytotoxic response.

A chronic alcohol-induced shift from a naïve CD8+ T cell phenotype to a memory cell CD8+ phenotype has been observed in both humans (Cook et al. 1994) and in mouse models (Song et al. 2002). Human chronic alcohol intake also leads to reduction in the expression of some selectins and CD11b (Song et al. 2001), molecules that interact with adhesion molecules. Reduction of selectin expression is also one of the strategies by which MDSCs promote tumor escape, inviting speculation about parallels between alcohol and MDSCs in altering tumor immunity.

Mounting an effective antitumor defense requires both effective antigen presentation and the capacity of the T cells to respond to the antigen priming. As was mentioned earlier, there is evidence that alcohol impairs antigen presentation by dendritic cells and monocytes. In addition, Gurung et al. (2009) report that chronic alcohol impairs the primary response of CD8+ cells to specific antigen priming in mice, but does not alter the CD4+ response to specific priming. After antigen priming, there are fewer antigen-specific CD8+ cells in ethanol-fed mice than in water-fed mice. The CD8+ cells from the ethanol-fed mice have clear intrinsic defects, including poorer proliferation and poorer IFNγ production after priming (Gurung et al. 2009). Thus, the immunodeficiency in the adaptive response of chronic alcoholics results both from impaired interactions between the antigen-presenting cells and the T cells (Cook et al. 2004) as well as from intrinsic defects in the T cells themselves (Gurung et al. 2009). The reduction in the capacity to raise antigen-specific CD8$^+$ T cells is consistent with the proposed, but as yet unproven, impaired immune surveillance in the context of chronic alcohol consumption. The relative contribution of an apparent generalized activation and heightened nonspecific T cell response to immunodeficiency is not yet clear.

Alcohol, Immune Function, and Cancer

Much of the current knowledge of the effects of alcohol on immune function is based on investigations carried out in cancer-free organs and organisms. More direct research focused on linking alcohol, immune function and cancer have employed the B16 melanoma model in the rodent (Ben-Eliyahu et al. 1996; Blank and Meadows 1996; Wu and Pruett 1999). Alcohol decreases host resistance to lung metastases of the B16F10 melanoma in female B6CF1 mice (Wu and Pruett 1999), and of the B16BL6 melanoma in C57/BL6 mice (Blank and Meadows 1996) following tail vein injections of the melanoma cells. Similarly, acute alcohol administration in male Fisher rats decreases resistance to metastasis of melanoma injected into the tail vein. By contrast, under more physiological conditions in which the melanomas are grown subcutaneously, metastasis is suppressed by chronic alcohol (Blank and Meadows 1996). The suppression of B16BL6 lung metastasis by alcohol is independent of NK cell activity (Spitzer et al. 2000).

Intriguingly, chronic alcohol consumption doubles the weight of B16F10 tumors in a mouse model, increases the vascularity of the tumors and stimulates expression of VEGF and its receptor in the tumors (Tan et al. 2007). The extent of tumor infiltration by immune cells was not reported, although the mice were immunocompetent. It remains to be determined whether the VEGF is of melanoma cell origin or is produced by adjacent cells in the microenvironment. Nevertheless, immunocytochemistry showed that the VEGF receptors are present on melanoma cells (Tan et al. 2007).

While metastasis and tumor vascularity are indications of cancer severity, host survival is perhaps the most pertinent reflection of host defense. Chronic alcohol consumption decreases the survival time in C57/BL6 mice bearing subcutaneous B16BL6 melanomas. Specific parameters that correlate with poorer survival include inhibition of the expansion of antigen-specific CD8$^+$ cells, acceleration of the decay of splenic IFNγ-producing CD8$^+$ cells, and an increase in the percentage of MDSCs in circulation (Zhang and Meadows 2010). The effects of alcohol on antitumor immunity remain an underexplored area of research.

Alcohol Alters Immune Regulation

Interaction among different immune cells, via their cytokines, affects immunoregulation. NK cells regulate dendritic cell function, and the converse is also true (Cooper et al. 2004; Gerosa et al. 2005; Zitvogel et al. 2006). Unrestricted NK cell function is necessary for cell-mediated tumor immunity, as is dendritic cell function. Since alcohol disrupts both NK cell function and dendritic cell biology, the potential for alcohol to disrupt antitumor immune surveillance exists. The many immunoregulatory functions of NKT cells also impact the nature and direction of the immune response and also provide a potential target for alcohol's interference with immune surveillance. Furthermore, a full understanding of the problem must take into account the many subtypes of each immune cell type and their diverse functions (Godfrey et al. 2010).

Early suggestions that alcohol alters the immune regulatory balance, specifically, Th1/Th2 polarization, have been inconclusive. For example, it was reported that immune function in chronic alcoholics trends toward a Th2 response at the expense of the Th1 response, based in large part on the elevation of circulating immunoglobulins in alcoholics (Cook 1998; Szabo 1999; Spies et al. 2004). Short-term alcohol exposure in rodent models also seems to favor a Th2 response over a Th1 response (Starkenburg et al. 2001). However, no skewing in the expression of Th1/Th2 cytokines from antigen-specific T cells was observed in a well-designed mouse model of chronic alcohol exposure (Gurung et al. 2009). The implications of these alterations in the Th1/Th2 balance on immune surveillance are unclear.

The increase in MDSCs (Zhang and Meadows 2010) and the modification of macrophage function in other settings under the influence of chronic alcohol exposure (Cook 1998; Szabo 1999) raises the possibility, yet to be proved, that alcohol influences the lineage commitment of myeloid precursor cells or the phenotype selection of tissue resident macrophages. The functional heterogeneity (Fig. 10.2) of tissue-specific macrophages ranging from proinflammatory to immune suppressive phenotypes reflects the diverse roles that macrophages play in maintaining tissue homeostasis (Stout et al. 2009). Within the context of acute inflammation, macrophages perform two functions, an early phase of tissue destruction and phagocytosis, followed by the expression of cytokines that favor tissue repair. In healthy unperturbed tissue, by contrast, macrophages function is not limited to the two extremes, since tissue-resident macrophages perform functions all long this spectrum of activity (Fig. 10.2) to maintain homeostasis (Stout et al. 2009). Potential disruptions of macrophage phenotype by alcohol might impact immune surveillance. For example, an alcohol-associated failure of normal macrophage function might lead to a loss of tissue integrity allowing invasion of normal tissue by a nascent tumor. Alternatively, a subversion of the wound-healing functions mediated by macrophages could conceivably lead to renegade proliferation. In either case, disruption of macrophage homeostasis by alcohol might have tumor-supporting consequences.

Future Prospects

Incomplete knowledge of immune cell types that had not yet been described in previous decades complicates the interpretation of initial reports on effects of chronic alcohol exposure on specific lymphocyte or leukocyte classes. Advances in the understanding of alcohol's effects on immune surveillance and immune function will parallel advances in the knowledge of the multiplicity of immune cell types.

As new cell types and subtypes are identified and characterized, the mechanism of alcohol-induced immune dysfunction may be clarified. For example, in the case of naïve $CD4^+$ cell differentiation into the diverse helper T cell classes, an expanded understanding of the effect of alcohol on Treg function and location might provide insight into the effect of alcohol on immune surveillance, just as a better understanding of the effect of alcohol on MDSCs and Th17 cells may clarify specific details of the mechanism of alcohol-induced immune dysfunction.

Characterization of the many subtypes of NK cells and NKT cells and their corresponding function (Godfrey et al. 2010) must be taken into account when considering immune regulation. In addition, alternatives to the classical activation of macrophages may have parallels in neutrophil and dendritic cell populations (DeNardo et al. 2010); these can be characterized in the context of chronic alcohol exposure. Immune cell phenotype is strongly influenced by the local niche, so the effects of alcohol on interactions between immune and nonimmune compartments may be very important.

Furthermore, assuming that alcohol targets any single immune cell type may be too narrow, since it is likely that alcohol disrupts immune regulation globally. Rather than considering the dichotomy of immune activation and immune suppression, it may be more illuminating to consider that alcohol exposure leads to an altered course of immune activation, by modifying T helper cell commitment or by influencing the range of macrophage function. Thus, advancing the field also requires insight into the role that alcohol plays in disrupting or dysregulating the entire system. In any complex signaling network, altering one component of the network may disrupt a broad array of functional components. Alcohol's alteration of immune function, with its widespread distribution of effects, may simultaneously alter many complex and widespread aspects of antitumor immunity. Focusing at the network level will require a systems biology approach.

The system includes both the immune network and its corresponding niche. Since immune function is tissue-specific, differences in local immune surveillance may explain why alcohol-associated cancers occur in the liver, colon, esophagus, larynx, pharynx, mouth, and breast. It is conceivable that alcohol perturbation of the niche plays a role in nascent as well as established tumors. Alcohol-induced alterations of the composition and function of infiltrating immune cells in established tumors will provide insight into immune surveillance and tumor escape. Optimally, laboratory models of alcohol-immune interactions will focus on tumors originating in organs associated with alcohol-induced cancer.

References

Adkis CA, Blaser K (2001) Mechanisms of interleukin-10-mediated immune suppression. Immunology 103:131–6.

Algarra I, Collado A, Garrido F (1997) Altered MHC class I antigens in tumors. Int J Clin Lab Res 27:95–102.

Ben-Eliyahu S, Page GG, Yirmiya R, Taylor AN (1996) Acute alcohol intoxication suppresses natural killer cell activity and promotes tumor metastasis. Nat Med.2:457–60.

Bierie B, Moses HL (2010) Transforming growth factor beta (TGF-β) and inflammation in cancer. Cytokine Growth Factor Rev 21:49–59.
Blank SE, Meadows GG (1996) Ethanol modulates metastatic potential of B16BL6 melanoma and host responses. Alcohol Clin Exp Res 20:624–8.
Cabrera T, Angustias Fernandez M, Sierra A, Garrido A, Herruzo A, Escobedo A, Fabra A, Garrido F (1996) High frequency of altered HLA class I phenotypes in invasive breast carcinomas. Hum Immunol 50:127–34.
Cook RT (1998) Alcohol abuse, alcoholism, and damage to the immune system – a review. Alcohol Clin Exp Res 22:1927–42.
Cook RT, Garvey MJ, Booth BM, Goeken JA, Stewart B, Noel M (1991) Activated CD-8 cells and HLA DR expression in alcoholics without overt liver disease. J Clin Immunol 11:246–53.
Cook RT, Li F, Vandersteen D, Ballas ZK, Cook BL, LaBrecque DR (1997) Ethanol and natural killer cells. I. Activity and immunophenotype in alcoholic humans. Alcohol Clin Exp Res 21:974–80.
Cook RT, Waldschmidt TJ, Ballas ZK, Cook BL, Booth BM, Stewart BC, Garvey MJ (1994) Fine T-cell subsets in alcoholics as determined by the expression of L-selectin, leukocyte common antigen, and beta-integrin. Alcohol Clin Exp Res 18:71–80.
Cook RT, Zhu X, Coleman RA, Ballas ZK, Waldschmidt TJ, Ray NB, LaBrecque DR, Cook BL (2004) T-cell activation after chronic ethanol ingestion in mice. Alcohol 33:175–81.
Cooper MA, Fehniger TA, Fuchs A, Colonna M, Caligiuri MA (2004) NK cell and DC interactions. Trends Immunol 25:47–52.
Cretney EJ, Takeda K, Yagita H, Glaccum M, Peschon JJ, Smyth MJ (2002) Increased susceptibility to tumor initiation and metastasis in TNF-related apoptosis-inducing ligand-deficient mice. J Immunol 168:1356–61.
Curiel TJ (2007) Tregs and rethinking cancer immunotherapy. J Clin Invest. 117:1167–74.
DeNardo DG, Andreu P, Coussens LM (2010) Interactions between lymphocytes and myeloid cells regulate pro-versus anti-tumor immunity. Cancer Metastasis Rev 29:309–16.
Dunn GP, Bruce AT, Ikeda H, Old LJ, Schreiber RD (2002) Cancer immunoediting: from immunosurveillance to tumor escape. Nature Immunol 3:991–8.
Fuchs EJ, Matzinger P (1996) Is cancer dangerous to the immune system? Semin Immunol 8:271–80.
Galon J, Costes A, Sanchez-Cabo F, Kirilovsky A, Mlecnik B, Lagorce-Pages C, Tosolini M, Camus M, Berger A, Wind P, Zinzindohoue F, Bruneval P, Cugnenc P, Trajanoski Z, Fridman W, Pages F (2006) Type, density, and location of immune cells within human colorectal tumors predict clinical outcome. Science 313:1960–4.
Garrido F, Ruiz-Cabello F, Cabrera T, Pérez-Villar JJ, López-Botet M, Duggan-Keen M, Stern PL (1997) Implications for immunosurveillance of altered HLA class I phenotypes in human tumours. Immunol Today 18:89–95.
Gerosa F, Gobbi A, Zorzi P, Burg S, Briere F, Carra G, Trinchieri G (2005) The reciprocal interaction of NK cells with plasmacytoid or myeloid dendritic cells profoundly affects innate resistance functions. J Immunol 174:727–34.
Godfrey DI, Stankovic S, Baxter AG (2010) Raising the NKT cell family. Nature Immunol 11:197–206.
Gurung P, Young BM, Coleman RA, Wiechert S, Turner LE, Ray NB, Waldschmidt TJ, Legge KL, Cook RT (2009) Chronic ethanol induces inhibition of antigen-specific CD8+ but not CD4+ immunodominant T cell responses following Listeria monocytogenes inoculation. J Leukoc Biol 85:34–43.
Hanson EM, Clements VK, Sinha P, Ilkovitch D, Ostrand-Rosenberg S (2009) Myeloid-derived suppressor cells down-regulate L-selectin expression on CD4+ and CD8+ T cells. J Immunol 183:937–44.
Hayashi T, Faustman DL (2002) Development of spontaneous uterine tumors in low molecular mass polypeptide-2 knockout mice. Cancer Res 62:24–7.
Hofbauer GF, Kamarashev J, Geertsen R, Böni R, Dummer R. (1998) Melan A/MART-1 immunoreactivity in formalin-fixed paraffin-embedded primary and metastatic melanoma: frequency and distribution. Melanoma Res 8:337–43.

Hung K, Hayashi R, Lafond-Walker A, Lowenstein C, Pardoll D, Levitsky H (1998) The central role of CD4+ T cells in the antitumor immune response. J Exp Med 188:2357–68.
Irwin M, Miller C (2000) Decreased natural killer cell responses and altered interleukin-6 and interleukin-10 production in alcoholism: an interaction between alcohol dependence and African-American ethnicity. Alcohol Clin Exp Res 24:560–9.
Khong HT, Restifo NP (2002) Natural selection of tumor variants in the generation of "tumor escape" phenotypes. Nature Immunol 3:999–1005.
Korkolopoulou P, Kaklamanis L, Pezzella F, Harris AL, Gatter KC (1996) Loss of antigen-presenting molecules (MHC class I and TAP-1) in lung cancer. Br J Cancer 73:148–53.
Kortylewski M, Kujawski M, Wang T, Wei S, Zhang S, Pilon-Thomas S, Niu G, Kay H, Mule J, Kerr WG, Jove R, Pardoll D, Yu H (2005) Inhibiting Stat3 signaling in the hematopoietic system elicits multicomponent antitumor immunity. Nature Med 11:1314–21.
Laso FJ, Iglesias-Osma C, Ciudad J, López A, Pastor I, Orfao A (1999) Chronic alcoholism is associated with an imbalanced production of Th-1/Th-2 cytokines by peripheral blood T cells. Alcohol Clin Exp Res 23:1306–11.
Laso FJ, Almeida J, Torres E, Vaquero JM, Marcos M, Orfao A (2010) Chronic Alcohol Consumption Is Associated With an Increased Cytotoxic Profile of Circulating Lymphocytes That May Be Related With the Development of Liver Injury. Alcohol Clin Exp Res 34 [Epub ahead of print].
Lau AH, Abe M, Thomson AW (2006) Ethanol affects the generation, cosignaling molecule expression, and function of plasmacytoid and myeloid dendritic cell subsets in vitro and in vivo. J Leukoc Biol 79:941–53.
Leek RD, Harris AL (2002) Tumor-associated macrophages in breast cancer. J Mammary Gland Biol Neoplasia 7:177–89.
Mandrekar P, Catalano D, Dolganiuc A, Kodys K, Szabo G (2004) Inhibition of myeloid dendritic cell accessory cell function and induction of T cell anergy by alcohol correlates with decreased IL-12 production. J Immunol 173:3398–3407.
Matzinger P (2002) The danger model: a renewed sense of self. Science 296:301–5.
Mantovani A, Allavena P, Sica A, Balkwill F (2008) Cancer-related inflammation. Nature 454:436–44.
Mantovani A, Savino B, Locati M, Zammataro L, Allavena P, Bonecchi R (2010) The chemokine system in cancer biology and therapy. Cytokine Growth Factor Rev 21:27–39.
Minagawa M, Deng Q, Liu ZX, Tsukamoto H, Dennert G (2004) Activated natural killer T cells induce liver injury by Fas and tumor necrosis factor-alpha during alcohol consumption. Gastroenterology 126:1387–99.
Motivala SJ, Dang, J, Obradovic T, Meadows GG, Butch AW, Irwin MR (2003) Leptin and cellular and innate immunity in abstinent alcoholics and controls. Alcohol Clin Exp Res 27:1819–24.
Noonan DM, De Lerma Barbaro A, Vannini N, Mortara L, Albini A (2008) Inflammation, inflammatory cells and angiogenesis: decisions and indecisions. Cancer Metastasis Rev 27:31–40.
Restifo NP, Esquivel F, Kawakami Y, Yewdell JW, Mulé JJ, Rosenberg SA, Bennink JR (1993) Identification of human cancers deficient in antigen processing. J Exp Med 177:265–72.
Sawanobori Y, Ueha S, Kurachi M, Shimaoka T, Talmadge JE, Abe J, Shono Y, Kitabatake M, Kakimi K, Mukaida N, Matsushima K (2008) Chemokine-mediated rapid turnover of myeloid-derived suppressor cells in tumor-bearing mice. Blood 111:5457–66.
Seliger B, Höhne A, Jung D, Kallfelz M, Knuth A, Jaeger E, Bernhard H, Momburg F, Tampé R, Huber C (1997) Expression and function of the peptide transporters in escape variants of human renal cell carcinomas. Exp Hematol 25:608–14.
Serafini P, De Santo C, Marigo I, Cingarlini S, Dolcetti L, Gallina G, Zanovello P, Bronte V (2004) Derangement of immune responses by myeloid suppressor cells. Cancer Immunol Immunother 53:64–72.
Shankaran V, Ikeda H, Bruce AT, White JM, Swanson PE, Old LJ, Schreiber RD (2001) IFNγ and lymphocytes prevent primary tumour development and shape tumour immunogenicity. Nature 410:1107–11.

Shields JD, Kourtis IC, Tomei AA, Roberts JM, Swartz MA (2010) Induction of lymphoidlike stroma and immune escape by tumors that express the chemokine CCL21. Science 328:749–752.

Shojaei F, Wu X, Zhong C, Yu L, Liang XH, Yao J, Blanchard D, Bais C, Peale FV, van Bruggen N, Ho C, Ross J, Tan M, Carano RA, Meng YG, Ferrara N (2007) Bv8 regulates myeloid-cell-dependent tumour angiogenesis. Nature 450:825–31.

Sinha P, Clements VK, Bunt SK, Albelda SM, Ostrand-Rosenberg S (2007) Cross-talk between myeloid-derived suppressor cells and macrophages subverts tumor immunity toward a type 2 response. J Immunol 179:977–83.

Smyth MJ, Thia KYT, Street SEA, MacGregor D, Godfrey DI, Trapani JA (2000a) Perforin-mediated cytotoxicity is critical for surveillance of spontaneous lymphoma. J Exp Med 192:755–60.

Smyth MJ, Thia KYT, Street SEA, Cretney E, Trapani, JA, Taniguchi M, Kawano T, Pelikan SB, Crowe NY, Godfrey DI (2000b) Differential Tumor surveillance by natural killer (NK) and NKT cells. J Exp Med 191:661–68.

Song K, Coleman RA, Alber C, Ballas ZK, Waldschmidt TJ, Mortari F, LaBrecque DR, Cook RT (2001) TH1 cytokine response of CD57+ T-cell subsets in healthy controls and patients with alcoholic liver disease. Alcohol 24:155–67.

Song K, Coleman RA, Zhu X, Alber C, Ballas ZK, Waldschmidt TJ, Cook RT (2002) Chronic ethanol consumption by mice results in activated splenic T cells. J Leukoc Biol 72:1109–16.

Spies CD, von Dossow V, Eggers V, Jetschmann G, El-Hilali R, Egert J, Fischer M, Schröder T, Höflich C, Sinha P, Paschen C, Mirsalim P, Brunsch R, Hopf J, Marks C, Wernecke KD, Pragst F, Ehrenreich H, Müller C, Tonnesen H, Oelkers W, Rohde W, Stein C, Kox WJ. (2004) Altered cell-mediated immunity and increased postoperative infection rate in long-term alcoholic patients. Anesthesiology. 100:1088–100

Spitzer JH, Meadows GG (1999) Modulation of perforin, granzyme A, and granzyme B in murine natural killer (NK), IL2 stimulated NK, and lymphokine-activated killer cells by alcohol consumption. Cell Immunol 194:205–12.

Spitzer JH, Núñez NP, Meadows SA, Gallucci RM, Blank SE, Meadows GG (2000) The modulation of B16BL6 melanoma metastasis is not directly mediated by cytolytic activity of natural killer cells in alcohol-consuming mice. Alcohol Clin Exp Res 24:837–44.

Starkenburg S, Munroe ME, Waltenbaugh (2001) Early alteration in leukocyte populations and Th1/Th2 function in ethanol-consuming mice. Alcohol Clin Exp Res 25:1221–30.

Stout RD, Watkins SK, Suttles J. (2009) Functional plasticity of macrophages: in situ reprogramming of tumor-associated macrophages. J Leukoc Biol. 86:1105–9.

Street SEA, Trapani JA, MacGregor D, Smyth MJ (2002) Suppression of lymphoma and epithelial malignancies effected by interferon γ. J Exp Med 196:129–34.

Surman DR, Dudley ME, Overwijk WW, Restifo NP (2000) Cutting edge: $CD4^+$ T cell control of $CD8^+$ T cell reactivity to a model tumor antigen. J Immunol 164:562–5.

Swann JB, Uldrich AP, van Dommelen S, Sharkey J, Murray WK, Godfrey DI, Smyth MJ (2009) Type I natural killer T cells suppress tumors caused by p53 loss in mice. Blood 113:6382–5.

Szabo G (1999) Consequences of alcohol consumption on host defence. Alcohol Alcohol 34:830–41.

Szabo G, Catalano D, White B, Mandrekar P (2004) Acute alcohol consumption inhibits accessory cell function of monocytes and dendritic cells. Alcohol Clin Exp Res 28:824–8.

Szabo G, Mandrekar P (2009) A recent perspective on alcohol, immunity and host defense. Alcohol Clin Exp Res 33:1–13.

Tan W, Bailey AP, Shparago M, Busby B, Covington J, Johnson JW, Young E, Gu JW (2007) Chronic alcohol consumption stimulates VEGF expression, tumor angiogenesis and progression of melanoma in mice. Cancer Biol Ther 6:1211–17.

Trinchieri G, Pflanz S, Kastelein RA (2003) The IL-12 Family of heterodimeric cytokines: New players in the regulation of T cell responses. Immunity 19:641–4.

Wang T, Niu G, Kortylewski M, Burdeyla L, Shain K, Zhang S, Bhattacharya R, Gabrilovich D, Heller R, Coppola D, Dalton W, Jove R, Pardoll D, Yu H (2004) Regulation of the innate and adaptive immune responses by Stat-3 signaling in tumor cells. Nature Med 10:48–54.
Wu WJ, Pruett SB (1999) Ethanol decreases host resistance to pulmonary metastases in a mouse model: role of natural killer cells and the ethanol-induced stress response. Int J Cancer 82:886–92.
Xiang R, Lode HN, Gillies SD, Reisfeld RA (1999) T cell memory against colon carcinoma is long-lived in the absence of antigen. J Immunol 163:3676–83.
Yang L, Huang J, Ren X, Gorska AE, Chytil A, Aakre M, Carbone DP, Matrisian LM, Richmond A, Lin PC, Moses HL (2008) Abrogation of TGF beta signaling in mammary carcinomas recruits Gr-1+CD11b+ myeloid cells that promote metastasis. Cancer Cell 13:23–35.
Yang R, Roden RBS (2007) Re: The Terminology Issue for Myeloid-Derived Suppressor Cells. Cancer Res 67:426.
Yu H, Kortylewski M, Pardoll D (2007) Crosstalk between cancer and immune cells: role of STAT3 in the tumour microenvironment. Nature Rev Immunol 7:41–51.
Zhang H, Meadows GG (2005) Chronic alcohol consumption in mice increases the proportion of peripheral memory T cells by homeostatic proliferation. J Leukoc Biol 78:1070–80.
Zhang H, Meadows GG (2008) Chronic alcohol consumption perturbs the balance between thymus-derived and bone marrow-derived natural killer cells in the spleen. J Leukocyte Biol 83:41–47.
Zhang H, Meadows GG (2010) Chronic alcohol consumption enhances myeloid-derived suppressor cells in B16BL6 melanoma-bearing mice. Cancer Immunol Immunother Mar 13 [Epub ahead of print].
Zhou J, Meadows GG (2003) Alcohol consumption decreases IL-2-induced NF-kappaB activity in enriched NK cells from C57BL/6 mice. Toxicol Sci 73:72–9.
Zingoni A, Sornasse T, Cocks BG, Tanaka Y, Santoni A, Lanier LL (2005) NK cell regulation of T cell-mediated responses. Mol Immunol 42:451–4.
Zitvogel L, Terme M, Borg C, Trinchieri G (2006) Dendritic cell-NK cell cross-talk: regulation and physiopathology. Curr Top Microbiol Immunol 298:157–74.

Chapter 11
Stem Cells and Alcohol-Related Cancers

Zhigang (Peter) Gao and Q. Max Guo

Abbreviations

ADH	Alcohol dehydrogenase
AKT/PKB	AKT/protein kinase B
ALDH	Aldehyde dehydrogenase
BMP	Bone morphogenetic protein
CSC	Cancer stem cell
CXCR4	C-X-C chemokine receptor type 4
CYP2E1	Cytochrome P450 2E1
DAX1	Dosage-sensitive sex reversal, adrenal hypoplasia critical region, on chromosome X, gene 1
EGF	Epidermal growth factor
Eomes	Eomesodermin
ER	Estrogen receptor
ES	Embryonic stem (cell)
FACS	Fluorescence-activated cell sorting
Foxa2	Forkhead box A2
Gata6	GATA-binding protein 6
GH	Growth hormone
GI	Gastrointestinal
GKM	Gatekeeper mutation
Gsc	Goosecoid
GST	Glutathione S transferase
Hand1	Heart and neural crest derivatives-expressed 1
HBV	Hepatitis B virus

Q.M. Guo (✉)
Division of Metabolism and Health Effects, National Institute on Alcohol Abuse and Alcoholism, National Institutes of Health, Bethesda, MD, USA
e-mail: qmguo@mail.nih.gov

S. Zakhari et al. (eds.), *Alcohol and Cancer*, DOI 10.1007/978-1-4614-0040-0_11,
© Springer Science+Business Media, LLC 2011

HCV	Hepatitis C virus
HESX1	Homeobox expressed in ES cells 1
HoxB1	Homeobox protein Hox-B1
IGF	Insulin-like growth factor
iPS	Induced pluripotent stem (cell)
Lgr5	Leucine-rich-repeat-containing G-protein-coupled receptor 5
Lhx5	LIM homeobox 5
LIF	Leukemia inhibitory factor
miRNA	microRNA
MTHFR	Methylene-tetrahydrofolate reductase
Myf5	Myogenic factor 5
NANOG	Homeobox protein NANOG
NOD/SCID	Nonobese diabetic/severe combined immunodeficiency
OC	Oval cells
OCT4	Octamer-binding protein 4
ONC	Oncogenes
Otx1	Orthodenticle homologue 1
PcGs	Polycomb group proteins
REX1/ZPF42	Zinc finger protein 42
SALL4	Sal-like protein 4
SOX2	SRY box-containing factor 2
SP	Side population
Stat3	Signal transducer and activator of transcription 3
T	Brachyury protein homolog
TBX3	T-box transcription factor
TCF3	Transcription factor 3 (E2A immunoglobulin enhancer-binding factors E12/E47)
TPG	Tumor-progenitor genes
TSG	Tumor suppressor genes
ZIC3	Zinc finger protein ZIC 3

Stem Cells

Stem cells are populations of cells with the potential to develop into many different types of cells, tissues, and organs. Stem cells are characterized by their capacities of multipotency to differentiate or self-renew. They play a crucial role in many aspects of biology, from embryo development to tissue repair and maintenance. In many organs and tissues, they serve as an internal system for regeneration and repair. Stem cells divide essentially without limit to maintain the stem cell pool and replenish other cells as long as needed.

Stem cells are distinguished from other cell types by possessing two important characteristics. First, they are undifferentiated cells capable of self-renewing, sometimes after long periods of inactivity. Second, under certain conditions, they can

Table 11.1 Types of stem cells

Stem cell type	Origin	Differentiation potential
Embryonic stem cells (ES)	Embryo blastocyst, primordial germ cell	*Totipotent* – are capable of producing all embryonic and postembryonic cells, tissues, and organs.
Adult stem cells (including fetal stem cell and cord blood stem cells)	Bone marrow, muscle, skin, brain, liver, heart, adipose tissue, cord blood, fetal liver, etc	*Multipotent* – are capable of producing multiple but limited number of lineages of cells in a closely related family; may transdifferentiate from one lineage to another
Induced pluripotent stem cells (iPS)	Fibroblast, liver, pancreas, neuron, etc	*Pluripotent* – are capable of producing cells of any three germ layers (ectoderm, endoderm, and mesoderm)

differentiate into tissue- or organ-specific cells. In some organs, such as bone marrow and gut, stem cells regularly proliferate to regenerate, repair, and replace damaged or worn-out tissues. In other organs such as the pancreas and the heart, stem cells remain in a quiescent state and only proliferate or differentiate under special circumstances.

Stem cells were first described more than a century ago. Early studies of stem cells were mostly focused on embryogenesis and early development. Since the 1970s, hematopoietic stem cells have been successfully used in clinic for bone marrow transplantation to treat leukemia. The development of a method to culture human embryonic stem (ES) cells by Thomson and colleagues in 1998 overcame a critical technical barrier and brought unprecedented excitement to the stem cell field (Thomson et al. 1998). Since then, many research interests have been focused on ES cells and adult stem cells from several types of tissues (somatic stem cells; see Table 11.1). ES cells are usually derived from the inner cell mass of an early-stage embryo, called blastocyst, or from human primordial germ cells (Shamblott et al. 1998). They are totipotent and give rise to cells of all three primary germ layers during development: ectoderm, endoderm, and mesoderm, as well as extraembryonic cell types. Adult stem cells reside in various tissues during already differentiated developmental stages (including the prenatal and early postnatal stage, such as stem cells in cord blood and fetal liver). They are multipotent and can differentiate into tissue-committed cell types. Well-studied adult stem cells include hematopoietic stem cells in the bone marrow, neuronal stem cells in the central nervous system, bulge stem cell in hair follicles, crypt stem cells in gastrointestinal (GI) tract, and hepatic stem cells in the liver (Civin and Small 1995; Blanpain and Fuchs 2009; Barker et al. 2008). Throughout the lifetime, adult stem cells serve as a continuous supply of cells for tissue repair and regeneration via self-renewal and differentiation.

Another breakthrough for the stem cell field occurred in 2006 when Shinya Yamanaka's laboratory reprogrammed mouse adult cells into pluripotent stem cells by introducing only four key transcription factors (Oct3/4, Sox2, c-Myc, and Klf4), which had been known to play an important role in stem cell maintenance

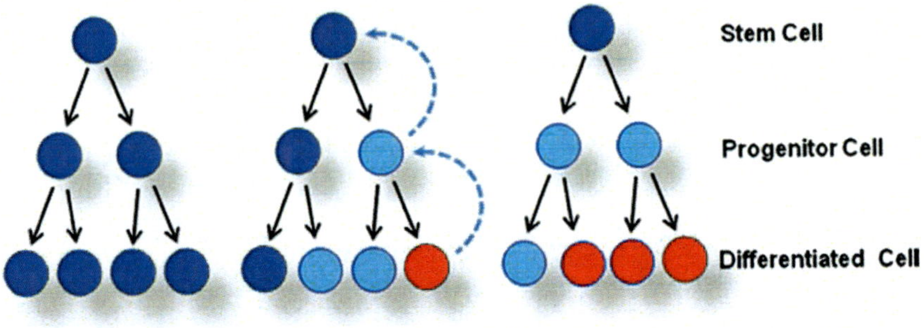

Fig. 11.1 Stem cell fates – self-renewal, differentiation, or dedifferentiation. *Dark blue* represents the undifferentiated state of stem cells (with stemness). *Turquoise* and *red* represent more highly differentiated cells

(Takahashi and Yamanaka 2006). A year later, the work was reproduced in human skin fibroblasts by Yamanaka's laboratory using the same combination of genes, and also independently by Thomson's laboratory by forcefully expressing OCT3/4, SOX2, NANOG, and LIN28 (Takahashi et al. 2007; Yu et al. 2007). This new category of stem cells is called *i*nduced *p*luripotent *s*tem (iPS) cells. This success of reprogramming terminally differentiated human somatic cells into iPS cells, which may have almost the same capacity as embryonic stem cells, has offered great opportunities for stem cell research and personalized regenerative medicine. For alcohol-induced tissue injury and alcohol-related cancers, iPS cells can be useful for exploring the biological mechanisms of these diseases and providing new therapeutic strategies for their treatment.

To maintain homeostasis of the stem cell pool, stem cells divide symmetrically or asymmetrically (Fig. 11.1). Asymmetric cell division produces two daughter cells: one self-renewed daughter stem cell remains the same as the parental cell, while the other is committed to lineage-specific differentiation. The lineage-specific progenitor cells further differentiate into mature cells. When the stem cell pool is used and reduced, stem cells can divide symmetrically to expand or recover the pool. In this case, the two daughter cells retain the same undifferentiated properties as the parental cell and maintain contact with the stem cell niche (Gao 2008). Not only could fully differentiated cells be induced to gain stemness and become stem cells (i.e., iPS cells) but also can be dedifferentiated back to a certain early progenitor stage (Zhou et al. 2008).

The above features of stem cells may have a close relationship with the development of cancers. Striking parallels can be found between stem cells and cancer cells. (1) Tumors may originate from the transformation of normal stem cells; (2) Similar signaling pathways are involved in regulating both self-renewal of stem cells and cancer cells; (3) Tumors may contain "cancer stem cells" – a minority of cells with indefinite potential for self-renewal that drive tumorigenesis. In addition, stem cells may be more susceptible than mature cells in the same tissue to accumulate genetic mutations and epigenetic changes because they live relatively longer and divide more times, and thus are more prone to tumorigenesis (Beachy et al. 2004; Fig. 11.2).

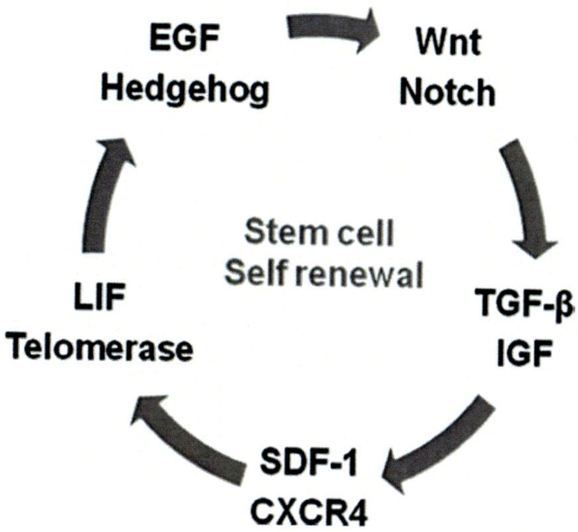

Fig. 11.2 Important pathways involved in stem cell self-renewal

The fate of stem cells is determined by genetic factors and environmental cues, which could consist of genetic and epigenetic regulation by stromal or accessory cells in a microenvironment, cytokines, and developmental growth factors (Gao 2008). Many players that regulate self-renewal and differentiation of stem cells are actually oncogenes or tumor suppressors. In many cases, the pathways regulating self-renewal of stem cells are also activated in various types of cancers (Beachy et al. 2004; Fig. 11.2). Dysregulated signaling pathways caused by changes in these genetic and environmental factors, including alcohol and its metabolites, may result in changes in cell fate.

Some transcription factors, such as the homeodomain transcription factors OCT4, NANOG, and SOX2, form a transcriptional module, which plays a central role in maintaining ES cell identity both in mice and humans (MacArthur et al. 2009). These three transcription factors regulate their own and each other's expression in a highly concerted manner. They co-occupy numerous developmentally important genes and repress the expression of the genes involved in lineage commitment of stem cells. The targets of these three transcription factors include *HAND1*, eomesodermin (*Eomes*), *LHX5*, *OTX1*, *HOXb1*, *MYF5*, T (brachyury protein homologue), *GSC* (goosecoid), *FOXA2*, and *GATA6*. At the same time, OCT4, NANOG, and SOX2 activate genes that are associated with self-renewal and pluripotency, including other ES cell-associated transcription factors such as *TC1*, *TBX3*, *REST*, *ZIC3*, *HESX1*, *STAT3*, *REX1* (also known as *ZPF42*), *SALL4*, *TCF3*, and *DAX1* (MacArthur et al. 2009).

Cancers can be initiated from a stem cell, a progenitor cell, or a mature cell. The accumulation of mutations in stem cells may lead to development of cancers, or cancerous stem cells. Normal and mutated progenitor cells can also acquire the capacity of self-renewal, but at the same time, they may lose their differentiation ability, and lose control for their proliferation. Thus, they become cancer-initiating cells and develop into tumors. For example, it has been recently demonstrated that stem cells in liver, the most important organ for alcohol metabolism, are responsible for the development of liver cancer in a mouse model (Rountree et al. 2009).

Cancer Stem Cells

Cancer Stem Cell Hypothesis

That a given cancer is comprised of a heterogeneous population of cells has been known for over a century (Vermeulen et al. 2008). These heterogeneous cell populations differ from each other in morphology, marker expression, differentiation grade, proliferation capacity, and tumor generation/initiation potential (Vermeulen et al. 2008). **The concept of cancer stem cells was first proposed 16 years ago based on** studies of leukemia stem cells (Lapidot et al. 1994). It was found that a small population of early progenitor cells with the expression pattern of $CD34^{+}CD38^{-}$, but not the cells with pattern of $CD34^{-}$ or $CD34^{+}CD38^{+}$, were actually leukemia initiation cells in a bone marrow transplantation model. Only these leukemia stem cells could engraft in the secondary transplanted animal and initiate leukemia. The idea was further developed in various solid tumors, especially in human breast and brain tumors (Bonnet and Dick 1997; Reviewed by Visvader and Lindeman 2008; Dalerba et al. 2007).

The cancer stem cell model hypothesizes that a small subset of cancer cells in a tumor, the cancer stem cells, constitutes a reservoir of self-sustaining cells with the exclusive ability to self-renew and maintain the tumor growth. Cancer stem cells (CSCs) in the tumor have the ability to divide and expand themselves. The other larger population of partially differentiated cancer cells derived from CSCs forms the bulk of the tumor (Clarke et al. 2006).

A tumor is hierarchically organized with two different cell populations: a small population of cancer stem cells (CSCs) with the ability to divide and expand the CSC pool, and a larger population of partially differentiated nontumorigenic cancer cells derived from CSCs, which form the bulk of the tumor. The model proposes that within the whole tumor bulk, only CSCs possess the distinct survival mechanism similar to stem cells. These stem cell properties are crucial for the maintenance and propagation of a tumor (Gupta et al. 2009; Visvader and Lindeman 2008).

Properties of Cancer Stem Cells

Five characteristics have been proposed for cancer stem cells (Gupta et al. 2009; Visvader and Lindeman 2008). These cells can (1) self-renew, (2) generate tumors in animal hosts, (3) differentiate into other cell types, (4) exist in a quiescent state

Table 11.2 Isolation of cancer stem cells in various malignancies

Cancer type	Markers for CSC
Colon carcinoma[a]	$CD133^+$, Lgr5, $CD44^+$/Lin-/ESA^+
Breast cancer[a]	CD24(–/low)/CD44+, ALDH1
Brain tumor	$CD133^+$
Lung cancer[a]	$CD133^+$
Pancreas carcinoma[a]	$CD44^+/CD24^+/ESA^+/CD133^+$
Hepatocellular carcinoma[a]	$CD133^+$, ALDH1
Ovarian carcinoma	Side population (SP)
Head and neck squamous cell carcinoma	$CD44^+$
Prostate carcinoma	$CD44^+/CD133^+$
Hematological malignancies	$CD34^+/CD38^-$

[a] Possibly alcohol-related

before generating tumors, and (5) generate tumors that are more resistant to a variety of conventional therapeutics than their counterparts generated from other cell types (Hanahan and Weinberg 2000). Therefore, cancers derived from stem cell are generally more difficult to treat using currently available therapeutics.

Stem Cells in Tumor Initiation and Progression

The cancer stem cell hypothesis can explain the whole tumor development process, from its initiation to its metastasis. Cancer stem cells (CSC) may also contribute significantly to the development of resistance to conventional chemotherapies for cancers. In the cancer stem cell model, intrinsic mutations are accumulated for oncogenes or tumor suppressor genes; epigenetic changes can also precipitate the process. All these may render the normal stem cells inside the tissue the loss of benign potential for differentiation. The CSC can develop into a tumor with cellular heterogeneity. CSCs can also initiate a new tumor (cancer-initiating cells), in places that may be distant from the original tumor (metastasis). Moreover, CSCs may provide the precursors of tumor stromal components, such as the precursors for tumor vasculogenesis (Gupta et al. 2009; Visvader and Lindeman 2008; Gao 2008).

Identification of the Cancer Stem Cell Population

Cell surface marker staining and fluorescence-activated cell sorting (FACS) by label retention and side population (SP) using the Hoechst 33342 exclusion are commonly used methods to identify stem cells. These methods can also be used for identifying the cancer stem cell population (Table 11.2). The alcohol-metabolizing enzyme aldehyde dehydrogenase (ALDH1) has been identified as a stem cell marker in two alcohol-related cancers: breast cancer and colon cancer (Ginestier et al. 2007; Huang et al. 2009; Moreb 2008; Zhou et al. 2009). CD133, CD44, CD24, and Lgr5 (Barker et al. 2010) are also commonly used cell surface markers to identify cancer stem cells in various tissues, such as breast cancer, brain tumors, and hepatocellular carcinoma. However, the above markers are also highly expressed in normal stem cells in the same tissues. For example, CD133 is not only enriched in brain tumor and liver cancer stem cells but also present in normal brain and liver stem cells (Rountree et al. 2009). The same is true for CD44, Sca1, Lgr5, and Thy1. In addition, markers used to identify stem cells from one organ are usually different from those used for identifying stem cells in other organs. Furthermore, a marker used to identify stem cells from a particular organ does not always work in different contexts. For example, culturing of stem cells, even for a short time, can drastically change their marker characteristics and protein expression profiles (Clarke et al. 2006). Since markers may or may not be useful for identifying stem cells from other organs or tumor types, a more reliable method to identify CSCs might be by using CSC's featured capacities of self-renewal and of causing the heterogeneous lineages of cancer cells in the tumor. CSC populations can be experimentally differentiated from other cancer cells (nontumorigenic) by examining their ability to regenerate a xenograft tumor in transplanted animals.

Epigenetic Regulation of Cancer Stem Cells

Epigenetic regulation plays a pivotal role in both stem cells and cancers. DNA methylation, histone modifications, and RNA-mediated silencing are the most widely studied epigenetic mechanisms (see Chap. 5 for more discussion). In the past few years, great advances have been made in characterizing epigenetic changes in stem cells and cancers. Global and gene-specific changes in DNA methylation can lead to chromosomal instability and increase tumorigenesis in various tissues and organs (Feinberg et al. 2006). Small RNAs (including microRNAs) are also integral elements in the posttranscriptional control of gene expression. MicroRNA (miRNA) plays an important role in determining stem cell fate by regulating several key genes involving stem cell renewal and differentiation, such as *OCT4*, *NANOG*, *SOX2*, and *SA114* (Inui et al. 2010). The Polycomb group proteins (PcGs) silence gene expression, allowing cells to both acquire and maintain stem cell or cancer stem cell identities (Gieni and Hendzel 2009). It has recently been found that epigenetic modifications of DNA could be kept in low-passage iPS cells (Kim et al 2010). It is of great interest to study alcohol's effects on epigenetic regulation (e.g., DNA methylation, histone modification, and miRNAs) of stem cells and cancer stem cells, and how these effects mediate alcohol-related cancer initiation and progression. New knowledge of epigenetic regulations of alcohol-related cancers may help to identify novel targets for therapeutic treatment of these cancers.

Implications for Cancer Therapy

The cancer stem cell hypothesis posits that cancer stem cells are a minority population of self-renewing cancer cells that fuel tumor growth and remain in patients after conventional chemotherapies. The hypothesis predicts that a complete eradication of a tumor requires agents that can target CSCs. In addition, since CSCs and regular stem cells share many characteristics, it is important that agents can discriminate between CSCs and normal stem cells. Therefore, a better understanding of stem cell biology as well as the genetics and epigenetics of CSCs in tumors is critical. In alcohol-related cancers, there is usually the additive or synergistic action between alcohol and other risk factors, such as carcinogens and virus infection, on stem cells and CSCs, and alcohol-induced compromise of the immune system. The impact of the therapy on CSCs should be carefully considered while these cancers are treated.

Stem Cells and Alcohol-Related Cancers

Chronic ethanol consumption may promote carcinogenesis through its metabolite **acetaldehyde, inflammation, increased oxidative stress, and induction of cytochrome** P4502E1 (*CYP2E1*), which can convert procarcinogens to carcinogens. Alcohol can interact with other risk factors, such as viral infection, smoking, obesity, and diabetes, on initiation and progression of cancers. Alcohol may affect the stem cell niche by perturbing many biochemical or signaling pathways known to be important for both stem cells and cancers. Examples of these pathways include Notch, Hedgehog, Wnt/β-catenin, EGF-like/EGFR/Neu, LIF, TGF-β, integrins, telomerase, SDF-1/CXCR4, prolactin/growth hormone (GH), the IGF-1, Estrogen Receptor (ER), and Stat3 pathways (Fig. 11.2). Alcohol and its metabolites may affect one or more of these pathways to interfere with the renewal or differentiation of stem cells or CSCs. **Alcohol may also have significant impact on endogenous stem cells in specific** organs or tissues (e.g., oral cavity, upper aerodigestive tract, stomach, colon, breast, liver, and pancreas), which may contribute to the development of cancers in these tissue. Polymorphisms in genes involved in alcohol metabolism, including alcohol dehydrogenase (*ADH*), aldehyde dehydrogenase (*ALDH*), *CYP2E1*, and methylene-tetrahydrofolate reductase (*MTHFR*) have been shown to be associated with certain alcohol-related cancers (Druesne-Pecollo et al. 2009; also see Chap. 4).

Liver

1. Hepatocytes, oval cells (OC), and bone marrow-derived cells may all be sources of liver progenitor/stem cells. Hepatic carcinogenesis can also originate from hepatocytes, oval cells, and bone marrow-derived cells (Williams et al. 1993; Li et al. 2009; Dumble et al. 2002; Ishikawa et al. 2004).

2. A close correlation has been observed between the degree of progenitor/stem cell activation and the severity of inflammation and fibrosis in chronic hepatitis. The major contributing factors include hepatitis C, hepatitis B, and alcohol (Pöschl and Seitz 2004).
3. Oval cells arise within the liver following certain types of liver injury. OC proliferation can be activated in a certain types of liver injury, especially when the proliferative capacity of hepatocytes is impaired.
4. Homing of adult bone marrow mesenchymal stem cells contributes to liver fibrosis. Myofibroblasts play a central role in the pathogenesis of liver fibrosis, and myofibroblasts from bone marrow have recently been identified in fibrotic livers. Bone marrow mesenchymal stem cells can migrate to the damaged liver and differentiate into myofibroblasts, and eventually develop into hepatocellular carcinoma (Li et al. 2009).

Pancreas

Pancreatic cancer stem cells represent less than 1% of all pancreatic cancer cells and express the surface markers CD44, CD24, and epithelial-specific antigen (Lee et al. 2008). CSCs identified by these markers have 100-fold higher tumorigenic potential than those without these markers. CSCs in pancreatic cancers also have the capacity to generate xenografts tumors in nonobese diabetic/severe combined immunodeficiency (NOD/SCID) mice. In comparison, other cancer cells devoid of these surface markers do not have such capacity. CSCs were found to be able to maintain their surface marker phenotype after repeated passages as xenografts (Lee et al. 2008).

Colorectal Tissue

Intestinal or crypt stem cells in small intestine and colon generate $>10^{10}$ new cells daily, which turn over the absorptive epithelium every 3–5 days (Barker et al. 2010). The dysregulation of AKT/PKB, Wnt, and/or BMP signaling pathways can disturb intestinal stem cell self-renewal (Lee et al. 2008). Colorectal carcinoma develops as a result of accumulated mutations during clonal expansion of stem cells. These mutations enhance stem cells' proliferative potential, independent from extrinsic growth signals and autonomous control of metabolic activities (van den Brink and Offerhaus 2007; Vogelstein and Kinzler 2004; Lee et al. 2008; Barker et al. 2010).

Breast

Like other cancer tissues, breast cancer contains a heterogeneous population of cells. Breast cancer stem cells may originate from normal breast stem cells that have undergone genetic and epigenetic alterations. Breast CSCs retain the ability of self-renewal and differentiation as normal breast stem cells, but lose the ability to form normal and functional mammary glands. A small population of tumorigenic cancer stem cells has the ability to self-renew and engraft in transplanted animals, whereas the large majority of more-differentiated cancer cells have limited proliferation potential and are weakly tumorigenic or nontumorigenic when injected into nude mice (Seitz and Stickel 2007; Dumitrescu and Shields 2005).

Future Directions

Recent advances in the fields of stem cells and cancer stem cells have provided great opportunities for understanding the underlying mechanisms of alcohol-induced tissue injury and alcohol-related cancers, and exploring new therapeutic strategies for their diagnosis and treatment. Pursuing such mechanistic insights of the pathological process of alcohol-related cancers can lead to new directions and novel targets in developing more effective treatment. In addition, stem cells can be used to (1) replace tissues/organs damaged by alcohol abuse, (2) deliver genetic therapies (gene therapy) for alcohol-related cancers, and (3) deliver chemotherapeutic agents for the treatment of alcohol-related cancers.

Of particular interest is the use of iPS cell lines to study the mechanisms involved in the pathogenesis of alcohol-induced cancers. There is a great need for iPS cells that mimic diverse human traits of alcohol metabolism and related cancers, such as esophageal cancers in individuals with defective ALDH2 enzymes. Investigating how transplanted stem cells (e.g., iPS cells) integrate into alcohol-damaged tissues and how they interact with the endogenous stem/progenitor cells (such as liver stem cells) is important. In addition, more characterization of cancer stem cells in alcohol-related cancers is also needed.

References

Barker N, Huch M, Kujala P, van de Wetering M, Snippert HJ, van Es JH, Sato T, Stange DE, Begthel H, van den Born M, Danenberg E, van den Brink S, Korving J, Abo A, Peters PJ, Wright N, Poulsom R, Clevers H (2010) Lgr5(+ve) stem cells drive self-renewal in the stomach and build long-lived gastric units in vitro. Cell Stem Cell 6:25–36.

Barker N, van de Wetering M, Clevers H (2008) The intestinal stem cell. Genes Dev 22:1856–64.

Beachy PA, Karhadkar SS, Berman DM (2004) Tissue repair and stem cell renewal in carcinogenesis. Nature 432:324–31.

Blanpain C and Fuchs E (2009) Epidermal homeostasis: a balancing act of stem cells in the skin. Nat Rev Mol Cell Biol 10:207–17.

Bonnet D, Dick JE (1997) Human acute myeloid leukemia is organized as a hierarchy that originates from a primitive hematopoietic cell. Nat Med 3:730–7.

Civin CI, Small D (1995) Purification and expansion of human hematopoietic stem/progenitor cells. Ann N Y Acad Sci 770:91–8.

Clarke MF, Dick JE, Dirks PB, Eaves CJ, Jamieson CHM, Jones DL, Visvader J, Weissman IL and Wahl GM (2006) Cancer stem cells – perspectives on current status and future directions: AACR workshop on cancer stem cells. Cancer Res 66:9339–44.

Dalerba P, Cho RW, Clarke MF (2007) Cancer Stem Cells: Models and Concepts. Annu Rev Med 58:267–84.

Druesne-Pecollo N, Tehard B, Mallet Y, Gerber M, Norat T, Hercberg S, Latino-Martel P (2009) Alcohol and genetic polymorphisms: effect on risk of alcohol-related cancer. Lancet Oncol 10:173–80.

Dumble ML, Croager EJ, Yeoh GC, Quail EA (2002) Generation and characterization of p53 null transformed hepatic progenitor cells: oval cells give rise to hepatocellular carcinoma. Carcinogenesis 23:435–45.

Dumitrescu RG, Shields PG (2005) The etiology of alcohol-induced breast cancer. Alcohol 35:213–25.

Feinberg AP, Ohlsson R, Henikoff S (2006) The epigenetic progenitor origin of human cancer. Nat Rev Genet 7:21–33.

Gao JX (2008) Cancer stem cells: the lessons from pre-cancerous stem cells. J Cell Mol Med 12:67–96.

Gieni RS, Hendzel MJ (2009) Polycomb group protein gene silencing, non-coding RNA, stem cells, and cancer. Biochem Cell Biol 87:711–46.

Ginestier C, Hur MH, Charafe-Jauffret E, Monville F, Dutcher J, Brown M, Jacquemier J, Viens P, Kleer CG, Liu S, Schott A, Hayes D, Birnbaum D, Wicha MS, Dontu G (2007) ALDH1 is a marker of normal and malignant human mammary stem cells and a predictor of poor clinical outcome. Cell Stem Cell 1:555–67.

Gupta PB, Chaffer CL, and Weinberg RA (2009) Cancer stem cells: mirage or reality? Nat Med 15:1010–2.

Hanahan D, Weinberg RA (2000) The hallmarks of cancer. Cell 100:57–70.

Huang EH, Hynes MJ, Zhang T, Ginestier C, Dontu G, Appelman H, Fields JZ, Wicha MS, Boman BM (2009) Aldehyde dehydrogenase 1 is a marker for normal and malignant human colonic stem cells (SC) and tracks SC overpopulation during colon tumorigenesis. Cancer Res 69:3382–9.

Kim K, Doi A, Wen B, Ng K, Zhao R, Cahan P, Kim J, Aryee MJ, Ji H, Ehrlich LI, Yabuuchi A, Takeuchi A, Cunniff KC, Hongguang H, McKinney-Freeman S, Naveiras O, Yoon TJ, Irizarry RA, Jung N, Seita J, Hanna J, Murakami P, Jaenisch R, Weissleder R, Orkin SH, Weissman IL, Feinberg AP, Daley GQ (2010) Epigenetic memory in induced pluripotent stem cells. *Nature*. 2010 Jul 19. [Epub ahead of print]

Inui M, Martello G, Piccolo S (2010) MicroRNA control of signal transduction. Nat Rev Mol Cell Biol 11:252–63.

Ishikawa H, Nakao K, Matsumoto K, Nishimura D, Ichikawa T, Hamasaki K, Eguchi K (2004) Bone marrow engraftment in a rodent model of chemical carcinogenesis but no role in the histogenesis of hepatocellular carcinoma. Gut 53:884–9.

Lapidot T, Sirard C, Vormoor J, Murdoch B, Hoang T, Caceres-Cortes J, Minden M, Paterson B, Caligiuri MA, Dick JE (1994) A cell initiating human acute myeloid leukaemia after transplantation into SCID mice. Nature 367:645–8.

Lee CJ, Dosch J, Simeone DM (2008) Pancreatic cancer stem cells. Journal of Clinical Oncology 26:2806–12.

Li C, Kong Y, Wang H, Wang S, Yu H, Liu X, Yang L, Jiang X, Li L, Li L (2009) Homing of bone marrow mesenchymal stem cells mediated by sphingosine 1-phosphate contributes to liver fibrosis. J Hepatol 50:1174–83.

MacArthur BD, Ma'ayan A, Lemischka IR (2009) Systems biology of stem cell fate and cellular reprogramming. Nat Rev Mol Cell Biol 10:672–81.

Moreb JS (2008) Aldehyde dehydrogenase as a marker for stem cells. Curr Stem Cell Res Ther 3:237–46.

Pöschl G, Seitz HK (2004) Alcohol and cancer. Alcohol Alcohol39:155–65.

Rountree CB, Ding W, He L, Stiles B (2009) Expansion of CD133-expressing liver cancer stem cells in liver-specific phosphatase and tensin homolog deleted on chromosome 10-deleted mice. Stem Cells 27:290–9.

Seitz HK, Stickel F (2007) Molecular mechanisms of alcohol-mediated carcinogenesis. Nat Rev Cancer 7:599–612.
Shamblott MJ, Axelman J, Wang S, Bugg EM, Littlefield JW, Donovan PJ, Blumenthal PD, Huggins GR, Gearhart JD (1998) Derivation of pluripotent stem cells from cultured human primordial germ cells. Proc Natl Acad Sci USA 95:13726–31.
Takahashi K, Tanabe K, Ohnuki M, Narita M, Ichisaka T, Tomoda K, Yamanaka S (2007) Induction of pluripotent stem cells from adult human fibroblasts by defined factors. Cell 131:861–72.
Takahashi K, Yamanaka S (2006) Induction of pluripotent stem cells from mouse embryonic and adult fibroblast cultures by defined factors. Cell 126:663–76.
Thomson JA, Itskovitz-Eldor J, Shapiro SS, Waknitz MA, Swiergiel JJ, Marshall VS, Jones JM (1998) Embryonic stem cell lines derived from human blastocysts. Science 282:1145–7.
van den Brink GR, Offerhaus GJ (2007) The morphogenetic code and colon cancer development. Cancer Cell 11:109–17.
Vermeulen L, Sprick MR, Kemper K, Stassi G and Medema JP (2008) Cancer stem cells - old concepts, new insights. Cell Death and Differentiation 15:947–58.
Visvader JE and Lindeman GJ (2008) Cancer stem cells in solid tumours: accumulating evidence and unresolved questions. Nat Rev Cancer 8:755–68.
Vogelstein B, Kinzler KW (2004) Cancer genes and the pathways they control. Nat Med 10:789–99.
Williams GM, Gebhardt R, Sirma H, Stenback F (1993) Non-linearity of neoplastic conversion induced in rat liver by low exposures to diethylnitrosamine. Carcinogenesis 14:2149–56.
Yu J, Vodyanik MA, Smuga-Otto K, Antosiewicz-Bourget J, Frane JL, Tian S, Nie J, Jonsdottir GA, Ruotti V, Stewart R, Slukvin II, Thomson JA (2007) Induced pluripotent stem cell lines derived from human somatic cells. Science 318:1917–20.
Zhou Q, Brown J, Kanarek A, Rajagopal J, Melton DA (2008) In vivo reprogramming of adult pancreatic exocrine cells to beta-cells. Nature 455:627–32.
Zhou P, Hohm S, Olusanya Y, Hess DA, Nolta J (2009) Human progenitor cells with high aldehyde dehydrogenase activity efficiently engraft into damaged liver in a novel model. Hepatology. 49:1992–2000.

Chapter 12
Epilogue, Consensus Recommendations: Alcohol and Cancer

Samir Zakhari

The National Institute on Alcohol Abuse and Alcoholism (NIAAA) provides leadership in the national effort to reduce alcohol-related diseases by conducting and supporting research in a wide range of scientific areas, including health risks and benefits of alcohol consumption. Excessive drinking is associated with an increased risk for cancers of several organs including the esophagus, oral cavity, liver, breast, and colon. Our knowledge of the mechanisms by which alcohol induces cancer is largely incomplete, and by understanding how alcohol causes cancer we can integrate this knowledge to design medications for cancer.

To address this issue, the staff in the Division of Metabolism and Health Effects (DMHE) thoroughly reviewed the current state-of-knowledge on alcohol and cancer, and presented their findings to the NIAAA Extramural Advisory Board (EAB; a working subgroup of the NIAAA National Advisory Council) and invited experts on June 8–9, 2010. This meeting was the first review of the biomedical aspects of alcohol and cancer in the NIAAA portfolio and will serve to guide future directions in developing NIAAA research goals in this area.

Extramural Advisory Board and Council Members

Fulton T. Crews, PhD
Chairman, EAB
Director, Bowles Center for Alcohol Studies
Professor, Pharmacology and Psychiatry
University of North Carolina School of Medicine

S. Zakhari (✉)
Division of Metabolism and Health Effects, National Institute on Alcohol Abuse and Alcoholism, National Institutes of Health, Bethesda, MD, USA
e-mail: szakhari@mail.nih.gov

S. Zakhari et al. (eds.), *Alcohol and Cancer*, DOI 10.1007/978-1-4614-0040-0_12,
© Springer Science+Business Media, LLC 2011

Thurston Bowles Building
Chapel Hill, NC 27599
ftcrews@med.unc.edu

David W. Crabb, MD
John B. Hickam Professor and Chairman
Department of Medicine
Indiana University Medical Center
545 Barnhall Drive
Indianapolis, IN 46202
dcrabb@iupui.edu

John C. Crabbe, PhD
Director, Portland Alcohol Research Center
Senior Research Career Scientist, Department of Veterans Affairs
Professor, Department of Behavioral Neuroscience
Oregon Health & Science University School of Medicine
3181 SW Sam Jackson Park Road
Portland, OR 97239
crabbe@ohsu.edu

Howard J. Edenberg, PhD
Distinguished Professor
Chancellor's Professor
Professor of Biochemistry and Molecular Biology
Professor, Medical and Molecular Genetics
Director, Center for Medical Genomics
Indiana University School of Medicine
635 Barnhill Drive
Indianapolis, IN 46202
edenberg@iupui.edu

Cindy L. Ehlers, PhD
Co-director, Scripps Alcohol Research Center
Professor, Department of Molecular and Integrative Neurosciences
Scripps Research Institute
10550 Torrey Pines Road
La Jolla, CA 92037
cindye@scripps.edu

Scott L. Friedman, MD
Professor of Medicine
Mount Sinai School of Medicine
Chief of the Division of Liver Diseases
Mount Sinai Hospital
1425 Madison Avenue
New York, NY 10029
scott.friedman@mssm.edu

Kathleen A. Grant, PhD
Professor, Department of Behavioral Neurosciences
Oregon Health and Science University
Senior Scientist, Division of Neuroscience, Oregon National Primate Research Center
505 NW 185th Avenue
Beaverton, OR 97006
grantka@ohsu.edu

Thomas K. Greenfield, PhD
Center Director, National Alcohol Research Center
Scientific Director, Alcohol Research Group, Public Health Institute
Adjunct Clinical Faculty, Department of Psychiatry
University of California-San Francisco
6475 Christie Avenue
Emeryville, CA 94608
tgreenfield@arg.org

R. Adron Harris, PhD
Director, Waggoner Center for Alcohol and Addiction Research
M. June and J. Virgil Waggoner Chair in Molecular Biology
University of Texas
2500 Speedway
Austin, TX 78712
harris@mail.utexas.edu

Deborah S. Hasin, PhD
Professor, Clinical Public Health
Professor, Department of Psychiatry, College of Physicians and Surgeons
Professor, Department of Epidemiology, Mailman School of Public Health
Columbia University
New York State Psychiatric Institute
New York, NY 10032
dsh2@columbia.edu

Andrew C. Heath, PhD
Director, Midwest Alcoholism Research Center
Spencer T. Olin Professor of Psychology
Washington University School of Medicine
Professor of Psychology
University of Missouri
660 South Euclid Avenue
St. Louis, MO 63108
Andrew@matlock.wustl.edu

Bankole A. Johnson, DSc, MD, PhD, MPhil, FRCPsych.
Professor of Neuroscience
Professor of Medicine
Alumni Professor and Chairman, Department of Psychiatry
and Neurobehavioral Sciences
University of Virginia
P.O. Box 800623
Charlottesville, VA 22908
bj4x@virginia.edu

Lynell W. Klassen, MD
Chairman, Department of Internal Medicine
University of Nebraska Medical Center
983332 Nebraska Medical Center
Omaha, NE 68198
lklassen@unmc.edu

John H. Krystal, MD
Robert L. McNeil, Jr. Professor of Clinical Pharmacology
Deputy Chairman for Research, Department of Psychiatry
Yale University School of Medicine
34 Park Street
New Haven, CT 06519
john.krystal@yale.edu

Peter M. Monti, PhD
Donald G. Millar Distinguished Professor of Alcohol and Addiction
Studies Director, Center for Alcohol and Addiction Studies
Brown University
Senior Career Research Scientist, Department of Veterans Affairs
121 South Main Street
Providence, RI 02912
Peter_Monti@brown.edu

Edward P. Riley, PhD
Distinguished Professor, Department of Psychology
San Diego State University
6363 Alvarado Court
San Diego, CA 92120
eriley@mail.sdsu.edu

Kenneth J. Sher, PhD
Curators' Professor, Department of Psychology
University of Missouri
210 McAlester Hall
Columbia, MO 65211
sherk@missouri.edu

Linda P. Spear, PhD
Distinguished Professor of Psychology
Binghamton University, SUNY
P.O. Box 6000
Binghamton, NY 13902
lspear@binghamton.edu

Gyongyi Szabo, MD, PhD
Professor, Department of Gastroenterology
Professor, Department of Medicine
University of Massachusetts Medical School
364 Plantation Street, Room 215
Worcester, MA 01605-2324
gyongyi.szabo@umassmed.edu

Invited Experts

Philip J. Brooks, PhD
Acting Section Chief, Section of Molecular Neurobiology
Laboratory of Neurogenetics, NIAAA
5625 Fishers Lane
Rockville, MD 20852
pjbrooks@mail.nih.gov

Curt I. Civin, MD
Associate Dean for Research
Director, Center for Stem Cell Biology & Regenerative Medicine
Professor, Pediatrics
University of Maryland School of Medicine
655 West Baltimore Street
Baltimore, MD 21201-1559
ccivin@som.umaryland.edu

Stephen J. Elledge, PhD
Department of Genetics
Center for Genetics and Genomics
Harvard Medical School
Room 158D, NRB
77 Avenue Louis Pasteur
Boston, MA 02115
selledge@genetics.med.harvard.edu

Albert J. Fornace, MD
Professor
Molecular Cancer Research Chair
Lombardi Comprehensive Cancer Center
Georgetown University
3800 Reservoir Road
Washington, DC 20057
af294@georgetown.edu

Lorraine J. Gudas, PhD
Chairman and Revlon Pharmaceutical Professor, Department of Pharmacology
Cornell University
1300 York Avenue, Room E-409
New York, NY 10065
ljgudas@med.cornell.edu

Helmut K. Seitz, MD, PhD
Department of Medicine and Laboratory of Alcohol Research, Liver
Disease and Nutrition
Salem Medical Centre
University of Heidelberg
Zeppelinstraße 11-33, 69121
Heidelberg, Germany
helmut_karl.seitz@urz.uni-heidelberg.de

Hua Yu, PhD
Professor, Cancer Immunotherapeutics & Tumor Immunology
Beckman research institute at City of Hope
1500 East Duarte Road
Duarte, CA 91010
hyu@coh.org

During the meeting in June, 2010, DMHE staff presented their findings to the EAB and Council members and invited experts, who recommended the areas of research listed below. Their recommendations were presented to the full National Advisory Council in the September 22–23, 2010 meeting, who unanimously adopted the EAB recommendations.

The sense of the panel and EAB was to focus on tissues for which human epidemiological data suggests increased cancer risk. It is also recommended that an increased investment be made in public health awareness about alcohol and cancer risk. Recommendations are not listed in terms of priority.

1. Systems approaches to tissue-specific contributions of ethanol to the development and progression of cancer.
   (a) Comprehensive, coordinated, and systematic approach to understanding dose, time, sex, and tissue-specific differences in effects of alcohol and metabolites on cancer

(b) Tissue-specific metabolites
(c) Signaling pathways/targets
(d) Genetic interactions that underlie alcohol-specific responses
(e) Biomarkers
(f) Direct carcinogenic mechanisms (e.g., acetaldehyde)

- DNA mutation/loss/translocation
- Epigenetic effects
- Transcriptome
- Proteome
- Metabolome

2. Molecular mechanisms. Effects of alcohol and/or its metabolites on cancer development and progression. Roles of the following:

(a) Oxidative stress
(b) Inflammation/immunity
(c) Retinoid homeostasis
(d) Epithelial mesenchymal transition and fibrosis
(e) Ethanol metabolism – Cyp2E1, ADH, ALDH
(f) Stem cells

3. Adapt/exploit established preclinical cancer models for studying alcohol-related carcinogenesis, e.g.,

(a) P53 null mouse, MMTV-WNT, C-MYC HCC, RIP-Tag
(b) Stem cells

4. Cell and molecular basis for enhanced cancer risks of alcohol with other agents. Mechanism underlying relationships with the following:

(a) Viruses
(b) Tobacco
(c) Obesity
(d) Ovarian hormones
(e) Microbes

5. Epidemiology and genotype–phenotype correlations

(a) Work with other institutes pursuing cancer-related studies by exploiting technologies and resources to address alcohol-related cancer, e.g., large-scale genomics (GWAS). Correlate genotypes with large-scale epidemiologic studies.
(b) NIAAA should have input into larger cancer epidemiology and intervention studies to get good reliable information on alcohol consumption.
(c) Collect information on cancer in ongoing epidemiologic studies

(d) Construct studies in high-risk populations to address alcohol–cancer mechanisms and health disparities, e.g.,

- Esophageal cancer in ALDH2-deficient Asian individuals.
- ASPD in Koreans with ALDH2 allele encourages drinking could theoretically lead to cancer
- Hispanics, high rates of cirrhosis, high rates of hepatocellular carcinoma (HCC)
- Cancers in Native Americans with very high rates of alcoholism, smoking, and diabetes
- High cancer families, e.g., BRCA1 carriers.
- Collect cancer information in the Collaborative studies on Genetics of Alcoholism (COGA)

Index

S. Zakhari et al. (eds.), *Alcohol and Cancer*, DOI 10.1007/978-1-4614-0040-0,
© Springer Science+Business Media, LLC 2011

U

V